SECOND EDITION

ADVANCED CARDIAC LIFE SUPPORT:
Certification Preparation and Review

BRUCE R. SHADE, EMT/P

Commissioner
Cleveland Emergency Medical Service
Chairperson, Society of Instructor/Coordinators of NAEMT
Basic and Advanced Cardiac Life Support Affiliate Faculty
Member, Emergency Cardiac Care Subcommittee
Northeastern Ohio Affiliate (AHA)
Cleveland, Ohio

Joann Grif Alspach, R.N., M.S.N., CCRN

Consultant, Critical Care Nursing Education
Formerly
Clinical Nurse Educator, Critical Care, National Institutes of Health
Clinical Nurse Specialist Critical Care and Director of Critical Care
Nursing Internship Programs, Suburban Hospital, Bethesda, Maryland
Basic and Advanced Cardiac Life Support Affiliate Faculty
Maryland Affiliate (AHA)
Annapolis, Maryland

Michael J. Ballenger, R.N., M.S.N., CCRN

Clinical Nurse Specialist in Cardiothoracic Surgery
Fairview General Hospital
Advanced Cardiac Life Support Affiliate Faculty
Northeastern Ohio Affiliate (AHA)
Cleveland, Ohio

Victor A. Morant, M.D.

Cardiologist
Director, Ambulatory Electrocardiology
The Cleveland Clinic Foundation
Chairperson, ECC Subcommittee
Basic and Advanced Cardiac Life Support Affiliate Faculty
Northeastern Ohio Affiliate (AHA)
Cleveland, Ohio

A BRADY BOOK

Prentice Hall Building, Englewood Cliffs, N.J. 07632

Library of Congress Cataloging-in-Publication Data

ADVANCED CARDIAC LIFE SUPPORT.
    1. Cardiac arrest—Treatment—Problems, exercises,
etc.   2. Cardiac resuscitation—Problems, exercises,
etc.   I. Shade, Bruce R.   [DNLM: 1. Heart Arrest—
examination questions.   2. Life Support Care—examination
questions.   3. Resuscitation—examination questions.
WG 18 A244]
RC685.C173A36 1988   616.1′2062   87-7238
ISBN 0-89303-001-5

Editorial/production supervision and
  interior design: Tom Aloisi
Cover design: Lundgren Graphics, LTD.
Manufacturing buyer: Lorraine Fumoso

ISBN: 0-89303-001-5   025

Prentice-Hall International (UK) Limited, *London*
Prentice-Hall of Australia Pty. Limited, *Sydney*
Prentice-Hall Canada Inc., *Toronto*
Prentice-Hall Hispanoamericana, S.A., *Mexico*
Prentice-Hall of India Private Limited, *New Delhi*
Prentice-Hall of Japan, Inc., *Tokyo*
Simon & Schuster Pte. Ltd., *Singapore*
Editora Prentice-Hall do Brasil, Ltda., *Rio de Janeiro*

NOTICE

It is the intent of the authors and publishers that this textbook be used as an adjunct to formal Advanced Cardiac Life Support courses taught by qualified instructors. The care procedures presented here represent accepted practices that are taught in the ACLS curriculum and which are recommended by the American Heart Association in the United States. The procedures are not offered as a standard of care. ACLS is to be performed under the authority and guidance of a licensed physician. It is the reader's responsibility to know and follow accepted standards of practice as defined by the medical authority for the area to which he or she belongs. Also, it is the reader's responsibility to stay informed of ACLS care procedure changes.

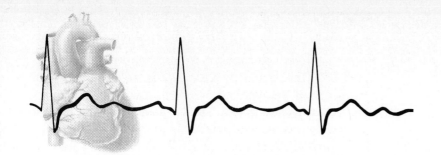

Contents

*For the precious gift of life, this book is dedicated to:
my wife Cheri, my daughter Katherine Ann,
and my mother and father, Lucille and Elmer Shade, Jr.*

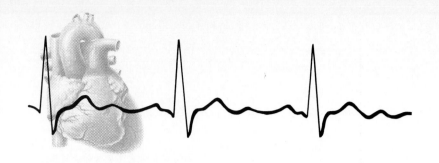

Preface

Cardiovascular disease knows no limitations; it strikes people regardless of sex, age, race, profession, or religion. In 1978 nearly one million people died from cardiovascular disease.

The American Heart Association (AHA) developed Basic and Advanced Cardiac Life Support courses (BCLS and ACLS) to educate the lay public and health care professionals in preventing premature death from cardiovascular disease. BCLS programs provide instruction in recognition and immediate management of cardiopulmonary arrest, whereas ACLS programs provide training in the more definitive aspects of emergency cardiac care.

The brief duration, weighty reference textbook, and comprehensive nature of ACLS training programs often pose problems for the busy health care professionals who comprise the course participants. *Advanced Cardiac Life Support: Certification Preparation and Review* was developed as a study manual to assist physicians, nurses, emergency medical technicians, paramedics, and other health care professionals in preparing for and successfully completing the ACLS course. It may also be useful to ACLS instructors and instructor-trainers to augment their teaching programs.

This self-paced review covers all essential content areas of the ACLS-course, including material necessary to pass both the written tests and performance test stations. A variety of study question formats and practice exercises are used to provide instruction and review in an easy-to-learn approach that presents content gradually and systematically. Each chapter begins with a set of instructional objectives, proceeds to a set of objective and subjective exercises, and ends with an answer key. In many instances the answer key offers additional instruction to reinforce and expand learning. Illustrations and tables are used liberally to enhance understanding and application of learning.

Chapter 1 affords a review of anatomy and physiology, the foundation of the entire course. The second chapter offers an overview of BCLS and its performance criteria. Chapter 3 contains a comprehensive review and a multitude of practice exercises in dysrhythmia interpretation and the basic tenets of electrocardiography for the many ACLS participants who need this supplemental instruction. Chapters 4 through 7 cover pharmacology, acid-base balance, airway management, IV cannulation, circulation support and defibrillation respectively. To avoid duplication and provide better application of content, chapters on myocardial infarction, sudden death, and neonatal and pediatric resuscitation follow as Chapters 8 through 10. Chapter 11 highlights additional perspectives and legal aspects which must be considered in ACLS. Chapter 12 culminates the review by providing 10 case history scenarios. They afford an opportunity for application and integration of all preceding chapters and help prepare for the Mega Code testing station. An appendix containing additional information regarding the most current ACLS standards supplements the text.

Advanced Cardiac Life Support: Certification Preparation and Review has evolved over a number of years as a study manual for hundreds of ACLS course participants and faculty who have assisted in its critique and refinement. We hope that you find it a useful adjunct in learning and welcome your comments and suggestions.

Bruce R. Shade, EMT/P
JoAnn Grif Alspach, R.N., M.S.N., CCRN
Michael J. Ballenger, R.N., M.S.N., CCRN
Victor A. Morant, M.D.

Contributors

We gratefully acknowledge the contributions of the following individuals:

Marilyn I. McNutt, EMT/P, R.N.M.T., A.R.R.T.
EMS Coordinator
Cleveland Emergency Medical Service
Basic and Advanced Cardiac Life Support Instructor
Northeastern Ohio Affiliate (AHA)
Cleveland, Ohio

Daniel Richard Beil, EMT/P
EMS Coordinator
Cleveland Emergency Medical Service
Basic and Advanced Cardiac Life Support Instructor
Northeastern Ohio Affiliate (AHA)
Cleveland, Ohio

Carla Streepy, M.D.
Director, Emergency Department
St. Vincent Charity Hospital
Advanced Cardiac Life Support Instructor
Northeastern Ohio Affiliate (AHA)
Cleveland, Ohio

Reviewers

John T. Sigafoos, R.N., EMT/P
Formerly:
Administrator
Emergency Medical Services
Ohio Board of Regents
Columbus, Ohio
Presently:
Director, Critical Care Transport
Riverside Methodist Hospital
Columbus, Ohio

Mary Ann Talley, R.N., M.P.A.
Director of Paramedic Education
University of South Alabama
Mobile, Alabama

Mitchell J. Brown
Formerly:
Commissioner
Cleveland Emergency Medical Service
Basic and Advanced Life Support Instructor
Presently:
Public Safety Director
City of Cleveland
Cleveland, Ohio

Bryan Bledsoe, EMT/P
Texas Osteopathic School of Medicine
Fort Worth, Texas

Mary Jackle, R.N., M.S.
Director
Critical Care Project
Metropolitan Medical Center
Minneapolis, Minnesota

For the cover design of the original workbook,

Andrew G. Rabatin, EMT/P, M.Ed.
Emergency Medical Services Coordinator
Richmond Heights General Hospital
Lieutenant/Paramedic
Willowick Fire Department
ACLS Instructor

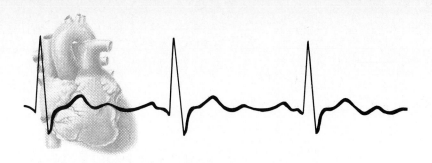

Special Thanks

Many people played a part in the conceptualization and production of this workbook.

Joseph Ezzie, Chief, Copley Fire Department, Akron: a fine friend who showed me the meaning of excellence and taught me that a picture, model, or live specimen is worth a thousand words. His inspiration lives on in this book.

Margo Kiraly, R.N., Paramedic Instructor for Cuyahoga Community College, Cleveland; tutored me through my first Advanced Cardiac Life Support Instructor Course, helped me to see the need for the workbook.

Pat Carr, Former Marketing Representative for Brady Communications Company; a good listener and "phone pal," encouraged me to submit the workbook for publication.

Richard Weimer, Former Editor for Brady Communications Company; a true gentleman and friend; was one of the first to recognize the potential for the workbook; continually harassed me to finish the manuscript.

Charles Mondin, Former Marketing Manager for Brady Communications Company; one of the most warmhearted individuals I have had the pleasure to be affiliated with, provided me with encouragement and support even as things looked most bleak.

Claire Merrick, Editor for the Brady products; one "neat lady" and dear friend; provided continual support and made me laugh as the project dragged on, was strong enough to say "enough is enough," otherwise the book would still be under revision.

Mary Ann Talley, R.N., MPA, Director Paramedic Training, University of South Alabama; "one-heck-of-a-lady," her initial, delightful review of the manuscript served as a source of support for me as I debated the worth of the document.

Mitchell J. Brown, Commissioner of Cleveland Emergency Medical Service; my mentor demanded excellence from me and allowed me to learn through my mistakes and accomplishments.

A special thanks goes to all the instructors and students who have used the workbook and provided feedback in order that it may be strengthened.

Tom Aloisi, Senior Production Editor at Prentice Hall, was assigned to put together the Second Edition of our manuscript, working with an accelerated schedule and changing content. Tom, like a painter of an exquisite picture, blended all the material to produce an outstanding work of art.

In Memory

Dale Eyerdom, Assistant Fire Chief, Granger Fire Department, Medina, Ohio.

Robert Coffman, EMT/Paramedic/Firefighter, Willowick Fire Department, Willowick, Ohio.

Dale and Bob, you are truly missed. . . .

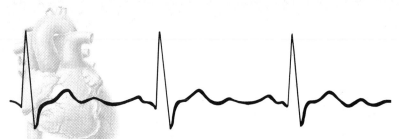

Directions for Use of This Manual

The *Review* manual may be used alone or in conjunction with the AHA *Textbook of Advanced Cardiac Life Support* to prepare for ACLS provider and instructor courses.

Start your review at least one to two weeks before participating in the course: allow more time if this material is unfamiliar to you. You will likely find it helpful to first review the foundational chapters (1, 2, 3) and then proceed to subsequent chapters according to your individual learning needs. It is not necessary to complete the chapters in sequence, though readers who are new to the ACLS content areas may find it easier to do this.

Begin by reading the objectives for the chapter. If you think you can already meet the objectives, complete all the review questions and exercises in the chapter before checking your answers in the answer key at the end. If you feel you need more practice and instruction before you can master the objectives, progress more gradually by answering the questions and verifying your answers on a one-by-one basis.

Seven types of review items are used in the study guide to accommodate various learning style preferences and to avoid the monotony of a single item format. Instructions for completing each item format follow:

MULTIPLE-CHOICE: Circle the letter of the correct/best response(s). In some instances, more than one response may be correct/best.

TRUE-FALSE: Circle "T" if the statement is true and "F" if the statement is false. When the statement is false, identify the reason why it is false.

MATCHING: Match the entries with the appropriate term, statement, or description. Some entries may have more than one correct response.

FILL-IN: Complete the statement or sentence with the correct/best word(s).

SEQUENCING: Number each entry to indicate the correct order in which it should be performed.

DESCRIPTION: Provide a brief explanation to the question posed.

SHADING: Darken the area(s) of the illustration to indicate your response.

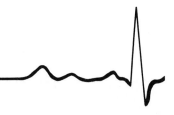

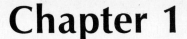

Chapter 1

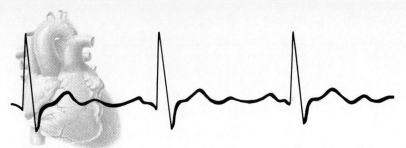

Anatomy and Physiology Review

OBJECTIVES

Upon completion of this chapter, you will be able to:

- Describe the major features of cardiac muscle contraction at the cellular level.
- Specify the role of calcium in cardiac muscle contraction.
- Explain each factor that regulates cardiac output.
- Calculate cardiac output values based on variable heart rates and stroke volumes.
- Recognize the clinical effects of inadequate cardiac output.
- Enumerate the sequence of events in ventricular systole and diastole.
- Distinguish among the physiological features of myocardial preload, afterload, and contractility.
- Contrast the cardiovascular influences of sympathetic and parasympathetic nervous system stimulation.
- Compare the cardiovascular effects of alpha and beta receptor stimulation.
- Identify the major features of coronary artery perfusion in normal and diseased states.

Instructions: For each of the following statements, circle T if the statement is true and F if the statement is false.

1. (T) F   The heart is the pump of the circulatory system; without its pumping action, no blood would be circulated.

2. (T) F   Cardiac muscle contraction produces the pumping action of the heart.

3. (T) F   Heart muscle is composed of a few large muscle fibers.

4. T   F   Cardiac muscle fibers are composed of tiny, tubelike structures called myofibrils.

5. (T) F   Myofibrils contain two protein filaments, actin and myosin, which connect by cross bridges.

6. T   (F)   *sliding* Cardiac muscle contraction and relaxation result from shortening and lengthening of the actin and myosin filaments.

7. T   F   Regulatory proteins inhibit the formation of cross bridges between actin and myosin filaments, thereby preventing muscle contraction.

8. T   F   Cardiac muscle contraction results in muscle depolarization.

9. T   F   Prior to stimulation of a cardiac muscle fiber, calcium ions are stored only in the extracellular space.

10. T   F   Following stimulation of a cardiac muscle fiber, calcium ions are transferred to the actin–myosin interaction sites, where they bind the inhibitory proteins and effect muscle contraction.

11. T   F   Cardiac muscle contraction can occur without calcium ions.

12. Describe how the normal cardiac electrical impulse spreads through the heart to depolarize the cardiac muscle fibers.

_____

_____

_____

_____

_____

_____

13. Number each of the following statements to indicate the normal sequence of cardiac muscle stimulation and contraction.

   2_____ Calcium slowly enters depolarized muscle cells during the plateau phase of the action potential.

   1_____ Depolarization originates spontaneously in the SA node and spreads through the cardiac conduction system to the individual muscle cells.

   4_____ The intracellular movement of calcium triggers calcium release from the sarcoplasmic reticulum to the actin–myosin interaction sites in the sarcomere.

   7_____ Cross bridges are formed and muscle fiber shortening (contraction) ensues.

   8_____ Calcium returns to its predepolarization locations, and the regulatory proteins prevent muscle contraction again.

   5 _____ Calcium ions bind the regulatory proteins that inhibit the formation of cross bridges between the contractile filaments.

   3_____ Calcium ions enter the sarcoplasmic reticulum from the extracellular space.

   6_____ Calcium removes the inhibitory effect of the regulatory proteins on the formation of cross bridges.

14. Match the following terms with their appropriate description.

   Terms

   _____ cardiac output

   _____ stroke volume

   _____ heart rate

   _____ compliance

   _____ preload

   _____ end-diastolic

   _____ diastole

   _____ Frank–Starling law

   _____ contractility

   _____ resistance

   _____ afterload

Description

a. interference with the ease of fluid flow; increases in smaller lumens and decreases in larger lumens

b. number of times the heart contracts each minute; normally between 60 and 100

c. resistance to blood flow out of the ventricles; normally determined by vasoactive state of peripheral arterial system, chiefly in arterioles

d. amount of blood pumped to the tissues each minute; product of heart rate and stroke volume

e. ability of the heart to stretch; healthy heart muscle fibers stretch easily, whereas damaged muscle is less distensible

f. amount of blood in the ventricle at the end volume of ventricular filling, which causes the ventricular muscle to stretch; influences how the myocardium contracts with each beat

g. amount of stretch applied to a muscle fiber before it contracts; influences the strength of the next contraction

h. principle that states "the greater the presystolic fiber length (preload) up to a point, the stronger the subsequent muscle contraction"

i. phase in which the ventricles fill with blood

j. volume of blood pumped out of the ventricle with each contraction; averages 70 ml at rest

k. force or strength of systolic contraction; determined by the amount and speed of muscle fiber shortening

l. period during which blood flows out of the ventricle as a result of increased ventricular pressure

Circle the letter of the BEST response for each of the following items.

15. Cardiac output can be reduced by:
    a. decreasing afterload
    b. decreasing heart rate
    c. increasing stroke volume
    d. increasing end-diastolic volume

16. The average resting adult cardiac output is approximately _____ liter(s) per minute.
    a. 1
    b. 3
    c. 5
    d. 12

17. Calculate cardiac outputs for each of the following heart rates. (Assume the stroke volume is 70 ml in each case.)

    48 per minute _____

    82 per minute _____

    124 per minute _____

18. Calculate cardiac outputs for each of the following stroke volumes. (Assume the heart rate is 72 per minute in each case.)

    16 ml _____

    60 ml _____

    110 ml _____

19. Calculate cardiac outputs for each of the following sets of stroke volume and heart rate.

SV(ml)	HR	=	Cardiac output
40	160	=	_____
50	50	=	_____
70	66	=	_____

For each of the following statements, circle T if the statement is true and F if the statement is false.

20. T F Cardiac output may be decreased by a reduction in either heart rate or stroke volume.

21. T F Diminished cardiac output results in increased coronary, cerebral, and renal blood flow.

22. T F Clinical signs of inadequate cardiac output include disorientation, diaphoresis, pallor, hypotension, and shortness of breath.

23. T F All patients with heart rates less than 60 per minute should be medicated to increase their heart rate.

24. T F Relative or absolute hypovolemia results in decreased stroke volume.

25. T F Hypovolemia due to diminished blood volume can be corrected by increasing the heart rate.

26. Number the correct sequence of events in ventricular diastole.

    _____ Ventricles distend maximally and muscle fibers stretch to accommodate the incoming blood.

    _____ Blood flows from the great veins into the atria.

    _____ Atrial contraction forces 30% of diastolic blood volume into the ventricles.

    _____ Approximately 70% of diastolic blood volume flows passively from the atria into the ventricles.

27. Preload is a reflection of (circle one):

    a. ventricular systolic pressure
    b. atrial systolic pressure
    c. ventricular end-diastolic pressure
    d. atrial end-diastolic volume

True or False

28. T   F   The higher the end-diastolic volume up to a point, the more forceful will be the subsequent ventricular contraction.

29. T   F   Increasingly greater end-diastolic volumes will continue to strengthen ventricular contractility.

30. Number the correct sequence of events in ventricular systole.

    _____ Pressure in the ventricles exceeds pressures in the aorta and pulmonary artery.

    _____ Ventricular pressure rises quickly and dramatically.

    _____ Ejection of blood from the ventricle occurs.

    _____ Ventricular muscle walls contract and squeeze on the blood in the ventricular chamber.

True or False

31. T   F   The rate at which the pressure rises in the ventricles is determined by how much and how fast the muscle fibers shorten.

32. T   F   Healthy ventricular muscle fibers shorten slowly so that ventricular pressures gradually exceed pulmonary artery and aortic pressures.

33. T   F   Loss of normal ventricular contractility will increase both stroke volume and cardiac output.

34. T   F   Ventricular contractility determines the end-diastolic volume.

35. T   F   The rate of pressure rise in the ventricles influences both the force of contraction and the stroke volume.

36. T   F   Myocardial ischemia, infarction, acidosis, and aneurysm can all decrease contractility of the heart.

37. Which of the following is a true statement regarding AFTERLOAD?

    a. The higher the afterload, the easier blood flows out of the left ventricle.
    b. Increased afterload may be caused by vasodilation and low blood volumes.
    c. The lower the afterload, the higher the peripheral arterial pressure.
    d. Increased afterload raises myocardial demands for blood and oxygen.

38. For each of the following characteristics, write S if it describes a sympathetic nervous system characteristic and P if it describes a parasympathetic nervous system characteristic.

    _____ Stimulation slows the heart rate.

    _____ It has alpha and beta receptors.

    _____ Stimulation increases myocardial contractility.

    _____ It derives its fibers from the vagus nerve.

    _____ Stimulation reduces cardiac output.

    _____ Acetylcholine is its neurotransmitter.

    _____ Norepinephrine is its neurotransmitter.

    _____ Stimulation speeds impulse conduction.

    _____ Stimulation allows more ions to enter cells.

    _____ Stimulation slows spontaneous depolarization in the cell.

    _____ Stimulation causes peripheral vasoconstriction.

True or False

39. T   F   Alpha-1 receptor sites are located on vascular smooth muscle; their stimulation causes vasoconstriction.

40. T   F   Stimulation of beta-1 receptors will elicit tachycardia and increased contractility.

41. T   F   Stimulation of beta-2 receptors leads to vasoconstriction, as well as bronchial and gut smooth muscle constriction.

42. T   F   Stimulation of alpha-1 receptors will increase afterload, myocardial workload, and myocardial oxygen consumption.

43. T F Stimulation of beta-2 receptors will decrease myocardial workload and myocardial oxygen consumption.

44. T F Coronary arteries possess only alpha adrenergic receptors.

45. T F Stimulation of beta-1 receptors increases cardiac automaticity.

Circle the letter of the BEST response in the following item.

46. Stimulation of the parasympathetic nervous system will result in:

1. slower heart rate
2. increased contractility
3. increased automaticity
4. peripheral vasoconstriction
5. slower impulse conduction
6. bronchodilation

   Answers
   a. 1 and 5
   b. 2 and 3
   c. 3 and 4
   d. 5 and 6

47. Label the coronary arteries and their branches in Figure 1–1.

48. Which of the following organs has the greatest percentage of arterial oxygen extraction in a resting state?

   a. brain
   b. liver
   c. heart
   d. kidneys

49. During exercise or stress, the most effective way in which the myocardium increases its oxygen supply is by (circle the correct answer):

   a. increasing heart rate
   b. decreasing myocardial oxygen extraction
   c. increasing coronary blood flow
   d. decreasing myocardial contractility

50. During exercise or stress, patients with severe coronary artery disease [circle the correct answer(s)]:

   a. have decreased myocardial oxygen requirements
   b. compensate with increased coronary collateral circulation
   c. compensate by reducing their heart rate
   d. may not be able to meet the increased cardiac demands for oxygen

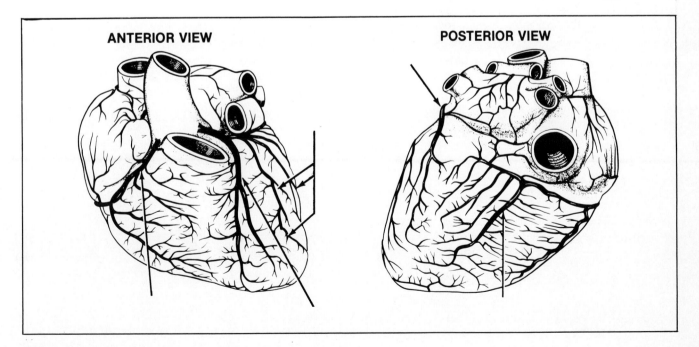

ANTERIOR VIEW   POSTERIOR VIEW

Figure 1–1

ANSWER KEY

1. TRUE: The heart normally pumps 60 to 100 times per minute. Variable tissue demands for blood may stimulate faster pumping via the sympathetic nervous system or slower pumping via the parasympathetic system.

2. TRUE: Wide bands of cardiac muscle layers provide effective contraction (Figure 1–2).

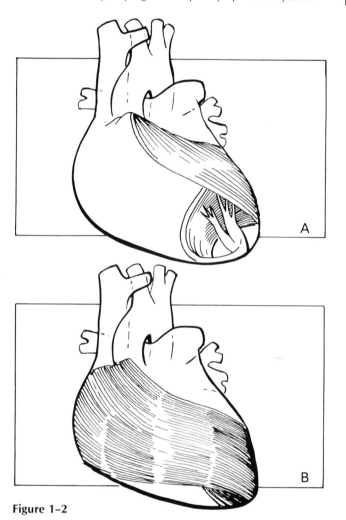
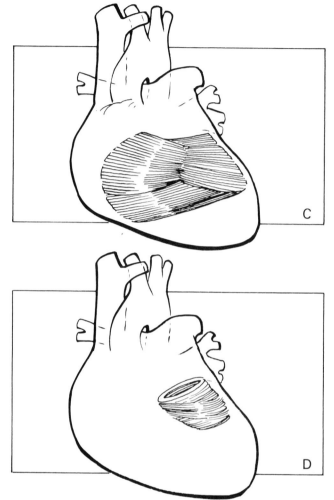

Figure 1–2

3. FALSE: Heart muscle is made up of numerous small muscle fibers that lie in series with one another, branching, spreading apart, and reconnecting. Individual fibers are separated from others by intercalated discs (Figure 1–3).

4. TRUE: See Figure 1–4.

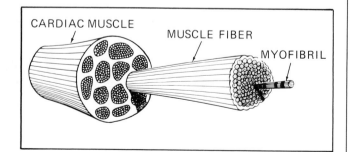

Figure 1–4

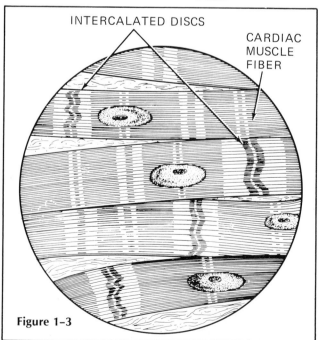

Figure 1–3

5. TRUE: Actin and myosin filaments lie in a parallel arrangement and are connected by cross bridges (Figure 1–5).

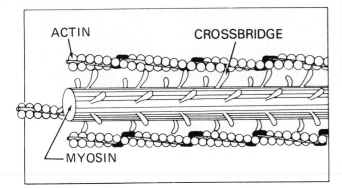

Figure 1–5

6. FALSE: Cardiac muscle contraction results from shortening of the muscle fiber due to increased overlap of the actin and myosin filaments. When the cross bridges pull on the filaments, the thin actin filaments slide over the thick myosin filaments (Figure 1–6a). During relaxation, the filament overlap decreases and results in return of the fiber to its original resting length. Release of the cross bridges allows the filaments to slide back to their resting position (Figure 1–6b).

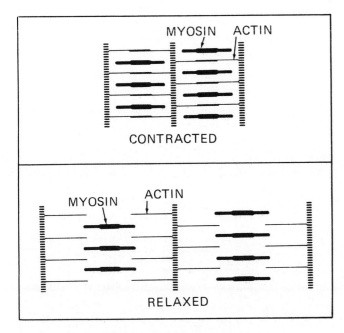

Figures 1–6a and 1–6b

7. TRUE: Troponin and tropomyosin are regulatory proteins that inhibit the formation of cross bridges between actin and myosin (Figure 1–7).

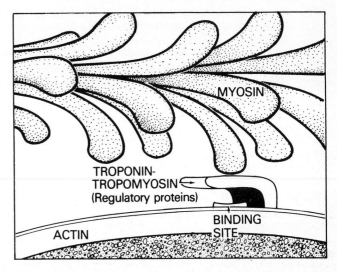

Figure 1–7

8. FALSE: For a muscle to contract, it must first be depolarized (electrically stimulated). Depolarization normally occurs when an impulse from the pacemaker of the heart spreads throughout the cardiac conduction system to reach all muscle fibers.

9. FALSE: Prior to stimulation of a cardiac fiber, calcium ions are stored in both the sarcoplasmic reticulum and the extracellular space.

10. TRUE: Calcium ions bind the regulatory proteins that inhibit the overlapping of actin and myosin. Removal of this inhibition allows muscle contraction to proceed (Figure 1–8).

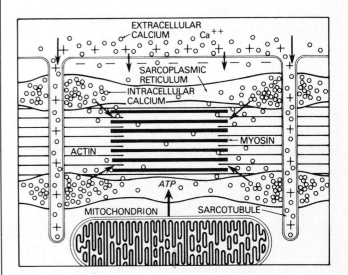

Figure 1–8

11. FALSE: Cardiac muscle contraction requires calcium ions to inhibit the regulatory proteins that prevent actin and myosin overlapping.

12. The normal cardiac electrical impulse travels as a wave of depolarization along the cell membrane of cardiac muscle cells. The speed of conduction is enhanced by the interconnected arrangement of muscle fibers and by areas of low electrical resistance between fibers called intercalated discs (Figure 1–9).

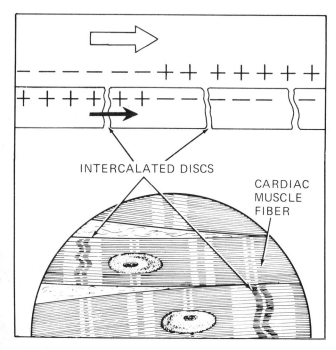

Figure 1–9

13. Sequence of cardiac muscle stimulation and contraction:

1st- Depolarization originates spontaneously in the SA node and spreads through the cardiac conduction system to the individual muscle cells (Figure 1–10).

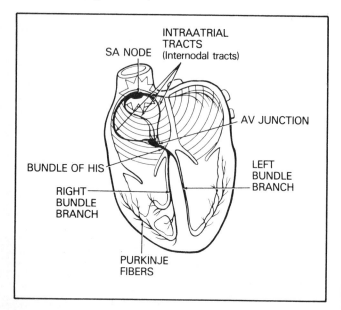

Figure 1–10

2nd- Calcium slowly enters depolarized muscle cells during the plateau phase of the action potential (Figure 1–11).

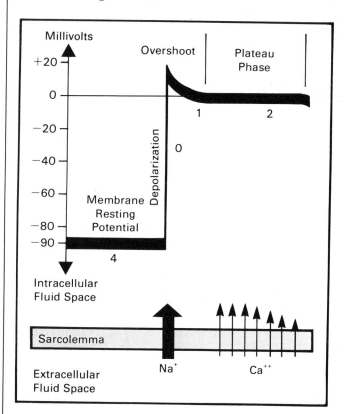

Figure 1–11

3rd- Calcium ions enter the sarcoplasmic reticulum from the extracellular space (Figure 1–12).

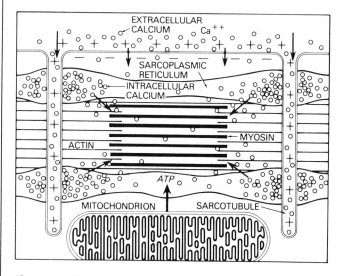

Figures 1–12

4th- The intracellular movement of calcium triggers calcium release from the sarcoplasmic reticulum to the actin–myosin interaction sites in the sarcomere (Figure 1–13).

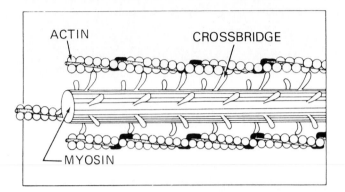

Figure 1–13

5th- Calcium ions bind the regulatory proteins that inhibit the formation of cross bridges between the contractile filaments (Figure 1–14).

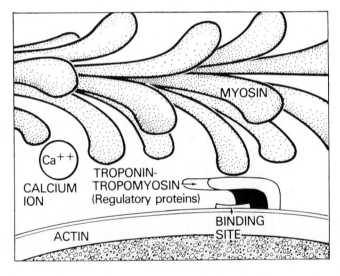

Figure 1–14

6th- Calcium removes the inhibitory effect of the regulatory proteins on the formation of cross bridges. Myofilament overlap requires the presence of calcium, oxygen, and energy (ATP) (Figure 1–15).

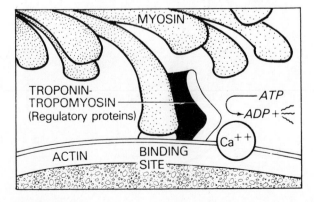

Figure 1–15

7th- Cross bridges are formed and muscle fiber shortening (contraction) ensues (Figure 1–16).

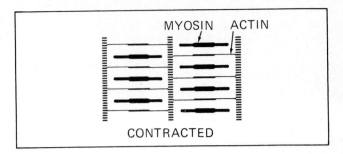

Figure 1–16

8th- Calcium returns to its predepolarization locations and the regulatory proteins prevent muscle contraction again (Figures 1–17 and 1–18).

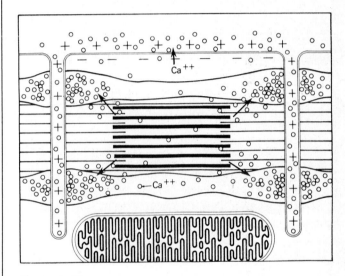

Figure 1–17

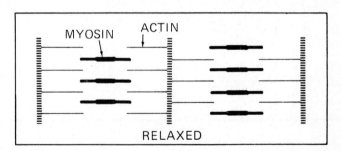

Figure 1–18

14. cardiac output: d
    stroke volume: j
    heart rate: b
    compliance: e
    preload: g
    end-diastolic volume: f
    diastole: i
    Frank–Starling law: h
    contractility: k
    resistance to flow: a
    afterload: c

15. b

16. c (70 ml SV × 72/minute heart rate = 5,040 ml/minute cardiac output)

17.   48 = 3360 ml/minute
   82 = 5740 ml/minute
  124 = 8680 ml/minute

18.   16 = 1152 ml/minute
   60 = 4320 ml/minute
  110 = 7920 ml/minute

19. 40 ml × 160 beats = 6400 ml/minute
  50 ml × 50 beats = 2500 ml/minute
  70 ml × 66 beats = 4620 ml/minute

20. TRUE

21. FALSE: Diminished cardiac output results in decreased coronary, cerebral, and renal blood flow.

22. TRUE

23. FALSE: Only patients who are symptomatic (hypotensive, ventricular ectopic beats) from bradycardia require therapy to increase heart rate.

24. TRUE

25. FALSE: Hypovolemia due to diminished blood volume (absolute hypovolemia) can only be corrected by increasing the blood volume.

26. Sequence of events in ventricular diastole:
   1st- Blood flows from the great veins into the atria (Figure 1-19).

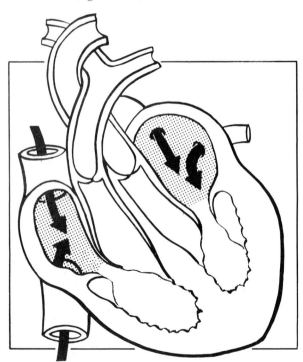

Figure 1-19

2nd- Approximately 70% of diastolic blood volume flows passively from the atria into the ventricles (Figure 1-20).

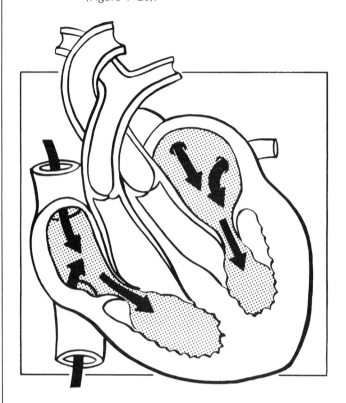

Figure 1-20

3rd- Atrial contraction forces 30% of diastolic blood volume into the ventricles (Figure 1-21).

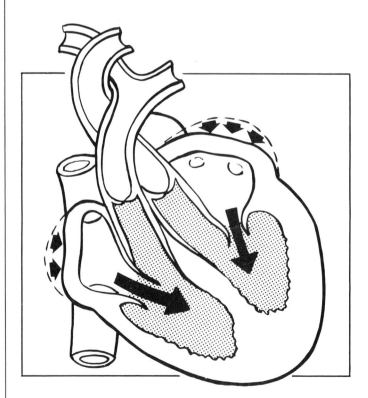

Figure 1-21

4th- Ventricles distend maximally and muscle fibers stretch to accommodate the incoming blood (Figure 1–22).

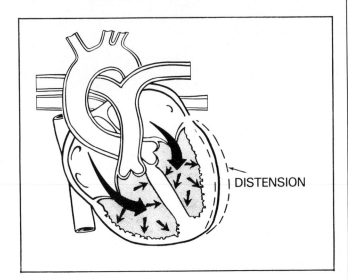

Figure 1–22

27. c

28. TRUE

29. FALSE: Beyond an optimal end-diastolic volume, stroke volume will decrease and ventricular contractility will be diminished (Figure 1–23).

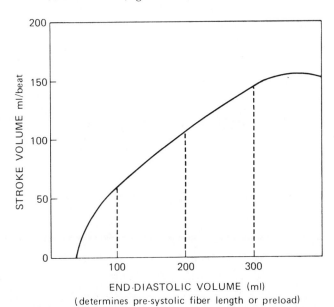

Figure 1–23

30. Sequence of events in ventricular systole (Figure 1–24):
  1st- The ventricular muscle walls contract and squeeze on the blood in the ventricular chamber.
  2nd- Ventricular pressure rises quickly and dramatically.
  3rd- Pressure in the ventricles exceeds pressures in the aorta and pulmonary artery.
  4th- Ejection of blood from the ventricle occurs.

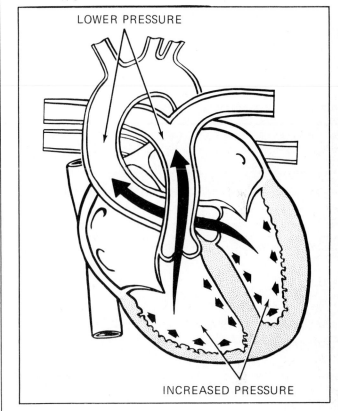

Figure 1–24

31. TRUE

32. FALSE: Healthy ventricular fibers shorten quickly; ventricular pressures rapidly exceed pulmonary artery and aortic pressures.

33. FALSE: Loss of normal ventricular contractility causes stroke volume and cardiac output to decrease.

34. FALSE: Ventricular contractility determines the end-systolic volume.

35. TRUE

36. TRUE

37. d

38. Autonomic nervous system characteristics:

S = it has alpha and beta receptors.
Stimulation increases myocardial contractility.
Norepinephrine is its neurotransmitter.
Stimulation speeds impulse conduction.
Stimulation allows more ions to enter cells.
Stimulation causes peripheral vasoconstriction.

P = stimulation slows the heart rate.
It derives its fibers from the vagus nerve.
Stimulation reduces cardiac output.
Acetylcholine is its neurotransmitter.
Stimulation slows spontaneous depolarization of the cell.
(See Figure 1–25.)

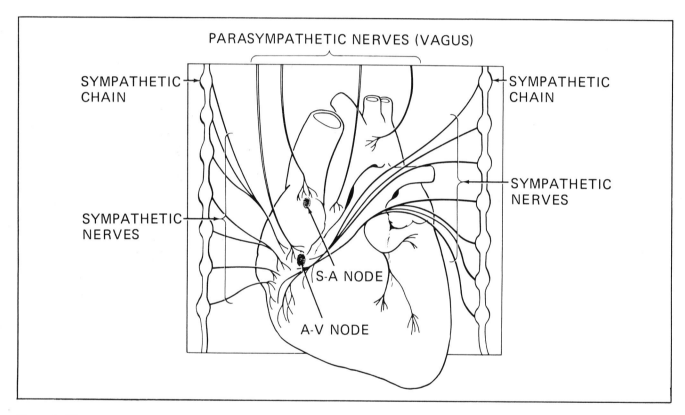

Figure 1–25

39. TRUE (Figure 1–26)

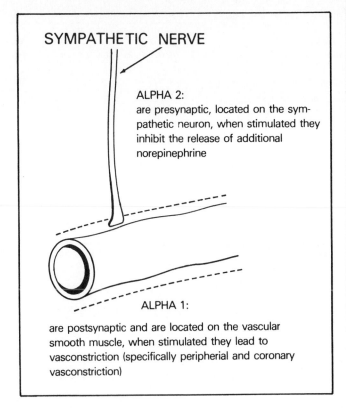

SYMPATHETIC NERVE

ALPHA 2:
are presynaptic, located on the sympathetic neuron, when stimulated they inhibit the release of additional norepinephrine

ALPHA 1:

are postsynaptic and are located on the vascular smooth muscle, when stimulated they lead to vasoconstriction (specifically peripherial and coronary vasconstriction)

Figure 1–26

40. TRUE (Figure 1–27)

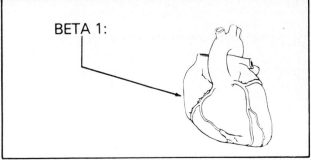

BETA 1:

when stimulated lead to an increase in automaticity, heart rate and myocardial contractility

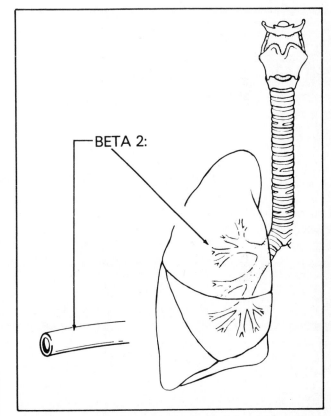

BETA 2:

when stimulated lead to relaxation of vascular smooth muscle in a number of circulations as well as relaxation of bronchial and gut smooth muscle

Figure 1–27

41. FALSE: Beta-2 receptor site stimulation results in peripheral vasodilation as well as bronchial and gut smooth muscle dilation (Figure 1–27).

42. TRUE

43. TRUE: Stimulation of beta-2 receptors decreases myocardial workload and myocardial oxygen consumption by decreasing afterload. The less resistance the heart has to pump against, the less its workload and oxygen requirement.

44. FALSE: The coronary arteries possess both alpha-1 and beta-1 receptors. Stimulation of alpha-1 receptors elicits coronary artery vasoconstriction, whereas stimulation of beta-1 receptors elicits coronary vasodilation.

45. TRUE

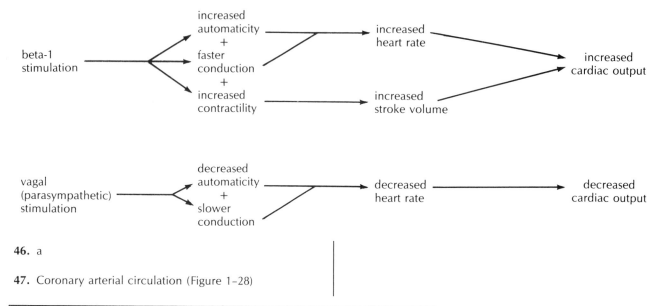

46. a

47. Coronary arterial circulation (Figure 1–28)

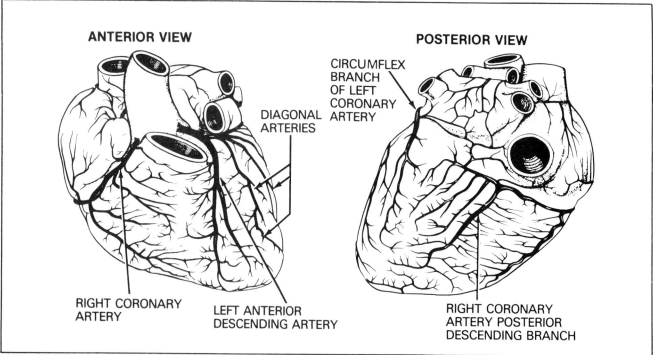

Figure 1–28

48. c: Even at rest, the myocardium normally extracts about 70% of its arterial oxygen supply, leaving a very small margin for further increasing myocardial oxygen supply through increased extraction. Additional demands for oxygen must be met through increased coronary blood flow (Figure 1–29).

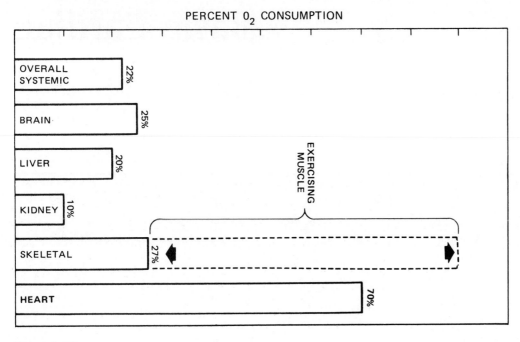

Figure 1–29

49. c

50. d

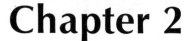

Chapter 2

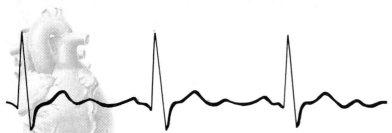

Basic Cardiac
Life Support Review

OBJECTIVES

Upon completion of this chapter, you will be able to:

- Recall the procedure for single-rescuer cardiopulmonary (CPR) on an adult victim.

- Specify the recommended procedures for providing two-rescuer CPR on an adult victim.

- Identify the correct procedure for two rescuers to switch positions during CPR on an adult victim.

- Recognize how to properly perform CPR pulse checks on infants, children, and adults.

- Distinguish among techniques appropriate for infant, child, and one- and two-rescuer adult CPR.

- Recall the procedures for relieving an obstructed airway in the infant, child, and adult victim.

1. Which of the following may be used to relieve an obstructed airway in the conscious adult?

   a. finger sweeps
   b. back blows
   c. subdiaphragmatic abdominal thrusts
   d. all the above

2. Number the following to indicate the correct sequence for performing abdominal thrusts when relieving an obstructed airway in a conscious, standing, or sitting victim.

   _____ Make a fist with one hand and place the thumb side against the victim's abdomen in the midline, slightly above the navel and well below the tip of the xiphoid.

   _____ Stand well behind the victim and wrap your arms around the victim's waist.

   _____ Press into the victim's abdomen with quick upward thrusts; each thrust should be distinct and delivered with the intent of relieving the airway obstruction.

   _____ Grasp the fist with the other hand.

   _____ Repeat the thrusts until either the foreign body is expelled or the victim becomes unconscious.

3. Chest thrusts would be used in place of abdominal thrusts when attempting to relieve an obstructed airway in a patient who:

   a. is experiencing a "cafe coronary"
   b. is pregnant
   c. is obese or too large to easily wrap your arms around
   d. is a small child or an infant
   e. has preexisting heart disease

For each of the following statements, circle T if the statement is true and F if the statement is false.

4. T   F   Backblows may be used for relieving an obstructed airway due to a foreign body in the child.

5. T   F   Blind finger sweeps are to be avoided in infants and small children when attempting to relieve a foreign-body airway obstruction.

6. T   F   The preferred technique for opening the airway in the unconscious patient is the head-tilt/chin-lift technique.

7. T   F   After determining breathlessness, the rescuer should deliver four ventilations at 1 to 1.5 seconds per breath.

8. T   F   The carotid pulse may be palpated on either side of the victim's neck.

9. T   F   The rescuer should allow 5 to 10 seconds for carotid pulse detection.

10. Once it has been determined that the victim is pulseless, the pulse should be checked again after the first [circle the correct answer(s)]:

    a. 15 compressions
    b. 30 seconds of CPR
    c. full minute of CPR and every few minutes thereafter
    d. 2 minutes of CPR and every 5 minutes thereafter

True or False

11. T   F   In two-rescuer CPR, the ventilator should deliver a ventilation after every fifth compression.

12. T   F   In two-rescuer CPR, the rescuer doing chest compressions should pause after every fifth compression to allow the ventilator to deliver a breath.

13. T   F   When performing two-rescuer CPR, chest compressions should be delivered at a rate of 80 to 100 per minute.

14. Number each drawing in Figure 2–1 to indicate the order in which the actions should be performed for one-rescuer cardiopulmonary resuscitation.

15. Number each drawing in Figure 2–2 to indicate the order in which the actions should be performed in two-rescuer CPR.

16. Number each drawing in Figure 2–3 to indicate the order in which the actions should be performed for two rescuers to switch positions during CPR.

17. For CPR on a five-year-old child, cardiac compressions should be performed with the [circle the correct answer(s)]:

    a. index and middle fingers of one hand
    b. heel of one hand
    c. fingers of both hands
    d. heels of both hands

ONE RESCUER CPR

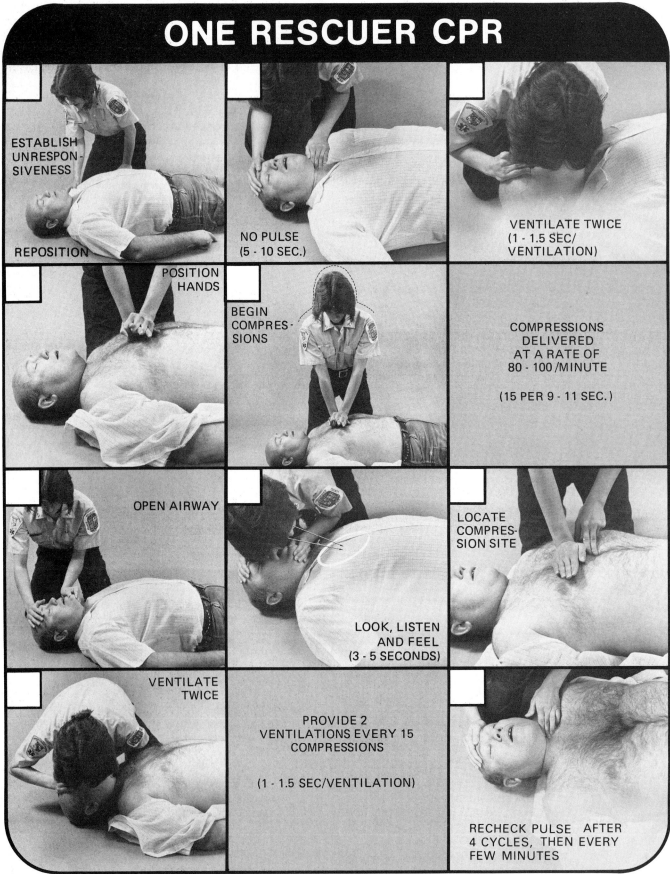

ESTABLISH UNRESPONSIVENESS

REPOSITION

NO PULSE (5 - 10 SEC.)

VENTILATE TWICE (1 - 1.5 SEC/ VENTILATION)

POSITION HANDS

BEGIN COMPRESSIONS

COMPRESSIONS DELIVERED AT A RATE OF 80 - 100 /MINUTE

(15 PER 9 - 11 SEC.)

OPEN AIRWAY

LOOK, LISTEN AND FEEL (3 - 5 SECONDS)

LOCATE COMPRESSION SITE

VENTILATE TWICE

PROVIDE 2 VENTILATIONS EVERY 15 COMPRESSIONS

(1 - 1.5 SEC/VENTILATION)

RECHECK PULSE AFTER 4 CYCLES, THEN EVERY FEW MINUTES

NOTE: WHEN ALONE CALL OUT FOR HELP IF PATIENT IS UNRESPONSIVE.
IF OFF DUTY, HAVE SOMEONE CALL DISPATCH AFTER CHECKING FOR PULSELESSNESS.

Figure 2-1

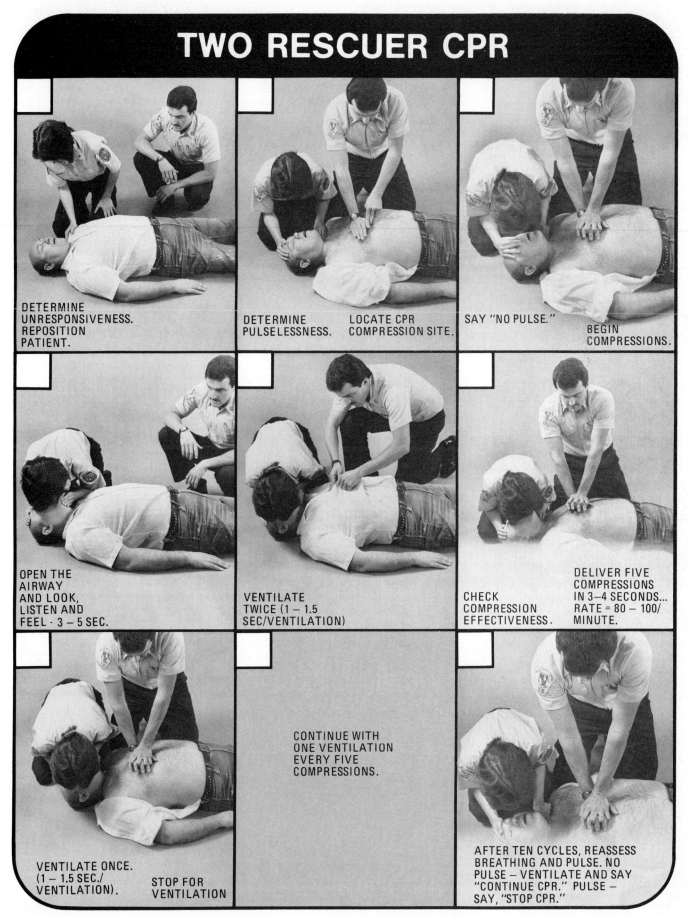

TWO RESCUER CPR

DETERMINE UNRESPONSIVENESS. REPOSITION PATIENT.

DETERMINE PULSELESSNESS.   LOCATE CPR COMPRESSION SITE.

SAY "NO PULSE."   BEGIN COMPRESSIONS.

OPEN THE AIRWAY AND LOOK, LISTEN AND FEEL - 3 – 5 SEC.

VENTILATE TWICE (1 – 1.5 SEC/VENTILATION)

CHECK COMPRESSION EFFECTIVENESS.   DELIVER FIVE COMPRESSIONS IN 3–4 SECONDS... RATE = 80 – 100/ MINUTE.

VENTILATE ONCE. (1 – 1.5 SEC./ VENTILATION).   STOP FOR VENTILATION

CONTINUE WITH ONE VENTILATION EVERY FIVE COMPRESSIONS.

AFTER TEN CYCLES, REASSESS BREATHING AND PULSE. NO PULSE – VENTILATE AND SAY "CONTINUE CPR." PULSE – SAY, "STOP CPR."

Figure 2–2

CHANGING POSITIONS

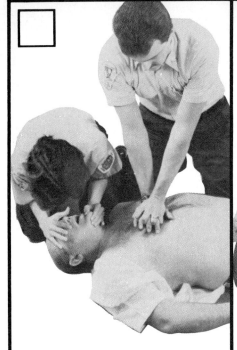

WHEN FATIGUED, THE COMPRESSOR CALLS FOR THE SWITCH. GIVE A CLEAR SIGNAL TO CHANGE.

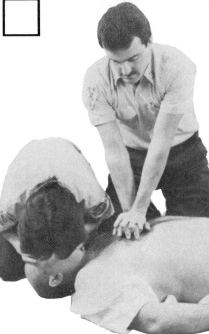

COMPRESSOR COMPLETES FIFTH COMPRESSION. VENTILATOR PROVIDES ONE VENTILATION.

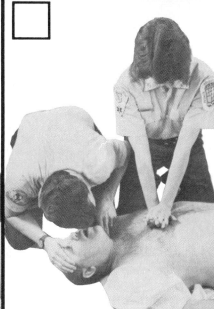

NEW COMPRESSOR DELIVERS FIVE COMPRESSIONS (3–4 SECONDS) AT A RATE OF 80–100 PER MINUTE. NEW VENTILATOR ASSESSES COMPRESSIONS.

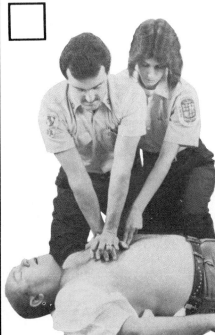

VENTILATOR MOVES TO CHEST AND BEGINS TO LOCATE COMPRESSION SITE. COMPRESSOR BEGINS MOVE TO HEAD.

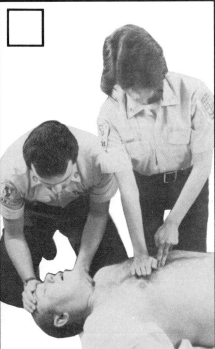

NEW COMPRESSOR FINDS SITE. NEW VENTILATOR CHECKS CAROTID PULSE (5 SECONDS)

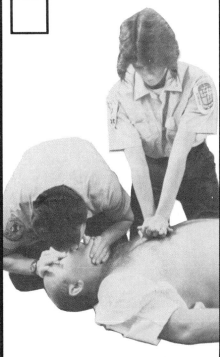

NEW VENTILATOR SAYS, "NO PULSE" AND VENTILATES ONCE (1–1.5 SECONDS).

Figure 2–3

18. The correct depth of cardiac compressions for a five-year-old child is _____ to _____ inch(es).

a. $\frac{1}{2}$ to 1
b. 1 to $1\frac{1}{2}$
c. $1\frac{1}{2}$ to 2
d. 2 to $2\frac{1}{2}$

True or False

19. T   F   If a child is large or older than 8 years old, the method for performing CPR is the same as for adults.

20. T   F   The correct rate for cardiac compressions in the child is 60 to 80 per minute.

21. Number the following to indicate the correct sequence for infant CPR.

_____ Establish pulselessness

_____ Deliver two slow breaths (1.0 to 1.5 seconds per breath)

_____ Begin cardiac compressions at a rate of 100 per minute

_____ Check for a pulse after 1 minute of CPR

_____ Establish unresponsiveness

_____ Open the airway

_____ Continue CPR at a ratio of five compressions to one ventilation

_____ Check for breathlessness

True or False

22. T   F   The rescuer should seal both the nose and mouth of the infant when providing rescue breathing.

23. T   F   The head-tilt/chin-lift technique for opening the airway is contraindicated in the infant.

24. T   F   The rescuer's thumb should be used to locate an infant's pulse.

25. T   F   In infant resuscitation, pulselessness should be established before attempts are made to ventilate the infant.

26. In Table 2–1, fill in the appropriate information for infant, child, one-rescuer, and two-rescuer adult CPR techniques.

TABLE 2–1

	Infant	Child	Adult, One Rescuer	Adult, Two Rescuers
Head Position to Open Airway				
Ventilation Rate (per minute)				
Pulse Check Site				
Cardiac Compression Site				
Perform Chest Compressions with:				
Depth of Cardiac Compressions (inches)				
Compression Rate (per minute)				
Compression-to-Ventilation Ratio				

ANSWER KEY

1. c: Subdiaphragmatic abdominal thrusts are used to relieve an obstructed airway in the conscious adult. Finger sweeps may be used to relieve an obstructed airway when the patient is unconscious. Back blows are no longer recommended for relieving an obstructed airway in the adult or child.

2. The correct sequence for performing abdominal thrusts when relieving an obstructed airway in a conscious, standing, or sitting victim.
   1st- Stand well behind the victim and wrap your arms around the victim's waist.
   2nd- Make a fist with one hand and place the thumb side against the victim's abdomen in the midline, slightly above the navel and well below the tip of the xiphoid.
   3rd- Grasp the fist with the other hand.
   4th- Press into the victim's abdomen with quick upward thrusts; each thrust should be distinct and delivered with the intent of relieving the airway obstruction.
   5th- Repeat the thrusts until either the foreign body is expelled or the victim becomes unconscious.

3. b, c, d: Chest thrusts would be used in place of abdominal thrusts when attempting to relieve an obstructed airway in a patient who is pregnant, is obese or too large to easily wrap your arms around, or is a small child or infant.

4. FALSE: Backblows are not recommended for the child. As in the adult, subdiaphragmatic abdominal thrusts are recommended in the child experiencing an obstructed airway due to a foreign body.

5. TRUE: It is felt that blind finger sweeps may push the foreign body back into the airway, causing further airway obstruction, and thus should be avoided in the infant.

6. TRUE: The preferred technique for opening the airway is the head-tilt/chin-lift technique. An exception would be when there is suspected neck injury. In that case, the jaw thrust without head tilt should be employed.

7. FALSE: The rescuer should deliver two ventilations.

8. FALSE: The carotid pulse should be checked only on the side where the rescuer is positioned. The rationale for this is that the rescuer could inadvertently collapse the victim's airway by reaching across the neck; additionally, bilateral carotid compression could result in vagal stimulation with bradycardia or asystole.

9. TRUE: This is sufficient time for detecting a very slow or weak, thready pulse.

10. c

11. TRUE: In two-rescuer CPR, the ventilator should deliver a ventilation after every fifth breath.

12. TRUE: In two-rescuer CPR, the rescuer doing chest compressions should pause after every fifth compression to allow the ventilator to deliver a breath.

13. TRUE: With two-rescuer CPR, the compression rate is 80 to 100 per minute.

14. The correct sequence for one-rescuer CPR is shown in Figure 2–4.

15. The correct sequence for two-rescuer CPR is shown in Figure 2–5.

16. The correct sequence for switching positions while performing two-rescuer CPR is shown in Figure 2–6.

17. b: Two fingers are used for infant cardiac compressions; the heels of both hands are used for adult compressions.

18. b: For the infant, the chest should be compressed 0.5 to 1.0 inch, and for the adult, the chest should be compressed 1.5 to 2 inches.

19. TRUE: If a child is larger or older than 8 years old, the method for performing CPR is the same as for adults.

20. FALSE: The correct rate of compressions in the child is 80 to 100 per minute.

21. The correct sequence for performing infant CPR:
    1st- Establish unresponsiveness.
    2nd- Open the airway.
    3rd- Check for breathlessness.
    4th- Deliver two slow breaths (1.0 to 1.5 seconds per breath).
    5th- Establish pulselessness.
    6th- Begin cardiac compressions at a rate of 100 per minute.
    7th- Continue CPR at a ratio of five compressions to one ventilation.
    8th- Check for a pulse after 1 minute of CPR.

22. TRUE: The rescuer should seal both the nose and mouth of the infant when providing rescue breathing.

23. FALSE: The head-tilt/chin-lift technique for opening the airway may be used in the infant. The head should be gently tilted back into a sniffing or neutral position in the infant.

24. FALSE: The rescuer should use the first two or three fingers to palpate a pulse to avoid sensing his or her own pulse in his or her own thumb.

25. FALSE: As in the adult, the pulse is checked after the airway is opened and the initial ventilations have been delivered.

ONE RESCUER CPR

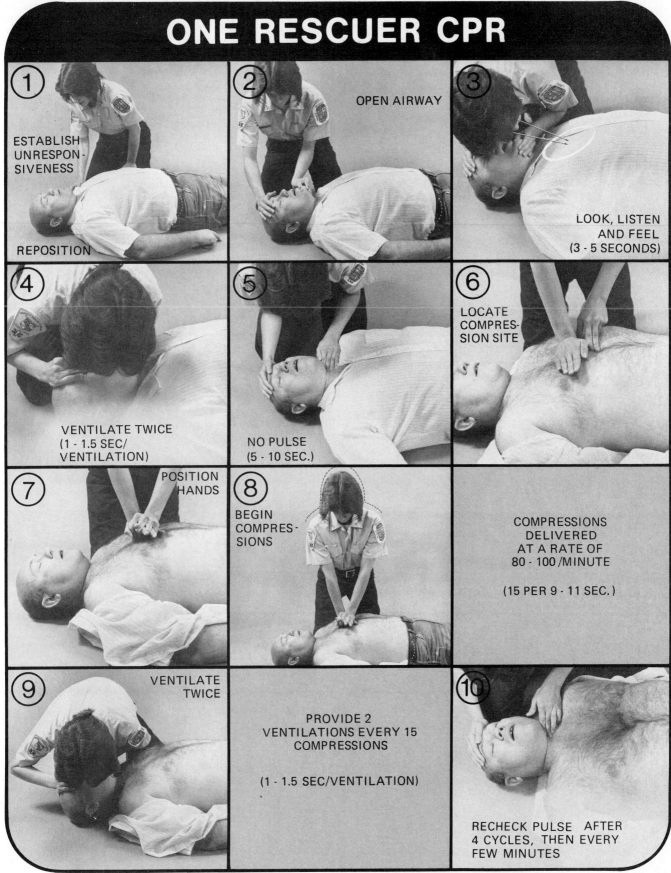

Figure 2–4

TWO RESCUER CPR

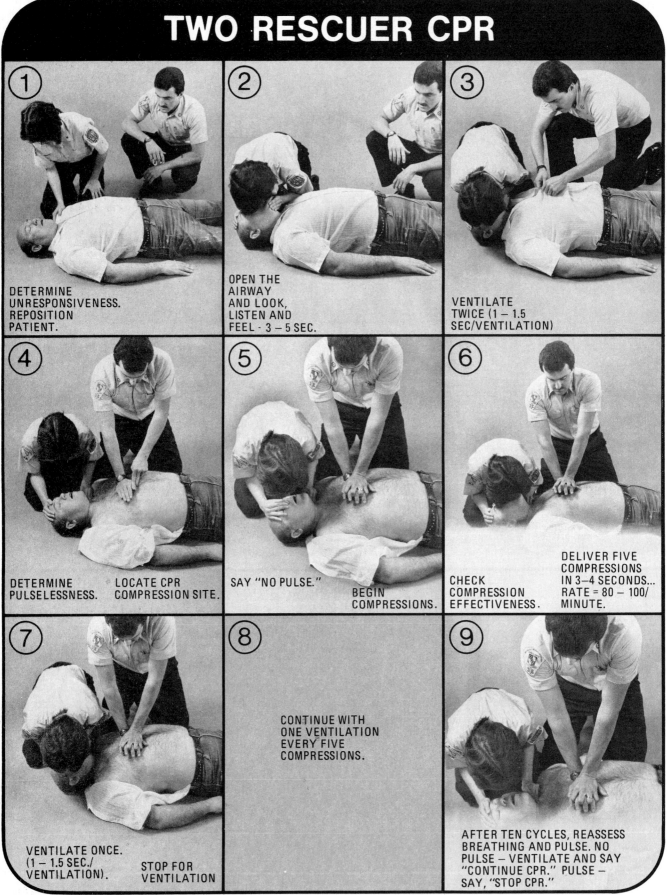

① DETERMINE UNRESPONSIVENESS. REPOSITION PATIENT.

② OPEN THE AIRWAY AND LOOK, LISTEN AND FEEL - 3 – 5 SEC.

③ VENTILATE TWICE (1 – 1.5 SEC/VENTILATION)

④ DETERMINE PULSELESSNESS. LOCATE CPR COMPRESSION SITE.

⑤ SAY "NO PULSE." BEGIN COMPRESSIONS.

⑥ CHECK COMPRESSION EFFECTIVENESS. DELIVER FIVE COMPRESSIONS IN 3–4 SECONDS... RATE = 80 – 100/ MINUTE.

⑦ VENTILATE ONCE. (1 – 1.5 SEC./ VENTILATION). STOP FOR VENTILATION

⑧ CONTINUE WITH ONE VENTILATION EVERY FIVE COMPRESSIONS.

⑨ AFTER TEN CYCLES, REASSESS BREATHING AND PULSE. NO PULSE – VENTILATE AND SAY "CONTINUE CPR." PULSE – SAY, "STOP CPR."

NOTE: ASSESS FOR SPONTANEOUS BREATHING AND PULSE FOR 5 SECONDS AT THE END OF THE FIRST MINUTE, THEN EVERY FEW MINUTES THEREAFTER.

Figure 2–5

CHANGING POSITIONS

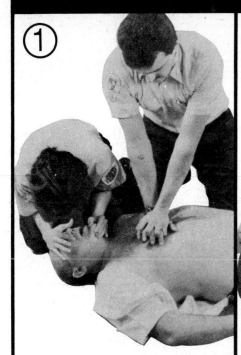

① WHEN FATIGUED, THE COMPRESSOR CALLS FOR THE SWITCH. GIVE A CLEAR SIGNAL TO CHANGE.

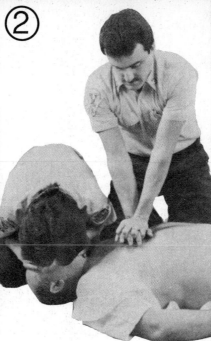

② COMPRESSOR COMPLETES FIFTH COMPRESSION. VENTILATOR PROVIDES ONE VENTILATION.

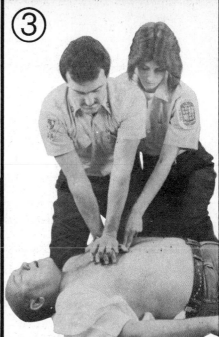

③ VENTILATOR MOVES TO CHEST AND BEGINS TO LOCATE COMPRESSION SITE. COMPRESSOR BEGINS MOVE TO HEAD.

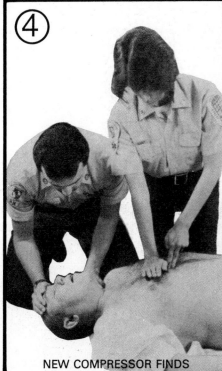

④ NEW COMPRESSOR FINDS SITE. NEW VENTILATOR CHECKS CAROTID PULSE (5 SECONDS)

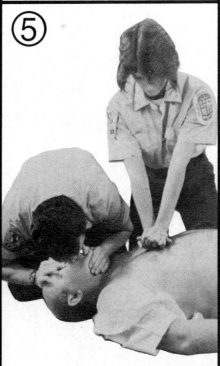

⑤ NEW VENTILATOR SAYS, "NO PULSE" AND VENTILATES ONCE (1-1.5 SECONDS).

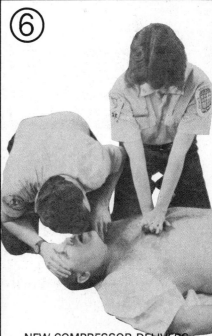

⑥ NEW COMPRESSOR DELIVERS FIVE COMPRESSIONS (3-4 SECONDS) AT A RATE OF 80-100 PER MINUTE. NEW VENTILATOR ASSESSES COMPRESSIONS.

NOTE: BOTH RESCUERS SHOWN ON THE SAME SIDE OF THE PATIENT FOR PURPOSE OF CLARITY.

Figure 2-6

26.

TABLE 2-2

	Infant	Child	Adult, One Rescuer	Adult, Two Rescuers
Head Position to Open Airway	Slight head tilt	Full hyperextension	Full hyperextension	Full hyperextension
Ventilation Rate (per minute)	20	15	12	12
Pulse Check Site	Brachial	Carotid	Carotid	Carotid
Cardiac Compression Site	One finger width below the intermammary line	Midsternum	Lower half of the sternum	Lower half of the sternum
Perform Chest Compressions with:	2 fingers	Heel of one hand	2 hands	2 hands
Depth of Cardiac Compressions (inches)	$\frac{1}{2}$ to 1	1 to $1\frac{1}{2}$	$1\frac{1}{2}$ to 2	$1\frac{1}{2}$ to 2
Compression Rate (per minute)	100	80 to 100	80 to 100	80 to 100
Compression-to-Ventilation Ratio	5 : 1	5 : 1	15 : 2	5 : 1

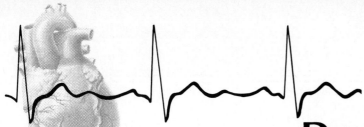

Chapter 3

Dysrhythmia Review and Interpretation

OBJECTIVES

Upon completion of this chapter, you will be able to:

- Identify the physiologic anatomy of the cardiac conduction system.

- Explain the major elements of cardiac electrophysiology.

- Distinguish between the properties of pacemaking and nonpacemaking cardiac cells.

- Correlate ECG waveforms and intervals with the physiologic events each represents.

- Differentiate between primary and escape pacemakers.

- Specify the characteristics of all ECG waveforms and intervals.

- Analyze ECG strips in a systematic and thorough manner.

- Correctly interpret ECG rhythm strips of the following dysrhythmias and AV conduction defects: sinus rhythm, sinus tachycardia, sinus bradycardia, wandering atrial pacemaker, atrial tachycardia, atrial flutter, atrial fibrillation, PACs, PJCs, PVCs, junctional escape rhythm, accelerated junctional rhythms, ventricular tachycardia, ventricular fibrillation, idioventricular rhythm, agonal rhythm, Torsade de Pointes, paroxysmal supraventricular tachycardia, first-degree AV block, second-degree AV block (Mobitz types I and II), and third-degree AV block.

- Compare and contrast the ECG characteristics of various cardiac dysrhythmias and AV conduction defects.

- State the clinical significance of commonly encountered cardiac dysrhythmias and conduction defects.

For each of the following statements, circle T if the statement is true and F is the statement is false.

1. T   F   The heart has two types of cells, electrical cells that initiate and conduct impulses, and muscle cells that contract in response to stimulation.

2. T   F   The pulse represents the electrical activity of the heart.

3. T   F   In the heart, electrical activity precedes mechanical activity.

4. T   F   If individual cardiac muscle fibers depolarize and contract in an uncoordinated manner, the heart beat will be strong and forceful.

5. Match the following terms with their appropriate description.

Terms

a. pacemaker cells
b. cardiac conduction system
c. automaticity

Description

_____ initiate cardiac electrical impulse

_____ ability to generate a spontaneous electrical impulse

_____ transmits cardiac impulse

6. Label the structures of the cardiac conduction system in Figure 3–1.

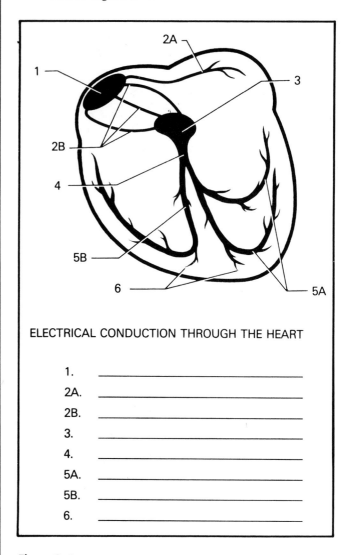

ELECTRICAL CONDUCTION THROUGH THE HEART

1.   _____
2A.   _____
2B.   _____
3.   _____
4.   _____
5A.   _____
5B.   _____
6.   _____

Figure 3–1

True or False

7. T   F   Pacemaker cells cannot depolarize spontaneously.

8. T   F   Each pacemaker site has its own inherent rate of automaticity.

9. T   F   Since the SA node has the fastest inherent rate of automaticity, it is normally the dominant pacemaker of the heart.

10. T   F   If the SA node fails to initiate an impulse, a lower pacemaker may initiate the impulse; this phenomenon is called an escape mechanism.

11. Match the following pacemaking sites with their respective characteristics:

Pacemaking Site

a. SA node
b. AV junction
c. ventricular conduction system

Description

_____ normal cardiac pacemaker

_____ rate of automaticity is 40 to 60 per minute

_____ rate of automaticity is less than 40/minute

_____ rate of automaticity is 60 to 100 per minute

_____ potential escape pacemaker

_____ pacemaker only when higher pacemaker fails or if its own rate of automaticity exceeds that of higher pacemakers

_____ initiates a beat/rhythm if an impulse fails to reach the ventricles within 1.5 seconds

12. Once the cardiac impulse leaves the SA node, it will [circle the correct answer(s)]:

a. proceed directly to the ventricles
b. travel through the atrial internodal pathways
c. travel directly to the AV junction
d. immediately enter the Purkinje fibers

13. Depolarization (electrical stimulation) of the atrial internodal pathways will result in [circle the correct answer(s)]:

a. ventricular contraction
b. AV junctional block
c. atrial contraction
d. slowing of conduction between the SA node and AV junction

14. At the AV junction there is normally a (an) [circle the correct answer(s)]:

a. slight delay in impulse conduction
b. acceleration of impulse conduction
c. intermittent blockade of impulses
d. retrograde movement of the impulse

15. Stimulation of the bundle of His, bundle branches, and Purkinje fibers results in [circle the correct answer(s)]:

a. atrial contraction
b. AV block
c. slowing of conduction in the Purkinje fibers
d. ventricular contraction

16. Starting at the SA node on Figure 3–2, draw an arrow to indicate the major direction of depolarization in the heart.

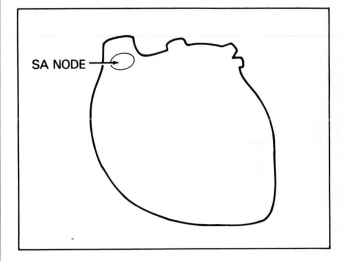

SA NODE

Figure 3–2

17. Label Figure 3–3 with the appropriate ECG waveforms and intervals.

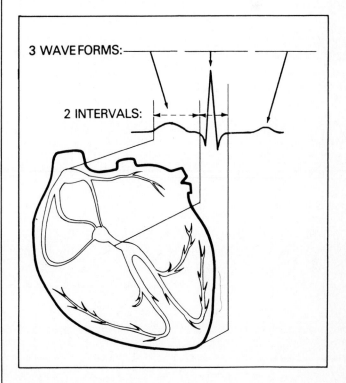

3 WAVEFORMS:

2 INTERVALS:

Figure 3–3

18. On the ECG graph paper in Figure 3–4, one small (1 mm) box measured from left to right represents _____ seconds; one large (5 mm) box represents _____ seconds.

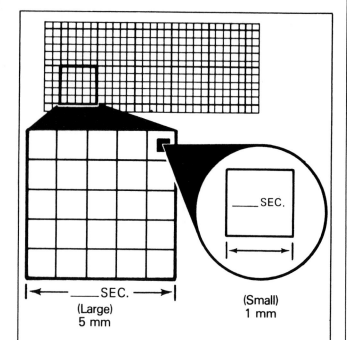

SEC.

SEC.
(Large)
5 mm

(Small)
1 mm

Figure 3–4

19. On the ECG graph paper (Figure 3–5), the space between two markers (interval A) represents _____ seconds; the space between three markers (interval B) represents _____ seconds.

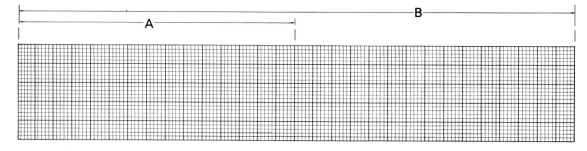

A   B

Figure 3–5

20. To calculate heart rate, multiply the number of QRS complexes in a 6-second rhythm strip by the number _____.

a. 5
b. 10
c. 15
d. 30

21. Match the two ECG intervals on Figure 3–6 with their respective normal limits.

   a. 0.02 to 0.04 second
   b. 0.04 to 0.10 second
   c. 0.12 to 0.20 second
   d. 0.24 to 0.28 second

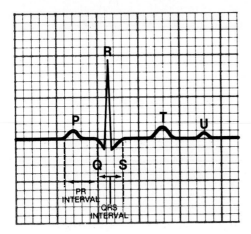

Figure 3–6

22. On Figure 3–7, label the proper locations for the positive, negative, and ground electrodes of lead II.

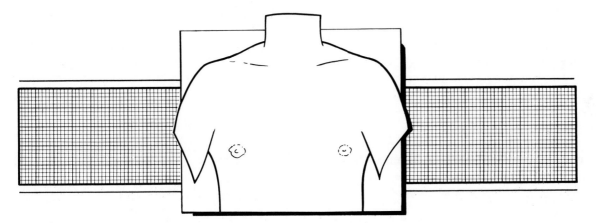

Figure 3–7

True or False

23. T F The P wave represents atrial depolarization.

24. T F The AV junction normally initiates atrial depolarization.

25. T F In lead II, P waves that originate in the SA node will be normal and positive deflections.

26. T F When P waves vary in size and/or configuration in the same lead, it may indicate that more than one pacemaker site is depolarizing the atria.

27. T   F   In lead II, an inverted (negative) P wave suggests that the impulse originated in the SA node.

28. Match the lead II ECG strips (Figures 3–8, 3–9, and 3–10) with the appropriate description.

ECG Strip

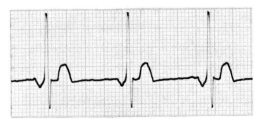

a. **Figure 3-8**

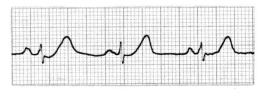

b. **Figure 3-9**

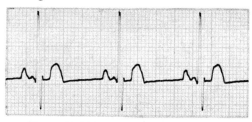

c. **Figure 3-10**

Description

_____ originated in the SA node

_____ originated in more than one location

_____ originated in region of AV junction

True or False

29. T   F   As the cardiac electrical impulse travels through the AV junction it is delayed slightly, allowing the atria to completely fill.

30. T   F   The P-R interval represents impulse delay at the AV junction.

31. T   F   P-R intervals greater than 0.20 second indicate an accentuation of normal impulse delay at the AV junction.

32. Match the lead II ECG strips (Figures 3–11, 3–12, and 3–13) with their appropriate description.

ECG Strip

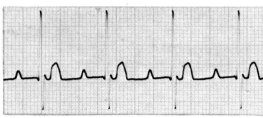

a. **Figure 3-11**

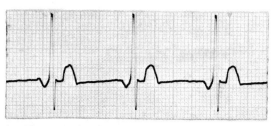

b. **Figure 3-12**

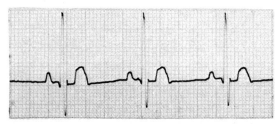

c. **Figure 3-13**

Description

_____ originated in region of AV junction

_____ originated in SA node and traveled normally through the AV junction

_____ originated in SA node, but was abnormally delayed at the AV junction

33. The QRS complex of Figure 3–14 represents [circle the correct answer(s)]:

  a. atrial depolarization
  b. atrial repolarization
  c. ventricular depolarization
  d. ventricular repolarization

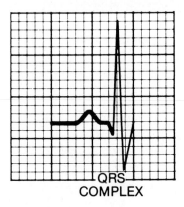

Figure 3–14

34. QRS complexes of greater than 0.12-second duration indicate that the impulse [circle the correct answer(s)]:

  a. originated from or was delayed within the ventricles
  b. terminated in the AV junction
  c. originated from or was delayed within the AV junction
  d. bypassed the normal delay at the AV junction

35. Match the QRS complexes in Figures 3–15, 3–16, and 3–17 with the appropriate description.

ECG Strip

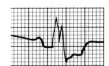

a. **Figure 3-15**

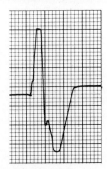

b. **Figure 3-16**

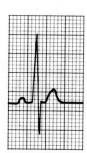

c. **Figure 3-17**

Description

_____ impulse traveled normally through the ventricles

_____ impulse originated in the ventricles

_____ impulse originated in the SA node, but was abnormally delayed in the AV junction

36. The T wave in Figure 3–18 represents [circle the correct answer(s)]:

  a. atrial depolarization
  b. delay of the impulse in the ventricles
  c. ventricular depolarization
  d. ventricular repolarization

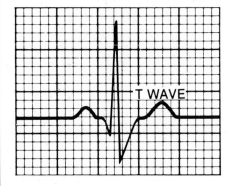

Figure 3–18

37. Atrial repolarization is hidden within the [circle the correct answer(s)]:

  a. P wave
  b. QRS complex
  c. ST segment
  d. T wave

38. The term dysrhythmia refers to a (an):

  a. abnormal blood pressure
  b. weak, irregular pulse
  c. erratic breathing pattern
  d. abnormal heart rhythm

39. Dysrhythmias may be caused by:

  a. acid–base imbalances
  b. electrolyte imbalances
  c. myocardial ischemia or infarction
  d. increased automaticity or reentry
  e. all the above

40. A normal heart rate is between

_____ and _____ beats per minute.

  a. 20 and 40
  b. 40 and 60
  c. 60 and 100
  d. 110 and 150

41. All heart rates faster than _____ beats per minute are considered a tachycardia.

   a. 50

   b. 75

   c. 90

   d. 100

42. Which of the following heart rates would be considered a bradycardia?

   a. 46 beats per minute

   b. 62 beats per minute

   c. 88 beats per minute

   d. 100 beats per minute

43. Match the following ECGs (Figures 3–19, 3–20, and 3–21) with the appropriate description:

ECG Strip

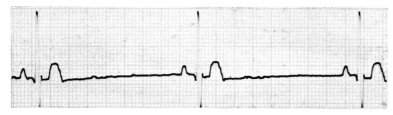

a. **Figure 3–19**

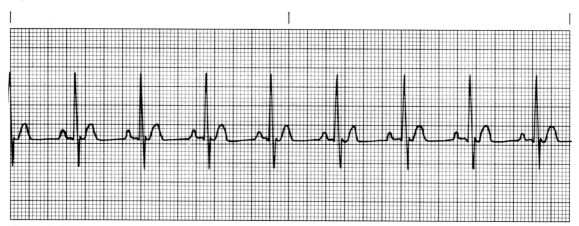

b. **Figure 3–20**

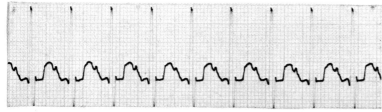

c. **Figure 3–21**

Description

_____ a tachycardia

_____ a normal heart rate

_____ a bradycardia

True or False

44. T   F   Slow heart rates are associated with accelerated conduction of the electrical impulse.

45. T   F   AV heart blocks, sinus arrest, and vagal stimulation may produce bradycardias.

46. T   F   Slow heart rates may result in inadequate cardiac output, decreased myocardial perfusion, and hypotension.

47. T   F   Heart rates between 100 and 150 beats per minute are usually the result of compensatory cardiovascular changes.

48. T   F   Heart rates between 100 and 180 beats per minute usually do not affect myocardial oxygen consumption.

49. T   F   Heart rates above 180 beats per minute will improve cardiac output and increase cerebral, pulmonary, renal, and myocardial perfusion.

50. Which of the following usually produce an irregular ventricular rhythm?

a. sinus tachycardia and bradycardia
b. premature ventricular ectopic beats and atrial fibrillation
c. junctional rhythm and ventricular tachycardia
d. first- and third-degree AV block

DIRECTIONS FOR ECG CHARACTERISTICS REVIEW

The next section contains questions regarding the characteristics of various dysrhythmias. You may find it helpful to refer to the following points as preparation for answering the items in this section. These are questions you should ask yourself to identify the correct interpretation of the rhythm strip.

1. WHAT HEART RATE IS TYPICALLY ASSOCIATED WITH THAT DYSRHYTHMIA OR CONDUCTION DEFECT?

   20 to 40 per minute?   60 to 100 per minute?
   40 to 60 per minute?   over 100 per minute?

2. ARE THE ATRIAL AND VENTRICULAR RATES THE SAME?

   YES: There are as many P waves as there are QRS complexes.

   NO: There are more P waves than QRS complexes, or vice versa.

3. IS THE P-P INTERVAL REGULAR?

   YES: The distances between consecutive P waves remain constant.

   NO: The distances between consecutive P waves vary.

4. IS THE R-R INTERVAL REGULAR?

   YES: The distances between consecutive R waves remain constant.

   NO: The distances between consecutive R waves vary.

5. IS THE VENTRICULAR RHYTHM REGULAR OR IRREGULAR?

   REGULAR: R-R intervals remain constant.

   ESSENTIALLY REGULAR: R-R intervals vary slightly but not usually by more than 0.04 second.

   REGULARLY IRREGULAR: R-R intervals contain an irregular cycle that repeats itself in some recognizable pattern. Examples include a premature beat that alternates with a normal beat (bigeminy) or the Wenckebach pattern of group beating.

   OCCASIONALLY IRREGULAR: In general the rhythm is regular, with occasional shortened or lengthened R-R intervals. The irregularity is random rather than patterned.

   IRREGULARLY IRREGULAR: The R-R intervals vary in length in every cycle, making the ventricular rhythm totally irregular.

6. WHAT DO P WAVES LOOK LIKE IN THIS RHYTHM? HOW ARE THEY RELATED TO THE QRS COMPLEXES?

7. ARE THE P-R INTERVALS WITHIN NORMAL LIMITS?

   YES: The P-R is between 0.12 and 0.20 second in duration.

   NO: The P-R is either less than 0.12 or greater than 0.20 second in duration.

8. ARE THE QRS INTERVALS WITHIN NORMAL LIMITS?

   YES: The QRS duration is less than 0.10 second.

   NO: The QRS duration is greater than 0.10 second.

9. WHERE IS THE PRIMARY PACEMAKER LOCATED?

   Is it in the SA node, atria, AV junction, or ventricles?

10. ARE ANY PREMATURE ECTOPIC BEATS PRESENT?

    How does the premature impulse affect the R-R interval?

    What type of P wave is associated with the premature impulse?

    What type of QRS complex is associated with the premature impulse?

    Are the ectopic premature beats PACs, PJCs, or PVCs?

51. (Normal) Sinus Rhythm

RATE: _____   ATRIAL vs. VENTRICULAR RATES: _____

P-P INTERVALS: _____   R-R INTERVALS: _____   RHYTHM: _____

P WAVES: _____   P-R INTERVALS: _____   QRS INTERVALS: _____

(PRIMARY) PACEMAKER SITE: _____

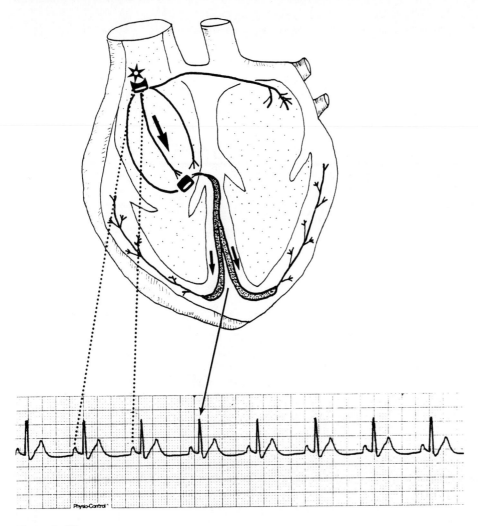

Figure 3–22

52. Sinus Bradycardia

RATE: _____   ATRIAL vs. VENTRICULAR RATES: _____

P-P INTERVALS: _____   R-R INTERVALS: _____   RHYTHM: _____

P WAVES: _____   P-R INTERVALS: _____   QRS INTERVALS: _____

(PRIMARY) PACEMAKER SITE: _____

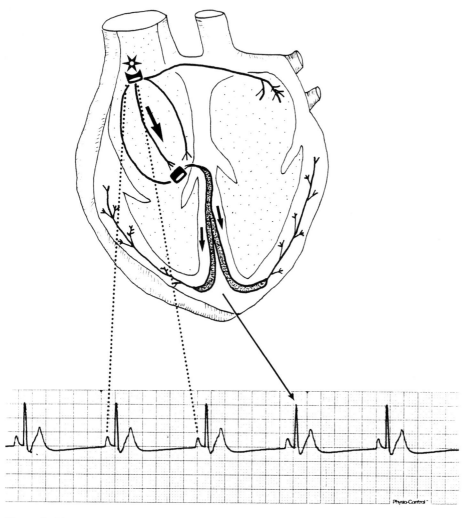

Figure 3–23

53. Sinus Tachycardia

RATE: _____ ATRIAL vs. VENTRICULAR RATES: _____

P-P INTERVALS: _____ R-R INTERVALS: _____ RHYTHM: _____

P WAVES: _____ P-R INTERVALS: _____ QRS INTERVALS: _____

(PRIMARY) PACEMAKER SITE: _____

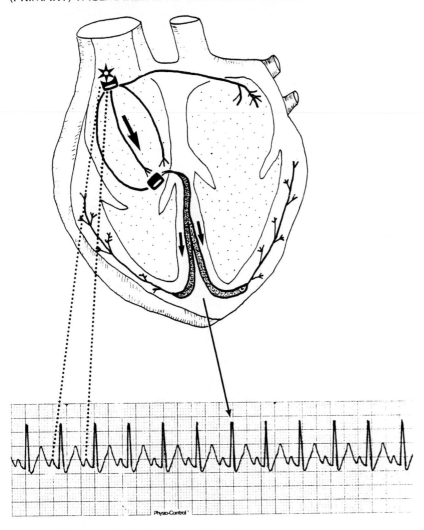

Figure 3–24

54. Wandering Atrial Pacemaker

RATE: _____   ATRIAL vs. VENTRICULAR RATES: _____

P-P INTERVALS: _____   R-R INTERVALS: _____   RHYTHM: _____

P WAVES: _____   P-R INTERVALS: _____   QRS INTERVALS: _____

(PRIMARY) PACEMAKER SITE: _____

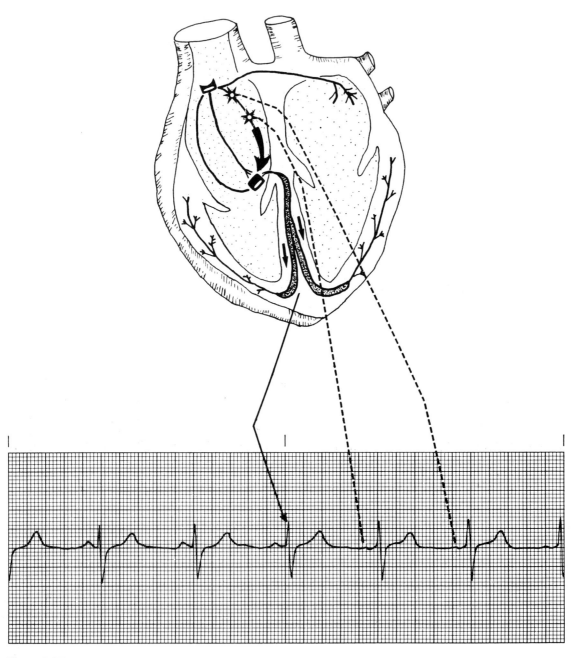

Figure 3-25

55. Atrial Tachycardia

RATE: _____   ATRIAL vs. VENTRICULAR RATES: _____

P-P INTERVALS: _____   R-R INTERVALS: _____   RHYTHM: _____

P WAVES: _____   P-R INTERVALS: _____   QRS INTERVALS: _____

(PRIMARY) PACEMAKER SITE: _____

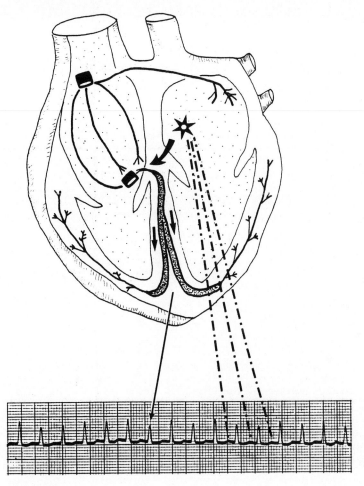

Figure 3-26

56. Atrial Flutter

RATE: _____ ATRIAL vs. VENTRICULAR RATES: _____

P-P INTERVALS: _____ R-R INTERVALS: _____ RHYTHM: _____

P WAVES: _____ P-R INTERVALS: _____ QRS INTERVALS: _____

(PRIMARY) PACEMAKER SITE: _____

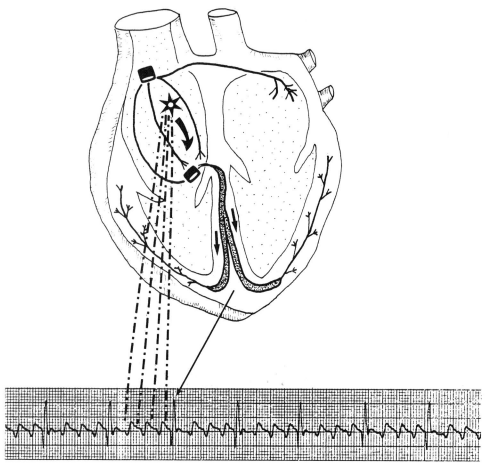

Figure 3–27

57. Atrial Fibrillation

RATE: _____   ATRIAL vs. VENTRICULAR RATES: _____

P-P INTERVALS: _____   R-R INTERVALS: _____   RHYTHM: _____

P WAVES: _____   P-R INTERVALS: _____   QRS INTERVALS: _____

(PRIMARY) PACEMAKER SITE: _____

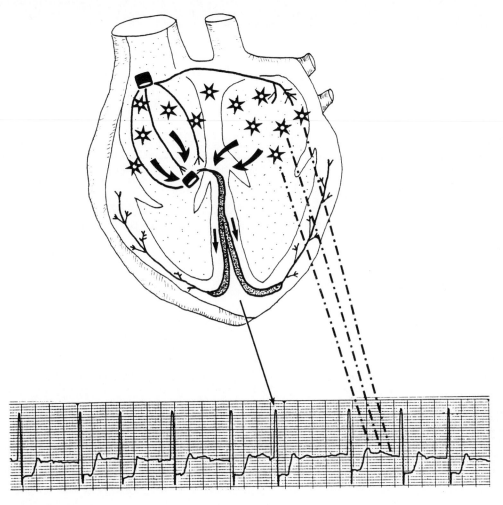

Figure 3–28

58. Premature Atrial Contractions (PACs)

RATE: _____   ATRIAL vs. VENTRICULAR RATES: _____

P-P INTERVALS: _____   R-R INTERVALS: _____   RHYTHM: _____

P WAVES: _____   P-R INTERVALS: _____   QRS INTERVALS: _____

(PRIMARY) PACEMAKER SITE: _____

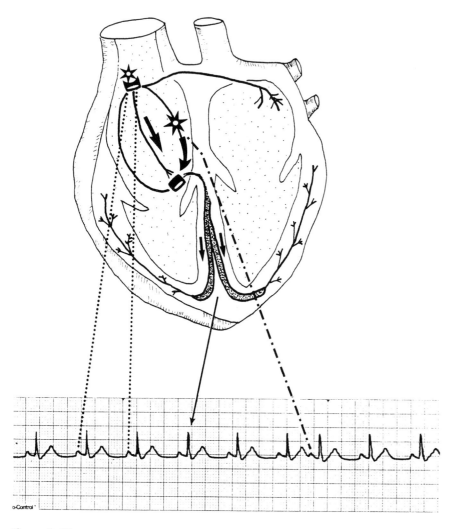

Figure 3–29

59. Premature Junctional Contractions (PJCs)

RATE: _____ ATRIAL vs. VENTRICULAR RATES: _____

P-P INTERVALS: _____ R-R INTERVALS: _____ RHYTHM: _____

P WAVES: _____ P-R INTERVALS: _____ QRS INTERVALS: _____

(PRIMARY) PACEMAKER SITE: _____

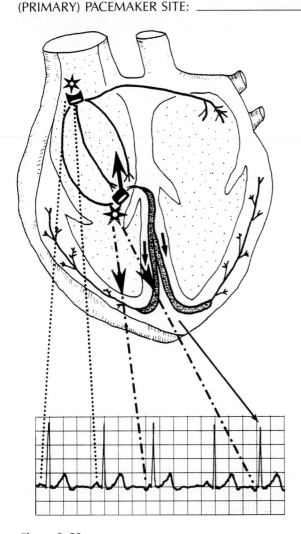

Figure 3–30

60. Premature Ventricular Contractions (PVCs)

RATE: _____ ATRIAL vs. VENTRICULAR RATES: _____

P-P INTERVALS: _____ R-R INTERVALS: _____ RHYTHM: _____

P WAVES: _____ P-R INTERVALS: _____ QRS INTERVALS: _____

(PRIMARY) PACEMAKER SITE: _____

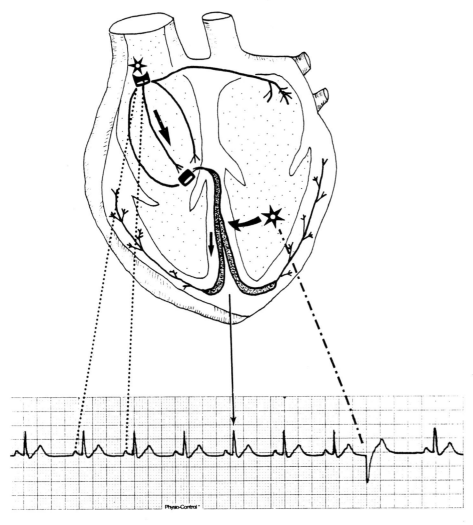

Figure 3–31

Multiform Premature Ventricular Contractions (PVCs)

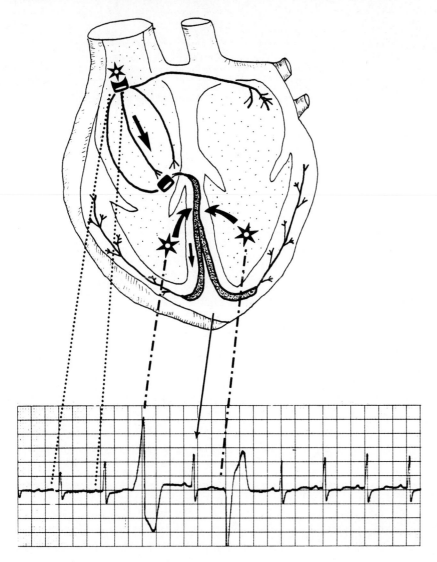

Figure 3–32

61. Junctional Escape Rhythm

RATE: _____   ATRIAL vs. VENTRICULAR RATES: _____

P-P INTERVALS: _____   R-R INTERVALS: _____   RHYTHM: _____

P WAVES: _____   P-R INTERVALS: _____   QRS INTERVALS: _____

(PRIMARY) PACEMAKER SITE: _____

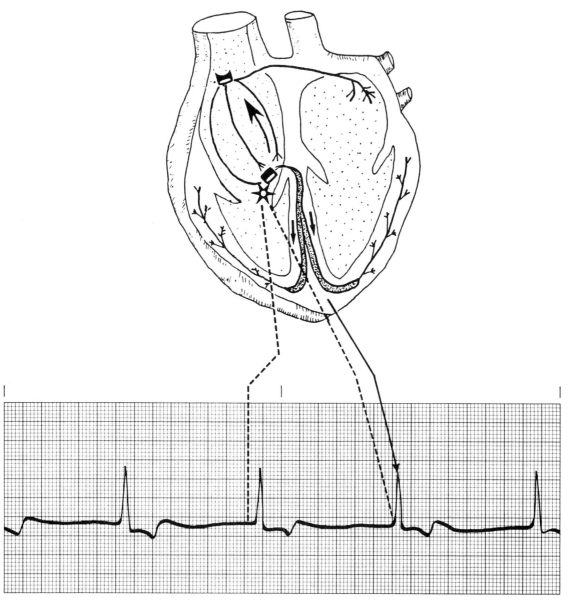

Figure 3–33

62. Accelerated Junctional Rhythm

RATE: _____ ATRIAL vs. VENTRICULAR RATES: _____

P-P INTERVALS: _____ R-R INTERVALS: _____ RHYTHM: _____

P WAVES: _____ P-R INTERVALS: _____ QRS INTERVALS: _____

(PRIMARY) PACEMAKER SITE: _____

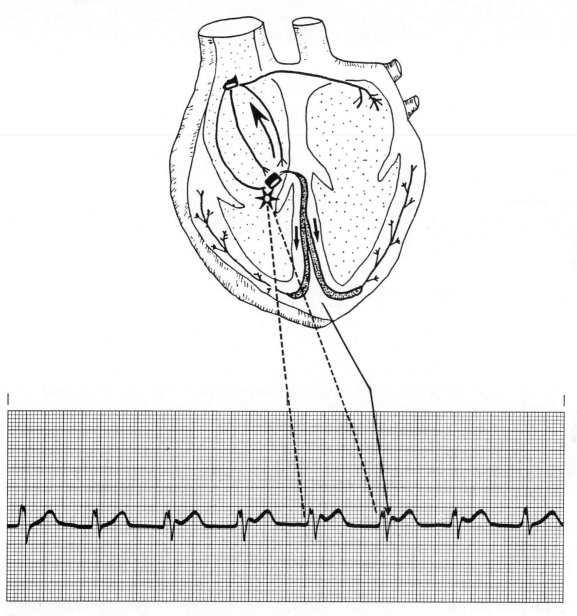

Figure 3-34

63. Ventricular Tachycardia

RATE: _____ ATRIAL vs. VENTRICULAR RATES: _____

P-P INTERVALS: _____ R-R INTERVALS: _____ RHYTHM: _____

P WAVES: _____ P-R INTERVALS: _____ QRS INTERVALS: _____

(PRIMARY) PACEMAKER SITE: _____

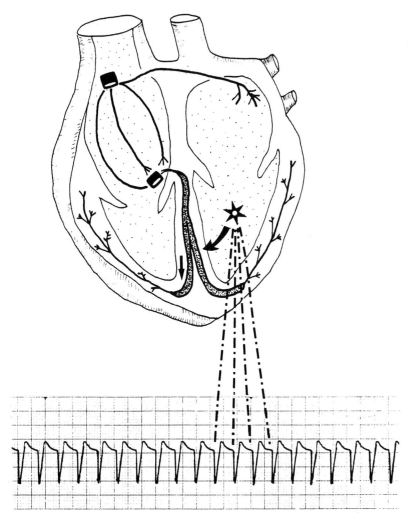

Figure 3–35

64. Ventricular Fibrillation

RATE: _____ ATRIAL vs. VENTRICULAR RATES: _____

P-P INTERVALS: _____ R-R INTERVALS: _____ RHYTHM: _____

P WAVES: _____ P-R INTERVALS: _____ QRS INTERVALS: _____

(PRIMARY) PACEMAKER SITE: _____

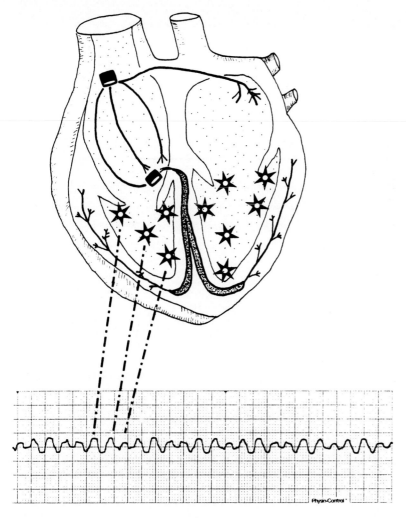

Figure 3–36

65. Idioventricular Rhythm

RATE: _____   ATRIAL vs. VENTRICULAR RATES: _____

P-P INTERVALS: _____   R-R INTERVALS: _____   RHYTHM: _____

P WAVES: _____   P-R INTERVALS: _____   QRS INTERVALS: _____

(PRIMARY) PACEMAKER SITE: _____

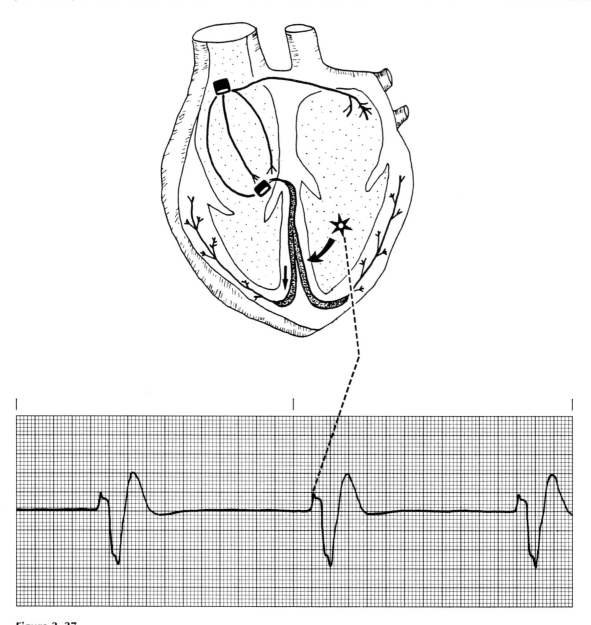

Figure 3–37

66. First-degree AV Block

RATE: _____   ATRIAL vs. VENTRICULAR RATES: _____

P-P INTERVALS: _____   R-R INTERVALS: _____   RHYTHM: _____

P WAVES: _____   P-R INTERVALS: _____   QRS INTERVALS: _____

(PRIMARY) PACEMAKER SITE: _____

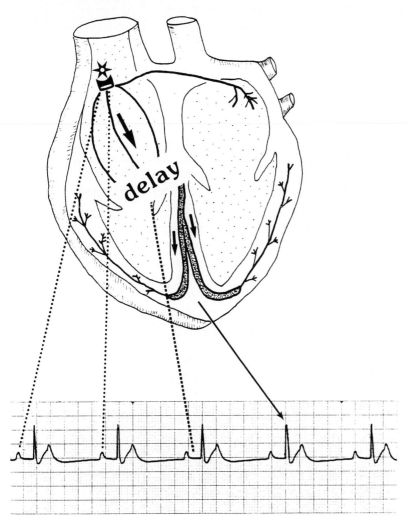

Figure 3–38

67. Second-degree AV Block, Mobitz I (Wenckebach)

RATE: _____   ATRIAL vs. VENTRICULAR RATES: _____

P-P INTERVALS: _____   R-R INTERVALS: _____   RHYTHM: _____

P WAVES: _____   P-R INTERVALS: _____   QRS INTERVALS: _____

(PRIMARY) PACEMAKER SITE: _____

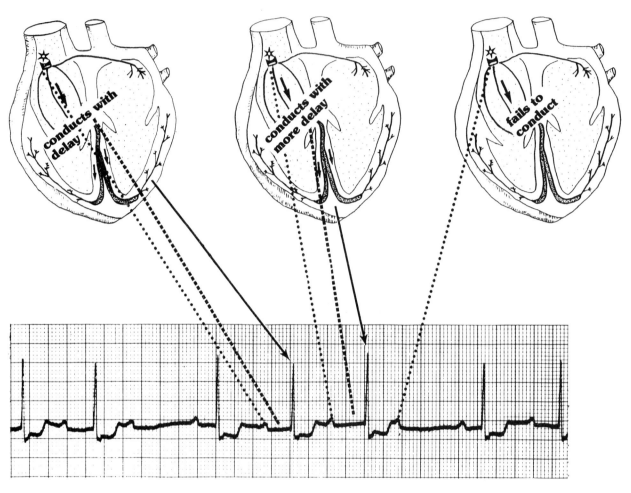

Figure 3–39

68. Second-degree AV Block, Mobitz II

RATE: _____ ATRIAL vs. VENTRICULAR RATES: _____

P-P INTERVALS: _____ R-R INTERVALS: _____ RHYTHM: _____

P WAVES: _____ P-R INTERVALS: _____ QRS INTERVALS: _____

(PRIMARY) PACEMAKER SITE: _____

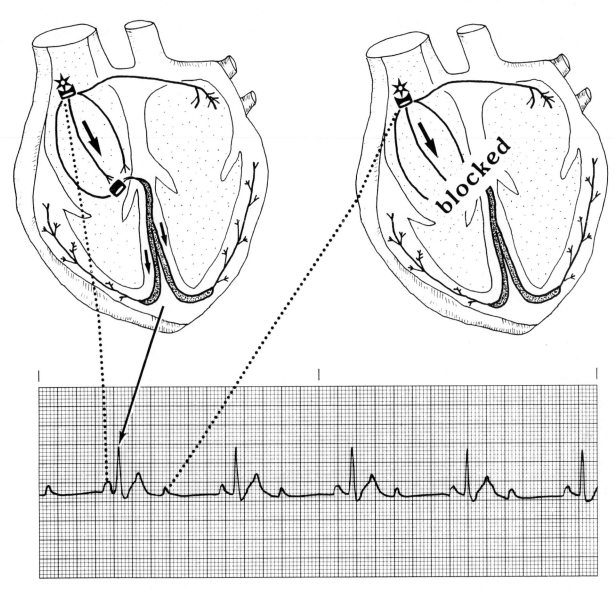

Figure 3–40

69. Third-degree (Complete) AV Block

RATE: _____ ATRIAL vs. VENTRICULAR RATES: _____

P-P INTERVALS: _____ R-R INTERVALS: _____ RHYTHM: _____

P WAVES: _____ P-R INTERVALS: _____ QRS INTERVALS: _____

(PRIMARY) PACEMAKER SITE: _____

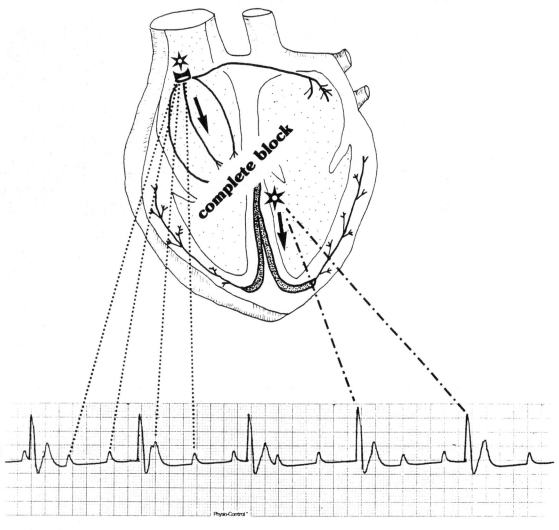

Figure 3-41

Directions: Fill in the characteristics of the rhythms given in Table 3-1.

TABLE 3-1

	Rate	Regularity	P Waves	QRS Complexes	Ratio of Atrial to Ventricular	P-R Interval	P to P Interval (regularity)	R to R Interval (regularity)	Clinical Significance of Rhythm
Sinus Rhythm									
Sinus Arrhythmia									
Sinus Bradycardia									
Sinus Tachycardia									
Atrial Flutter									
Atrial Fibrillation									
Atrial Tachycardia									

Directions: Fill in the characteristics of the rhythms given in Table 3–2.

TABLE 3–2

	Rate	Regularity	P Waves	QRS Complexes	Ratio of Atrial to Ventricular	P-R Interval	P to P Interval (regularity)	R to R Interval (regularity)	Clinical Significance of Rhythm
Wandering Atrial Pacemaker									
Junctional Escape Rhythm									
Accelerated Junctional Rhythm									
Junctional Tachycardia									
First-degree AV Block									
Mobitz I, Wenckebach									
Mobitz II, Second-Degree AV Block									

Directions: Fill in the characteristics of the rhythms given in Table 3–3.

TABLE 3–3

	Rate	Regularity	P Waves	QRS Complexes	Ratio of Atrial to Ventricular	P-R Interval	P to P Interval (regularity)	R to R Interval (regularity)	Clinical Significance of Rhythm
Complete AV Block									
Ventricular Tachycardia									
Ventricular Fibrillation									
Idioventricular Rhythm									
Agonal Rhythm									
Asystole									

Directions: Fill in the characteristics of the rhythms given in Table 3–4.

TABLE 3–4

	Site of Origin	P Wave	QRS Complexes	T Wave	Effect on R-R Interval	Compensatory Pause
Premature Atrial Contraction						
Premature Junctional Contraction						
Premature Ventricular Contraction						

ADDITIONAL ECG REVIEW

True or False

70. T   F   (Normal) sinus rhythm has a P-R interval between 0.12 and 0.20 second.

71. T   F   The pacemaker site of the ECG in Figure 3–42 is in the SA node.

72. T   F   The ECG rhythm in Figure 3–42 is sinus bradycardia.

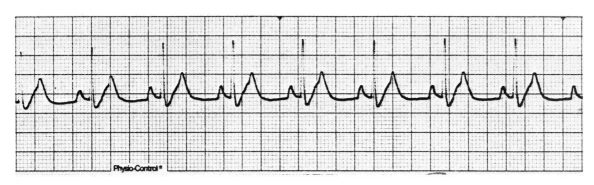

Figure 3–42

73. T   F   In sinus bradycardia, there is more than one P wave for every QRS complex.

74. T   F   In sinus bradycardia, the rhythm is essentially regular.

75. T   F   Sinus bradycardia may cause decreased cardiac output.

76. T   F   Sinus tachycardia is usually the result of severe coronary artery disease.

77. T   F   Atrial rhythms originate in the AV junction.

78. T   F   For an atrial rhythm to occur, an atrial pacemaker must initiate an impulse faster than the SA node.

79. T   F   Atrial rhythms have P waves and QRS complexes that are identical to those found in sinus rhythms.

80. T   F   A wandering atrial pacemaker has P waves that vary in size and configuration.

81. T   F   In wandering atrial pacemaker, the P-R interval remains constant.

82. T   F   The early beats on the rhythm strip (Figure 3–43) are premature atrial contractions.

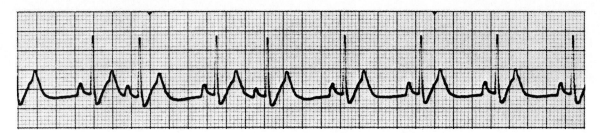

Figure 3–43

83. T   F   Atrial tachycardia may be caused by the rapid firing of one or several atrial pacemakers.

84. T   F   Atrial tachycardia usually has a rate between 160 and 220 beats per minute.

85. T   F   Atrial tachycardia rarely results in hemodynamic compromise.

86. T   F   In atrial tachycardia, the P waves are often buried in the T wave of the preceding beat.

87. T   F   In atrial tachycardia, the QRS complexes will usually be wide and bizarre in appearance.

88. T   F   Atrial tachycardia is characterized by sawtooth waveforms that replace normal P waves.

89. T   F   The rhythm strip in Figure 3–44 shows a variable AV conduction ratio.

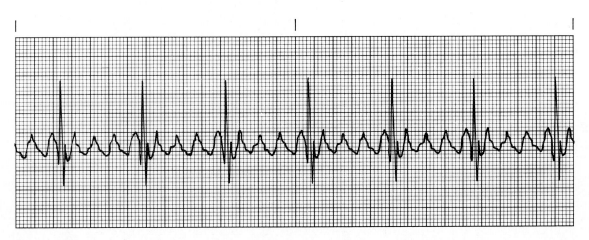

Figure 3–44

90. T   F   With the dysrhythmia in Figure 3–45, the atria are neither filling nor emptying effectively.

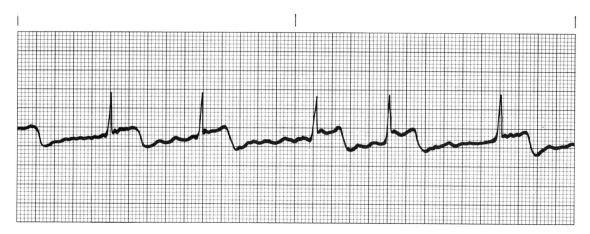

Figure 3–45

91. T   F   In atrial fibrillation, all the atrial impulses are conducted through to the ventricles.

92. T   F   There are no identifiable P waves in atrial fibrillation.

93. T   F   Retrograde atrial conduction indicates the presence of myocardial disease.

94. T   F   In junctional rhythms, the QRS complex is normal in duration and configuration.

95. T   F   The P wave of a PJC may precede, coincide with, or follow the QRS complex.

96. T   F   Rhythms that arise due to the failure (default) of higher pacemakers are called escape rhythms.

97. T   F   If the SA node stopped functioning, you would expect to see the ECG rhythm in Figure 3–46.

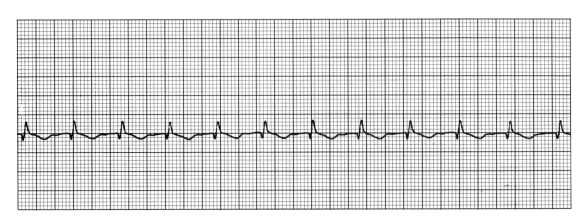

Figure 3–46

98. T   F   A junctional rhythm at 60 to 100 per minute is called an accelerated junctional rhythm; a junctional rhythm at 100 to 180 per minute is called a junctional tachycardia.

99. T   F   In both accelerated junctional rhythm and junctional tachycardia, P waves are not observable and QRS complexes are wide and bizarre.

100. T   F   AV blocks (conduction defects) result when an impulse that originated in the SA node is delayed or blocked as it passes through the AV junction.

101. T   F   All degrees of AV block have more P waves than QRS complexes.

102. T   F   The ECG in Figure 3–47 shows second-degree AV block, Mobitz II.

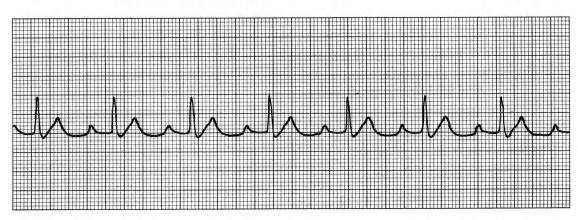

Figure 3–47

103. T   F   In the Wenckebach form of AV block, a QRS follows each P wave.

104. T   F   In the Wenckebach form of AV block, P-P intervals are regular.

105. T   F   In the Wenckebach form of AV block, there is a progressive lengthening of the P-R interval until a QRS complex is "dropped."

106. T   F   The Wenckebach phenomenon produces a rhythm that may be characterized as regularly irregular.

107. T   F   The ECG strip in Figure 3–48 shows second-degree AV block, Mobitz I (Wenckebach).

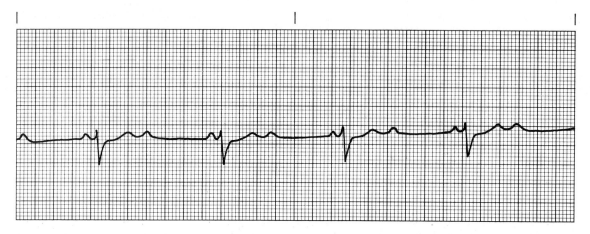

Figure 3–48

108. T   F   Second-degree AV block, Mobitz II, is characterized by more P waves than QRS complexes and a constant P-R interval in all conducted beats.

109. T   F   Second-degree AV block, Mobitz II, is an intermittent AV block.

110. T   F   In Mobitz II AV block, the AV junction blocks impulses at a constant ratio.

111. T   F   The ECG strip in Figure 3–49 shows third-degree (complete) AV block.

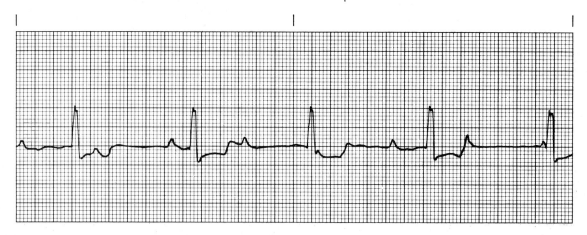

Figure 3–49

112. T   F   In complete AV block, the P-P and R-R intervals are each regular.

113. T   F   In complete AV block, the P-R interval remains constant.

114. T   F   The QRS complex may be of junctional or ventricular origin in third-degree AV block.

115. T   F   Third-degree AV block may be classified as an intermittent block in AV conduction.

116. T   F   Ventricular rhythms have QRS complexes longer than 0.12 second in duration.

117. T   F   When a beat that originated above the ventricles has an associated QRS greater than 0.12 second in duration, there is a problem with conduction through the ventricular pathways.

118. T   F   Ventricular escape rhythms usually have a rate between 40 and 60 beats per minute.

119. T   F   Premature ventricular contractions (PVCs) have a bizarre QRS greater than 0.12 second in duration and an ST segment and T wave opposite in polarity to the major QRS deflection.

120. T   F   An interpolated PVC is one that does not interrupt the normal R-R interval and has no compensatory pause.

121. T   F   An R-on-T phenomenon occurs when the R wave of a PVC falls on or near the T wave of the preceding cycle.

122. T   F   A PVC that falls on the "vulnerable period" of the preceding T wave is of little clinical concern.

123. T   F   PVCs that occur in succession (pairs) are more likely to precipitate ventricular fibrillation than occasional, single PVCs.

124. T   F   When PVCs alternate with normal sinus beats, the resulting dysrhythmia is called ventricular trigeminy.

125. T   F   Bigeminal, trigeminal, and quadrigeminal PVCs cause the ventricular rhythm to be regularly irregular.

126. T   F   Ventricular tachycardia is usually the result of increased ventricular ectopic automaticity or reentry.

127. T   F   Ventricular tachycardia usually has a rate of 20 to 40 per minute.

128. T   F   In ventricular tachycardia, QRS complexes are less than 0.12 second in duration and are preceded by a P wave.

129. T   F   The dysrhythmia illustrated in Figure 3–50 rarely results in hemodynamic compromise.

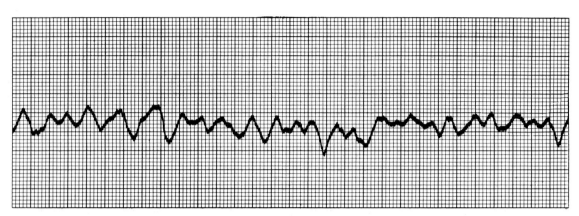

Figure 3–50

130. T   F   An idioventricular escape rhythm typically affords an inadequate cardiac output.

131. T   F   The ECG in Figure 3–51 shows an agonal rhythm.

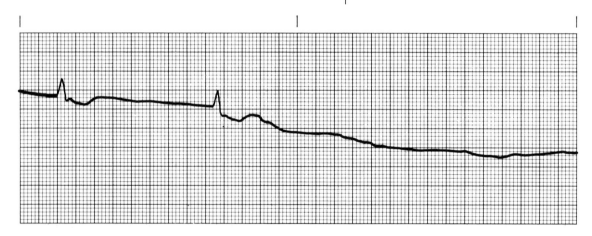

Figure 3–51

132. T   F   Ventricular asystole is evidenced as a continuous straight line on the ECG strip.

133. Place a check mark beside the dysrhythmias listed below that have more P waves than QRS complexes.

_____ sinus rhythm

_____ sinus bradycardia

_____ sinus tachycardia

_____ atrial tachycardia

_____ 1st-degree AV block

_____ 2nd-degree AV block, Type I (Wenckebach)

_____ 2nd-degree AV block, Type II

_____ 3rd-degree AV block

134. Place a check mark beside the dysrhythmias below that could result in an *irregular* R-R (ventricular) rhythm.

_____ sinus rhythm

_____ sinus bradycardia

_____ sinus tachycardia

_____ atrial tachycardia

_____ 1st-degree AV block

_____ 2nd-degree AV block, Type I (Wenckebach)

_____ 2nd-degree AV block, Type II

_____ 3rd-degree AV block

_____ ventricular tachycardia

_____ atrial fibrillation

_____ atrial flutter

_____ PACs

_____ PJCs

_____ PVCs

135. Match the following P-R intervals with the dysrhythmias and conduction defects they characterize:

P-R Interval

a. ranges between 0.12 and 0.20 second
b. usually less than 0.12 second
c. greater than 0.20 second
d. progressively lengthens
e. completely inconsistent

Dysrhythmia

_____ sinus rhythm

_____ sinus bradycardia

_____ sinus tachycardia

_____ atrial tachycardia

_____ 1st-degree AV block

_____ 2nd-degree AV block, Type I (Wenckebach)

_____ 2nd-degree AV block, Type II

_____ 3rd-degree AV block

_____ junctional escape rhythm

_____ accelerated junctional rhythm

ECG RHYTHM STRIP INTERPRETATION

Each rhythm strip in Figures 3–52 through 3–168 must be analyzed in a systematic fashion. The following questions are asked each time a dysrhythmia is analyzed:

RATE

What is the exact rate?
Is the atrial rate the same as the ventricular rate?

RHYTHM

Is it regular or irregular?
Are there any patterns to the irregularity?
Are there any ectopic beats? If so, are they early or late?

P WAVES

Are the P waves regular?
Is there one P wave for every QRS complex?
Is the P wave in front of or behind the QRS complex?

Is the P wave normal and upright in lead II?
Are there more P waves than QRS complexes?
Do all the P waves look alike?
Are the irregular P waves associated with ectopic beats?

P-R INTERVAL

Are all the P-R intervals constant?
Is the P-R interval within the normal range?
If the P-R interval varies, is there a pattern to the changing measurements?

QRS COMPLEX

What is the QRS duration?
Is the QRS duration within the normal range?
Are all QRS complexes equal in duration?
Do all the QRS complexes look alike?
Are the abnormal QRS complexes associated with ectopic beats?

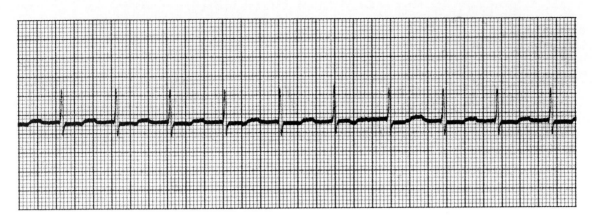

Figure 3–52

136. RATE: _____ RHYTHM: _____
  P WAVES: _____ P-R INTERVALS: _____
  QRS: _____ INTERPRETATION: _____

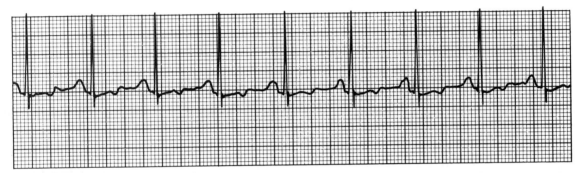

Figure 3–53

137. RATE: _____ RHYTHM: _____
  P WAVES: _____ P-R INTERVALS: _____
  QRS: _____ INTERPRETATION: _____

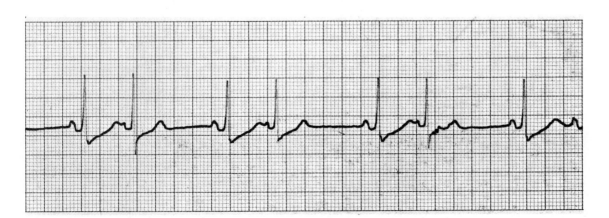

Figure 3–54

138. RATE: _____ RHYTHM: _____
  P WAVES: _____ P-R INTERVALS: _____
  QRS: _____ INTERPRETATION: _____

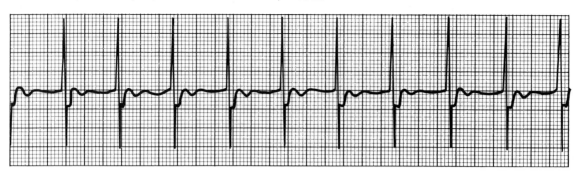

Figure 3–55

139. RATE: _____ RHYTHM: _____

      P WAVES: _____ P-R INTERVALS: _____

      QRS: _____ INTERPRETATION: _____

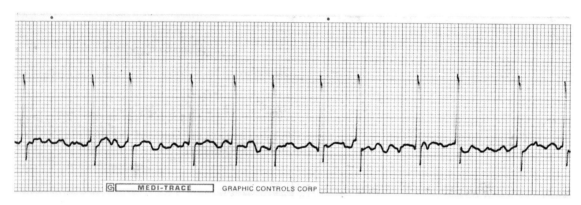

Figure 3–56

140. RATE: _____ RHYTHM: _____

      P WAVES: _____ P-R INTERVALS: _____

      QRS: _____ INTERPRETATION: _____

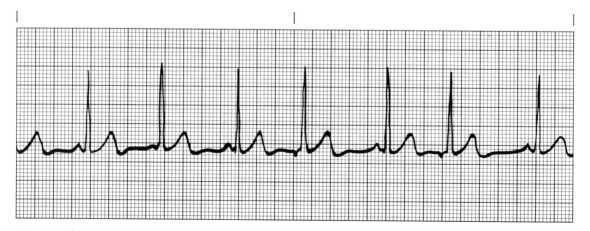

Figure 3–57

141. RATE: _____ RHYTHM: _____

      P WAVES: _____ P-R INTERVALS: _____

      QRS: _____ INTERPRETATION: _____

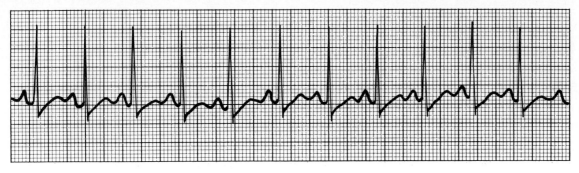

Figure 3–58

142. RATE: _____ RHYTHM: _____

P WAVES: _____ P-R INTERVALS: _____

QRS: _____ INTERPRETATION: _____

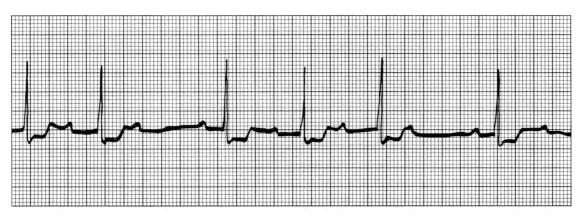

Figure 3–59

143. RATE: _____ RHYTHM: _____

P WAVES: _____ P-R INTERVALS: _____

QRS: _____ INTERPRETATION: _____

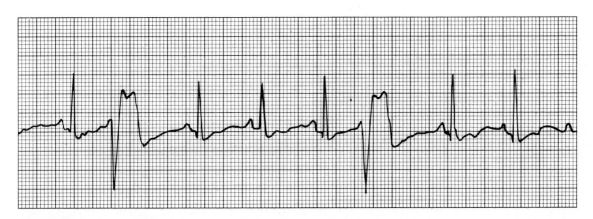

Figure 3–60

144. RATE: _____ RHYTHM: _____

P WAVES: _____ P-R INTERVALS: _____

QRS: _____ INTERPRETATION: _____

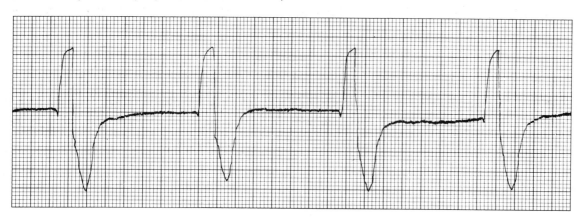

Figure 3–61

145. RATE: _____ RHYTHM: _____

     P WAVES: _____ P-R INTERVALS: _____

     QRS: _____ INTERPRETATION: _____

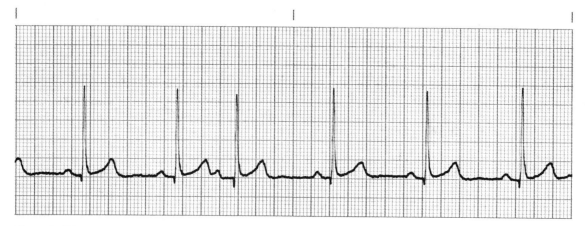

Figure 3–62

146. RATE: _____ RHYTHM: _____

     P WAVES: _____ P-R INTERVALS: _____

     QRS: _____ INTERPRETATION: _____

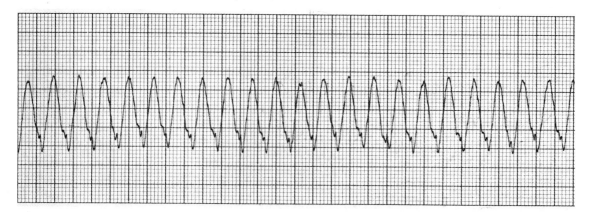

Figure 3–63

147. RATE: _____ RHYTHM: _____

     P WAVES: _____ P-R INTERVALS: _____

     QRS: _____ INTERPRETATION: _____

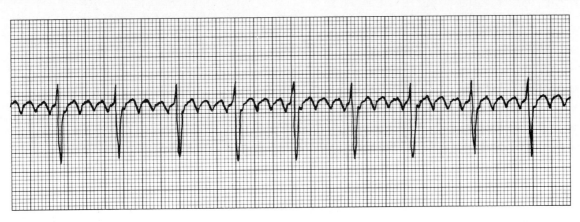

Figure 3–64

148. RATE: _____ RHYTHM: _____
P WAVES: _____ P-R INTERVALS: _____
QRS: _____ INTERPRETATION: _____

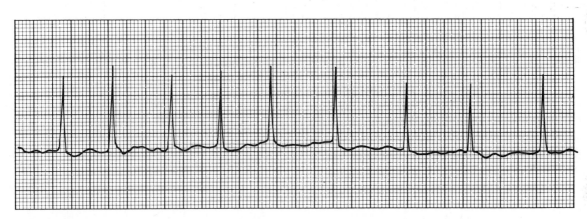

Figure 3–65

149. RATE: _____ RHYTHM: _____
P WAVES: _____ P-R INTERVALS: _____
QRS: _____ INTERPRETATION: _____

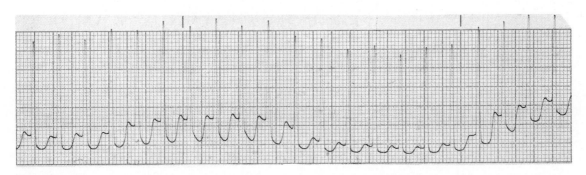

Figure 3–66

150. RATE: _____ RHYTHM: _____
P WAVES: _____ P-R INTERVALS: _____
QRS: _____ INTERPRETATION: _____

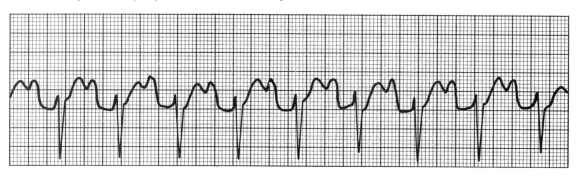

Figure 3-67

151. RATE: _____   RHYTHM: _____

   P WAVES: _____   P-R INTERVALS: _____

   QRS: _____   INTERPRETATION: _____

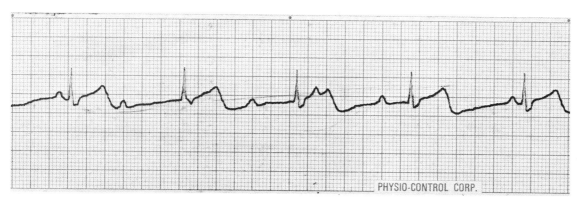

PHYSIO-CONTROL CORP.

Figure 3-68

152. RATE: _____   RHYTHM: _____

   P WAVES: _____   P-R INTERVALS: _____

   QRS: _____   INTERPRETATION: _____

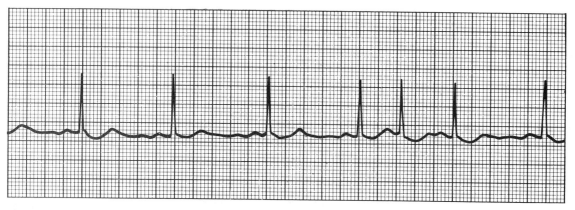

Figure 3-69

153. RATE: _____   RHYTHM: _____

   P WAVES: _____   P-R INTERVALS: _____

   QRS: _____   INTERPRETATION: _____

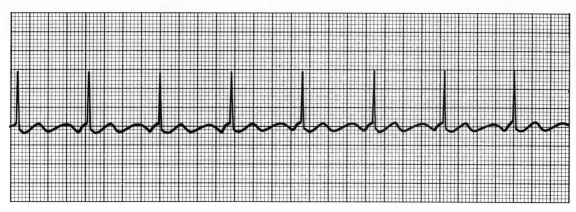

Figure 3–70

154. RATE: _____ RHYTHM: _____

     P WAVES: _____ P-R INTERVALS: _____

     QRS: _____ INTERPRETATION: _____

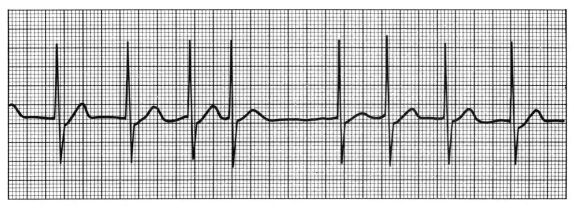

Figure 3–71

155. RATE: _____ RHYTHM: _____

     P WAVES: _____ P-R INTERVALS: _____

     QRS: _____ INTERPRETATION: _____

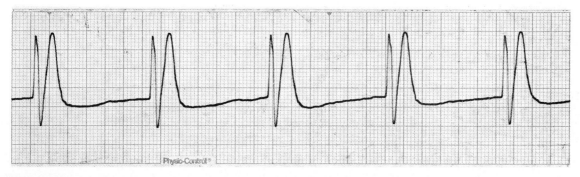

Figure 3–72

156. RATE: _____ RHYTHM: _____

     P WAVES: _____ P-R INTERVALS: _____

     QRS: _____ INTERPRETATION: _____

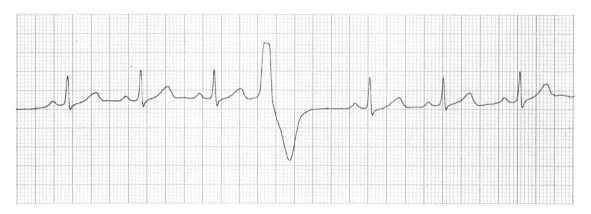

Figure 3–73

157. RATE: _____ RHYTHM: _____

   P WAVES: _____ P-R INTERVALS: _____

   QRS: _____ INTERPRETATION: _____

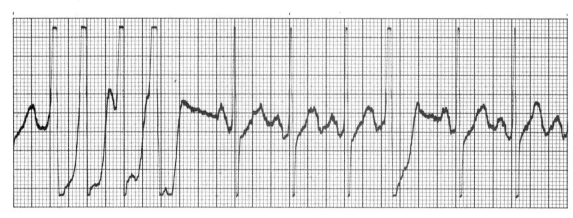

Figure 3–74

158. RATE: _____ RHYTHM: _____

   P WAVES: _____ P-R INTERVALS: _____

   QRS: _____ INTERPRETATION: _____

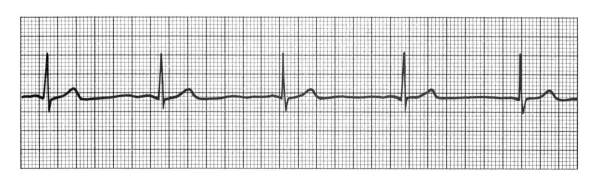

Figure 3–75

159. RATE: _____ RHYTHM: _____

   P WAVES: _____ P-R INTERVALS: _____

   QRS: _____ INTERPRETATION: _____

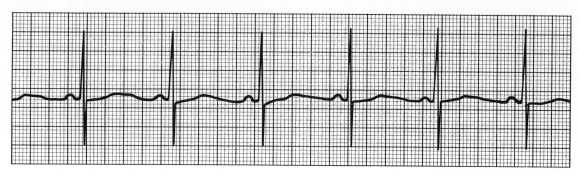

Figure 3–76

160. RATE: _____ RHYTHM: _____

P WAVES: _____ P-R INTERVALS: _____

QRS: _____ INTERPRETATION: _____

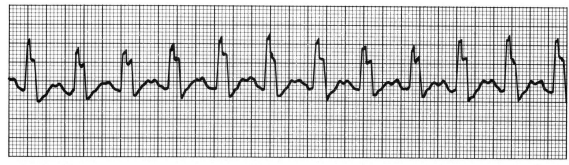

Figure 3–77

161. RATE: _____ RHYTHM: _____

P WAVES: _____ P-R INTERVALS: _____

QRS: _____ INTERPRETATION: _____

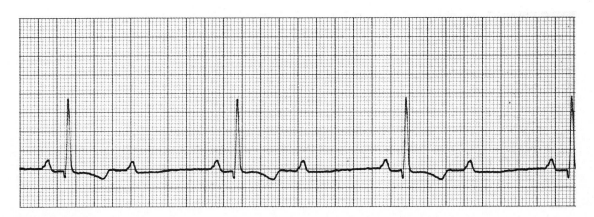

Figure 3–78

162. RATE: _____ RHYTHM: _____

P WAVES: _____ P-R INTERVALS: _____

QRS: _____ INTERPRETATION: _____

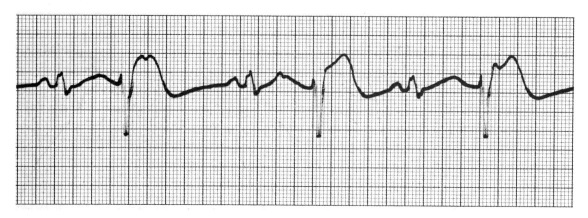

Figure 3–79

163. RATE: _____   RHYTHM: _____
    P WAVES: _____   P-R INTERVALS: _____
    QRS: _____   INTERPRETATION: _____

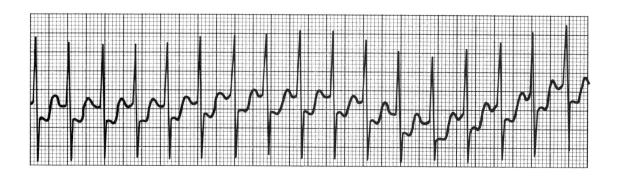

Figure 3–80

164. RATE: _____   RHYTHM: _____
    P WAVES: _____   P-R INTERVALS: _____
    QRS: _____   INTERPRETATION: _____

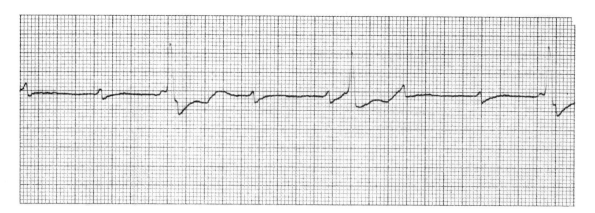

Figure 3–81

165. RATE: _____   RHYTHM: _____
    P WAVES: _____   P-R INTERVALS: _____
    QRS: _____   INTERPRETATION: _____

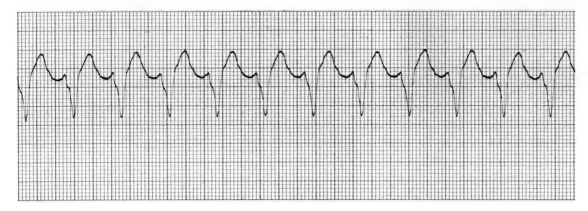

Figure 3–82

166. RATE: _____ RHYTHM: _____

P WAVES: _____ P-R INTERVALS: _____

QRS: _____ INTERPRETATION: _____

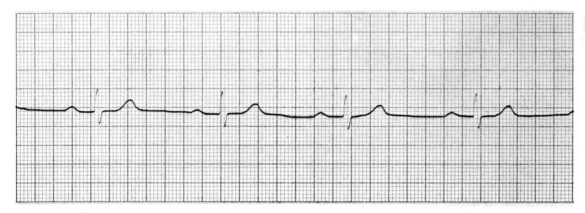

Figure 3–83

167. RATE: _____ RHYTHM: _____

P WAVES: _____ P-R INTERVALS: _____

QRS: _____ INTERPRETATION: _____

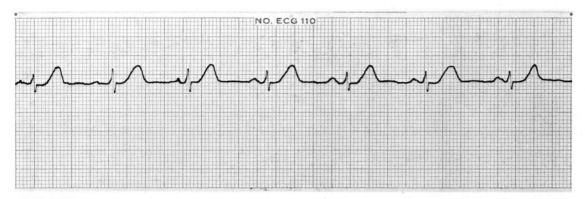

Figure 3–84

168. RATE: _____ RHYTHM: _____

P WAVES: _____ P-R INTERVALS: _____

QRS: _____ INTERPRETATION: _____

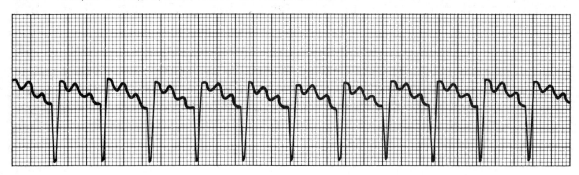

Figure 3–85

169. RATE: _____   RHYTHM: _____
  P WAVES: _____   P-R INTERVALS: _____
  QRS: _____   INTERPRETATION: _____

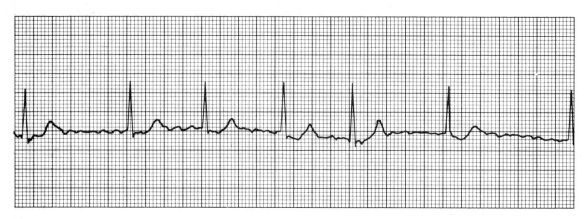

Figure 3–86

170. RATE: _____   RHYTHM: _____
  P WAVES: _____   P-R INTERVALS: _____
  QRS: _____   INTERPRETATION: _____

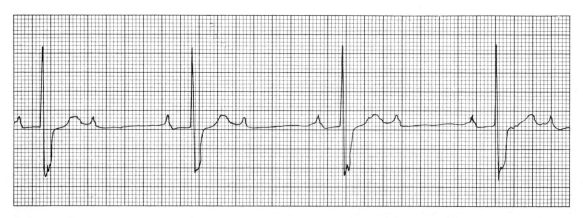

Figure 3–87

171. RATE: _____   RHYTHM: _____
  P WAVES: _____   P-R INTERVALS: _____
  QRS: _____   INTERPRETATION: _____

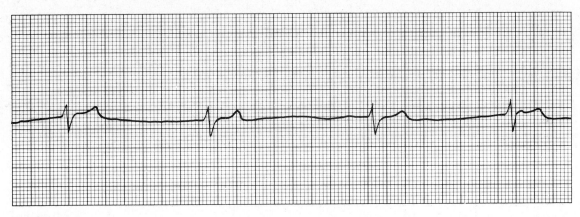

Figure 3–88

172. RATE: _____   RHYTHM: _____

P WAVES: _____   P-R INTERVALS: _____

QRS: _____   INTERPRETATION: _____

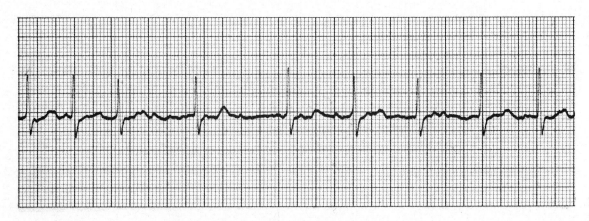

Figure 3–89

173. RATE: _____   RHYTHM: _____

P WAVES: _____   P-R INTERVALS: _____

QRS: _____   INTERPRETATION: _____

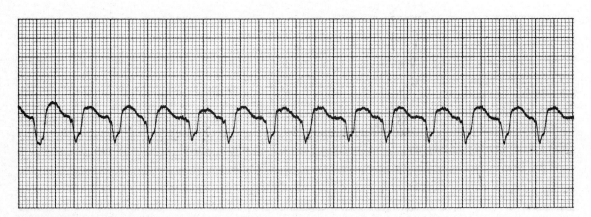

Figure 3–90

174. RATE: _____   RHYTHM: _____

P WAVES: _____   P-R INTERVALS: _____

QRS: _____   INTERPRETATION: _____

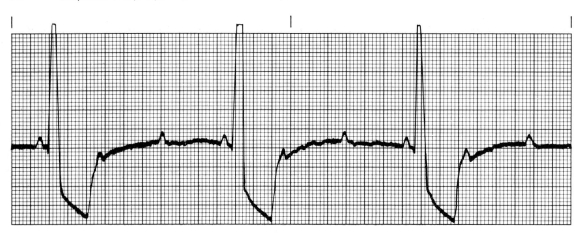

Figure 3–91

175. RATE: _____   RHYTHM: _____
      P WAVES: _____   P-R INTERVALS: _____
      QRS: _____   INTERPRETATION: _____

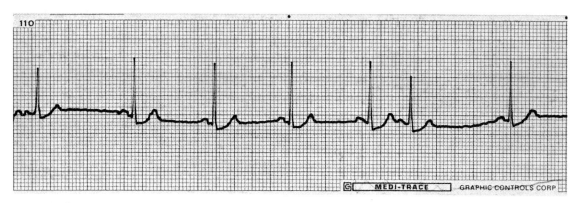

Figure 3–92

176. RATE: _____   RHYTHM: _____
      P WAVES: _____   P-R INTERVALS: _____
      QRS: _____   INTERPRETATION: _____

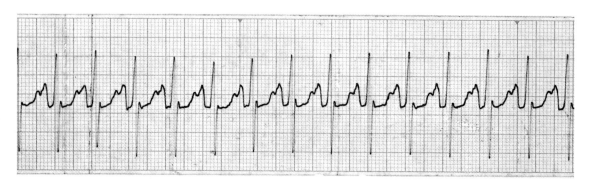

Figure 3–93

177. RATE: _____   RHYTHM: _____
      P WAVES: _____   P-R INTERVALS: _____
      QRS: _____   INTERPRETATION: _____

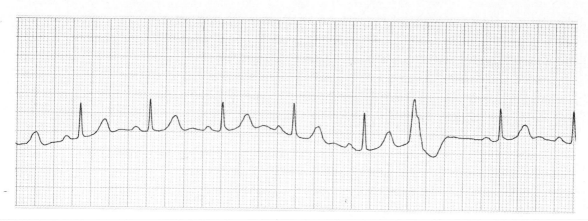

Figure 3–94

178. RATE: _____   RHYTHM: _____

     P WAVES: _____   P-R INTERVALS: _____

     QRS: _____   INTERPRETATION: _____

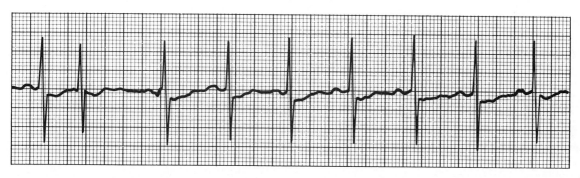

Figure 3–95

179. RATE: _____   RHYTHM: _____

     P WAVES: _____   P-R INTERVALS: _____

     QRS: _____   INTERPRETATION: _____

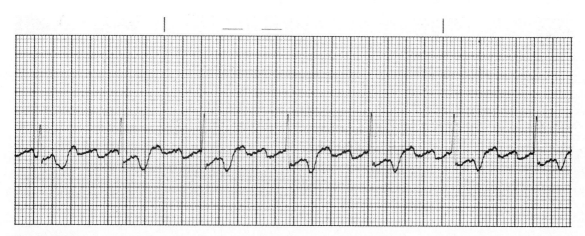

Figure 3–96

180. RATE: _____   RHYTHM: _____

     P WAVES: _____   P-R INTERVALS: _____

     QRS: _____   INTERPRETATION: _____

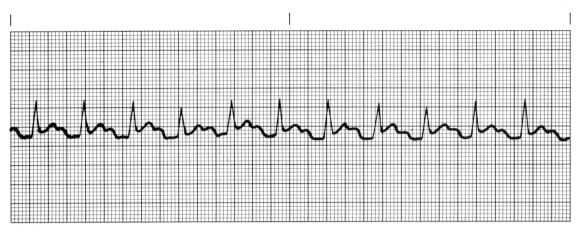

Figure 3–97

181. RATE: _____   RHYTHM: _____

    P WAVES: _____   P-R INTERVALS: _____

    QRS: _____   INTERPRETATION: _____

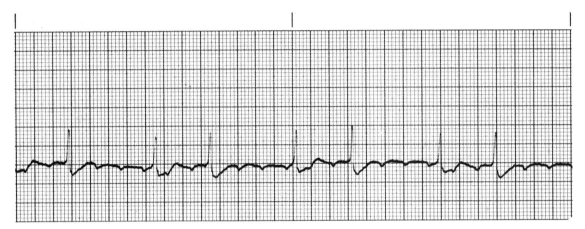

Figure 3–98

182. RATE: _____   RHYTHM: _____

    P WAVES: _____   P-R INTERVALS: _____

    QRS: _____   INTERPRETATION: _____

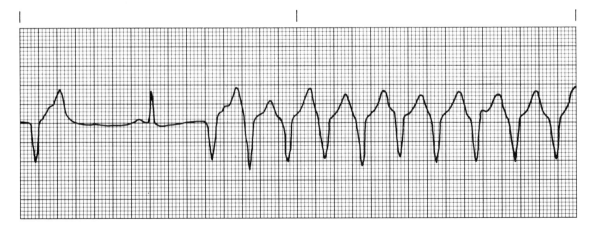

Figure 3–99

183. RATE: _____   RHYTHM: _____

    P WAVES: _____   P-R INTERVALS: _____

    QRS: _____   INTERPRETATION: _____

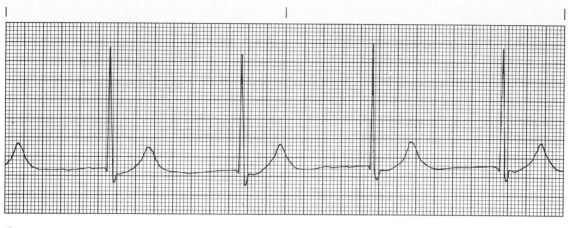

Figure 3–100

184. RATE: _____   RHYTHM: _____
      P WAVES: _____   P-R INTERVALS: _____
      QRS: _____   INTERPRETATION: _____

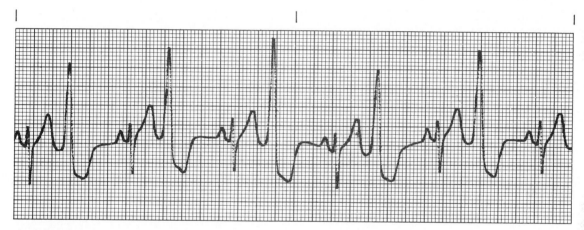

Figure 3–101

185. RATE: _____   RHYTHM: _____
      P WAVES: _____   P-R INTERVALS: _____
      QRS: _____   INTERPRETATION: _____

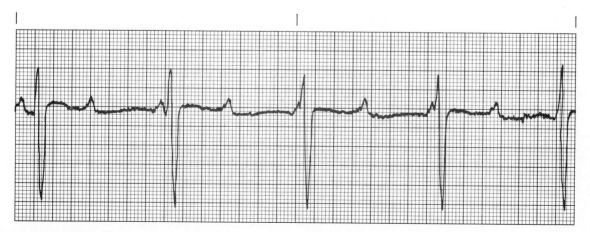

Figure 3–102

186. RATE: _____   RHYTHM: _____
      P WAVES: _____   P-R INTERVALS: _____
      QRS: _____   INTERPRETATION: _____

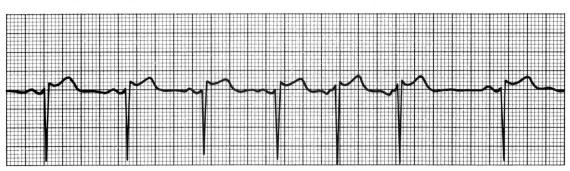

Figure 3–103

187. RATE: _____   RHYTHM: _____

       P WAVES: _____   P-R INTERVALS: _____

       QRS: _____   INTERPRETATION: _____

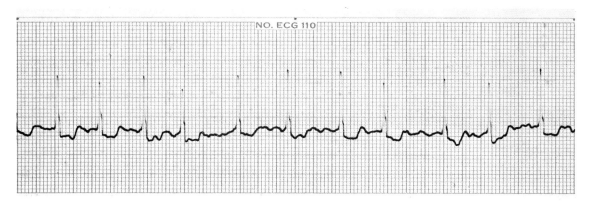

Figure 3–104

188. RATE: _____   RHYTHM: _____

       P WAVES: _____   P-R INTERVALS: _____

       QRS: _____   INTERPRETATION: _____

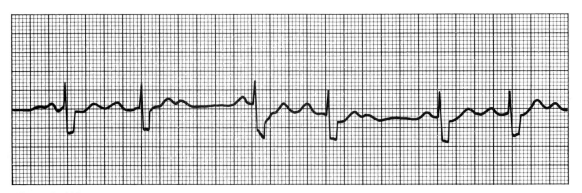

Figure 3–105

189. RATE: _____   RHYTHM: _____

       P WAVES: _____   P-R INTERVALS: _____

       QRS: _____   INTERPRETATION: _____

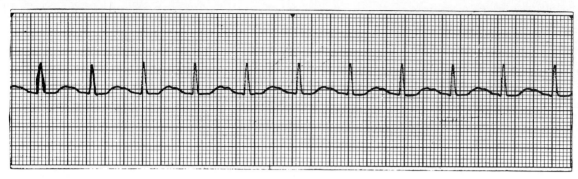

Figure 3-106

190. RATE: _____ RHYTHM: _____

　　　 P WAVES: _____ P-R INTERVALS: _____

　　　 QRS: _____ INTERPRETATION: _____

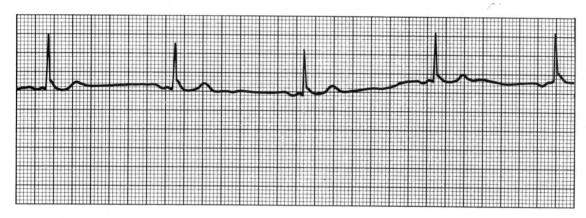

Figure 3-107

191. RATE: _____ RHYTHM: _____

　　　 P WAVES: _____ P-R INTERVALS: _____

　　　 QRS: _____ INTERPRETATION: _____

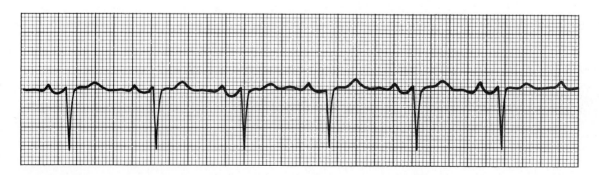

Figure 3-108

192. RATE: _____ RHYTHM: _____

　　　 P WAVES: _____ P-R INTERVALS: _____

　　　 QRS: _____ INTERPRETATION: _____

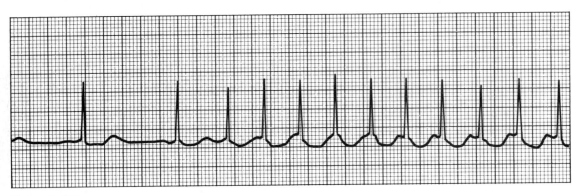

Figure 3–109

193. RATE: _____ RHYTHM: _____

P WAVES: _____ P-R INTERVALS: _____

QRS: _____ INTERPRETATION: _____

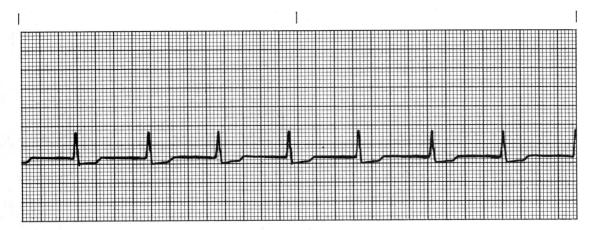

Figure 3–110

194. RATE: _____ RHYTHM: _____

P WAVES: _____ P-R INTERVALS: _____

QRS: _____ INTERPRETATION: _____

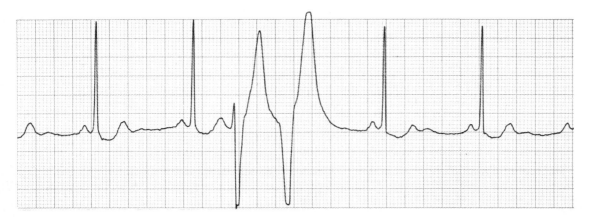

Figure 3–111

195. RATE: _____ RHYTHM: _____

P WAVES: _____ P-R INTERVALS: _____

QRS: _____ INTERPRETATION: _____

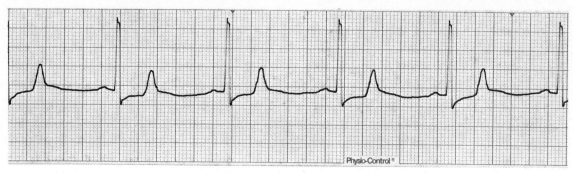

Figure 3–112

196. RATE: _____   RHYTHM: _____

P WAVES: _____   P-R INTERVALS: _____

QRS: _____   INTERPRETATION: _____

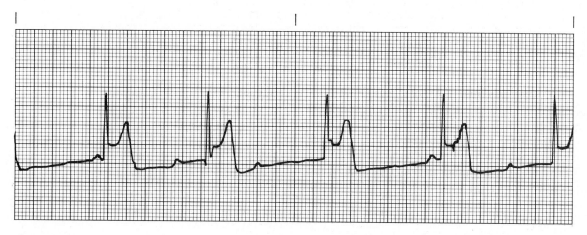

Figure 3–113

197. RATE: _____   RHYTHM: _____

P WAVES: _____   P-R INTERVALS: _____

QRS: _____   INTERPRETATION: _____

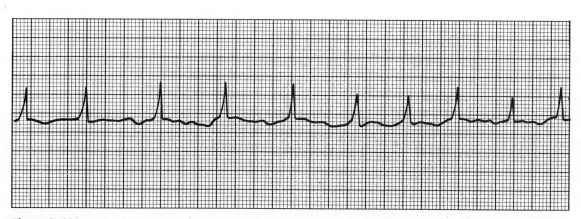

Figure 3–114

198. RATE: _____   RHYTHM: _____

P WAVES: _____   P-R INTERVALS: _____

QRS: _____   INTERPRETATION: _____

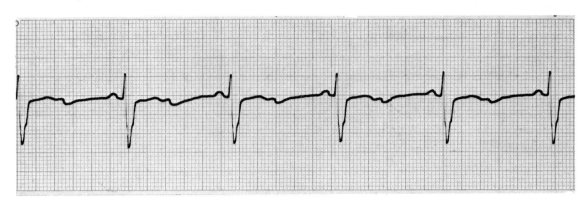

Figure 3-115

199. RATE: _____ RHYTHM: _____

P WAVES: _____ P-R INTERVALS: _____

QRS: _____ INTERPRETATION: _____

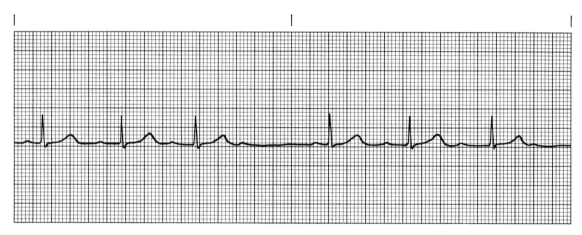

Figure 3-116

200. RATE: _____ RHYTHM: _____

P WAVES: _____ P-R INTERVALS: _____

QRS: _____ INTERPRETATION: _____

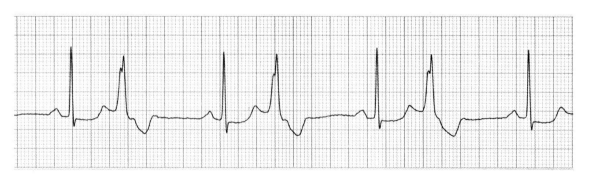

Figure 3-117

201. RATE: _____ RHYTHM: _____

P WAVES: _____ P-R INTERVALS: _____

QRS: _____ INTERPRETATION: _____

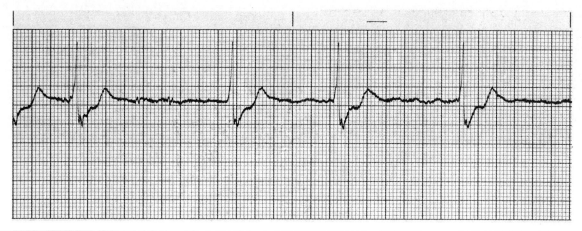

Figure 3–118

202. RATE: _____ RHYTHM: _____
　　　 P WAVES: _____ P-R INTERVALS: _____
　　　 QRS: _____ INTERPRETATION: _____

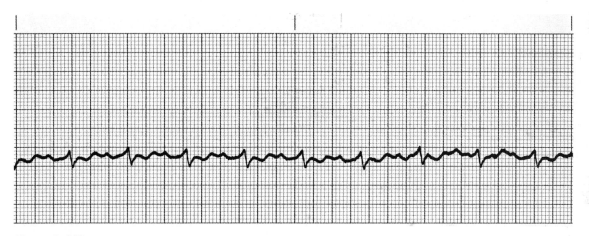

Figure 3–119

203. RATE: _____ RHYTHM: _____
　　　 P WAVES: _____ P-R INTERVALS: _____
　　　 QRS: _____ INTERPRETATION: _____

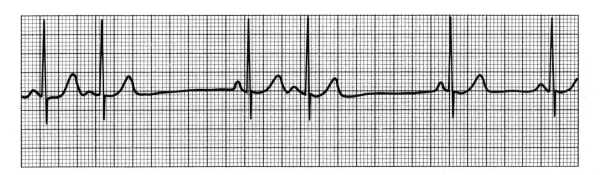

Figure 3–120

204. RATE: _____ RHYTHM: _____
　　　 P WAVES: _____ P-R INTERVALS: _____
　　　 QRS: _____ INTERPRETATION: _____

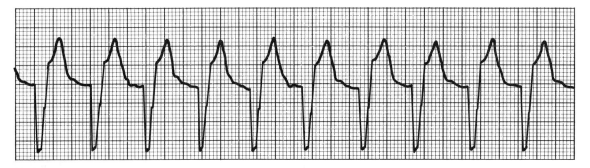

Figure 3–121

205. RATE: _____   RHYTHM: _____

P WAVES: _____   P-R INTERVALS: _____

QRS: _____   INTERPRETATION: _____

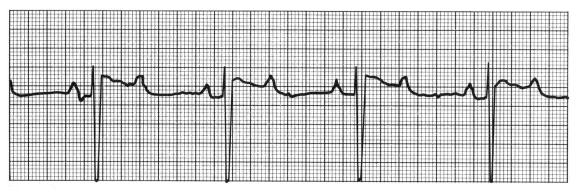

Figure 3–122

206. RATE: _____   RHYTHM: _____

P WAVES: _____   P-R INTERVALS: _____

QRS: _____   INTERPRETATION: _____

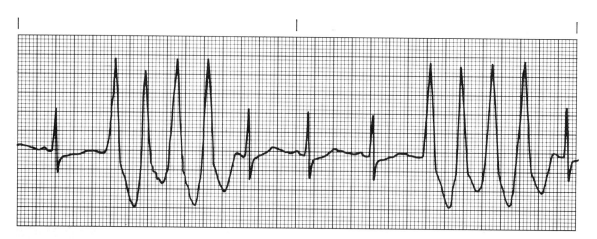

Figure 3–123

207. RATE: _____   RHYTHM: _____

P WAVES: _____   P-R INTERVALS: _____

QRS: _____   INTERPRETATION: _____

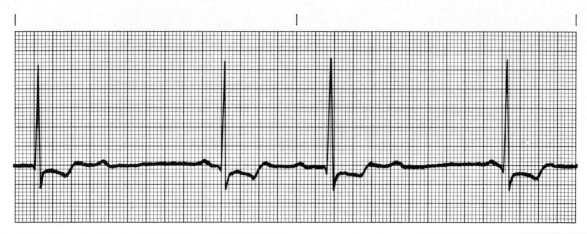

Figure 3–124

208. RATE: _____   RHYTHM: _____

P WAVES: _____   P-R INTERVALS: _____

QRS: _____   INTERPRETATION: _____

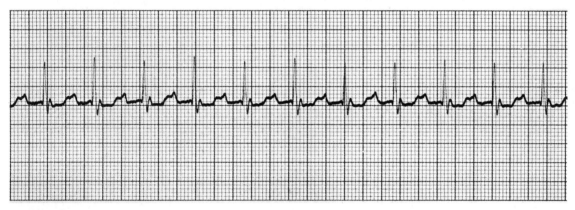

Figure 3–125

209. RATE: _____   RHYTHM: _____

P WAVES: _____   P-R INTERVALS: _____

QRS: _____   INTERPRETATION: _____

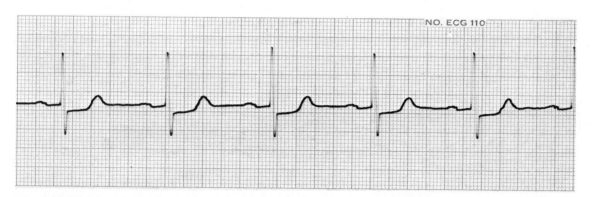

Figure 3–126

210. RATE: _____   RHYTHM: _____

P WAVES: _____   P-R INTERVALS: _____

QRS: _____   INTERPRETATION: _____

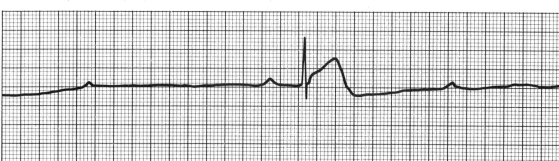

Figure 3–127

211. RATE: _____   RHYTHM: _____

P WAVES: _____   P-R INTERVALS: _____

QRS: _____   INTERPRETATION: _____

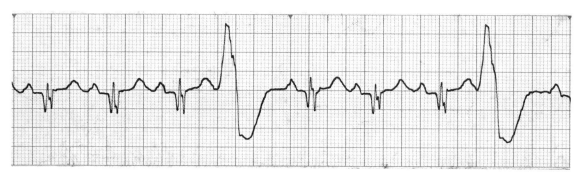

Figure 3–128

212. RATE: _____   RHYTHM: _____

P WAVES: _____   P-R INTERVALS: _____

QRS: _____   INTERPRETATION: _____

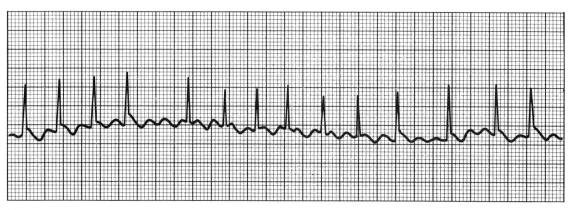

Figure 3–129

213. RATE: _____   RHYTHM: _____

P WAVES: _____   P-R INTERVALS: _____

QRS: _____   INTERPRETATION: _____

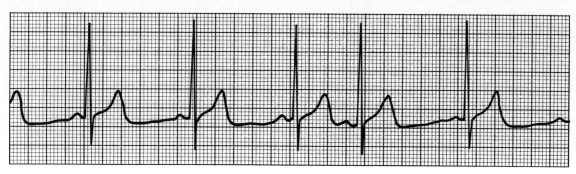

Figure 3–130

214. RATE: _____ RHYTHM: _____
   P WAVES: _____ P-R INTERVALS: _____
   QRS: _____ INTERPRETATION: _____

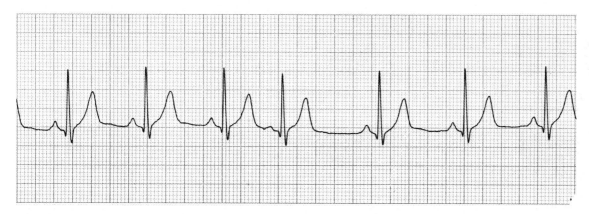

Figure 3–131

215. RATE: _____ RHYTHM: _____
   P WAVES: _____ P-R INTERVALS: _____
   QRS: _____ INTERPRETATION: _____

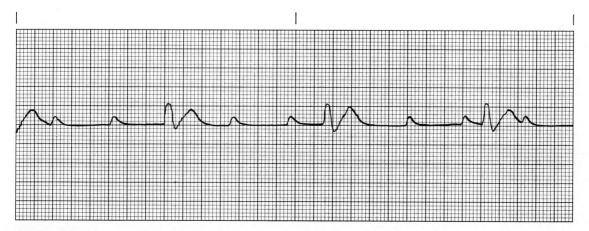

Figure 3–132

216. RATE: _____ RHYTHM: _____
   P WAVES: _____ P-R INTERVALS: _____
   QRS: _____ INTERPRETATION: _____

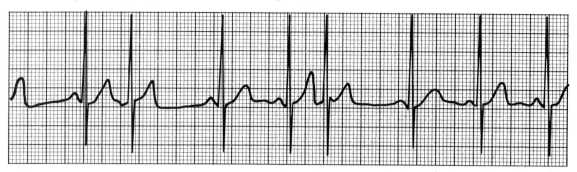

Figure 3–133

217. RATE: _____ RHYTHM: _____
 P WAVES: _____ P-R INTERVALS: _____
 QRS: _____ INTERPRETATION: _____

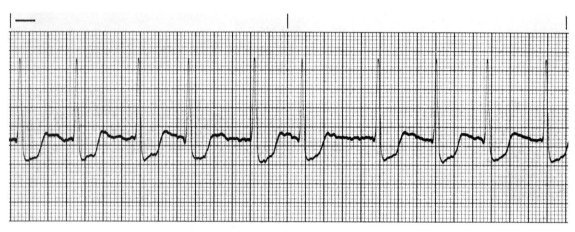

Figure 3–134

218. RATE: _____ RHYTHM: _____
 P WAVES: _____ P-R INTERVALS: _____
 QRS: _____ INTERPRETATION: _____

NO. ECG 110 ... MEDI-TRACE GRAPHIC CONT

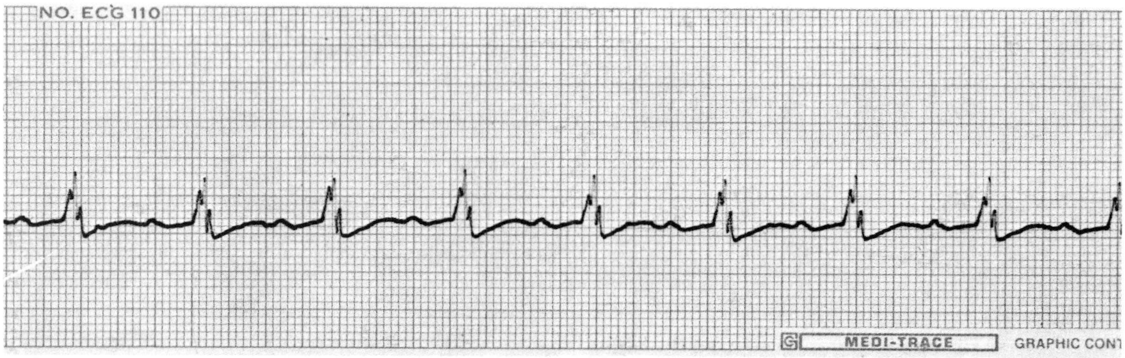

Figure 3–135

219. RATE: _____ RHYTHM: _____
 P WAVES: _____ P-R INTERVALS: _____
 QRS: _____ INTERPRETATION: _____

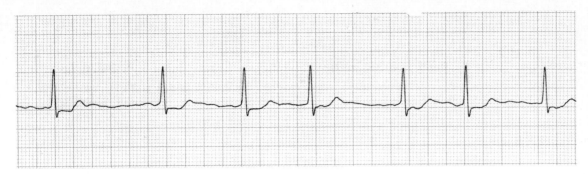

Figure 3–136

220. RATE: _____   RHYTHM: _____

P WAVES: _____   P-R INTERVALS: _____

QRS: _____   INTERPRETATION: _____

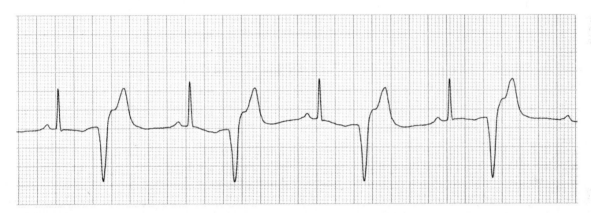

Figure 3–137

221. RATE: _____   RHYTHM: _____

P WAVES: _____   P-R INTERVALS: _____

QRS: _____   INTERPRETATION: _____

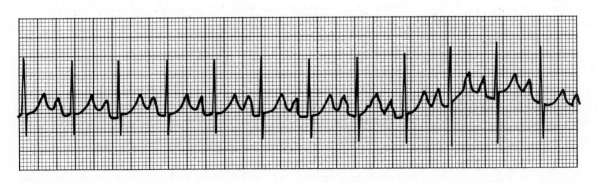

Figure 3–138

222. RATE: _____   RHYTHM: _____

P WAVES: _____   P-R INTERVALS: _____

QRS: _____   INTERPRETATION: _____

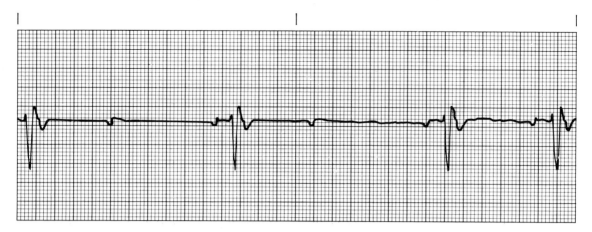

Figure 3–139

223. RATE: _____ RHYTHM: _____
        P WAVES: _____ P-R INTERVALS: _____
        QRS: _____ INTERPRETATION: _____

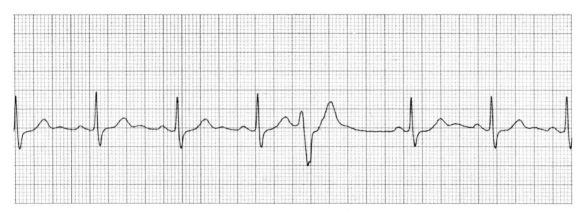

Figure 3–140

224. RATE: _____ RHYTHM: _____
        P WAVES: _____ P-R INTERVALS: _____
        QRS: _____ INTERPRETATION: _____

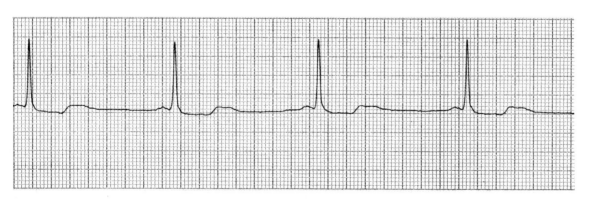

Figure 3–141

225. RATE: _____ RHYTHM: _____
        P WAVES: _____ P-R INTERVALS: _____
        QRS: _____ INTERPRETATION: _____

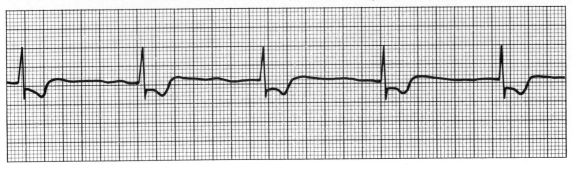

Figure 3–142

226. RATE: _____   RHYTHM: _____
P WAVES: _____   P-R INTERVALS: _____
QRS: _____   INTERPRETATION: _____

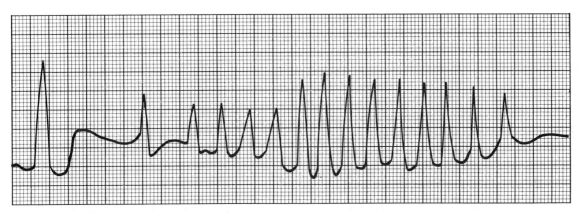

Figure 3–143

227. RATE: _____   RHYTHM: _____
P WAVES: _____   P-R INTERVALS: _____
QRS: _____   INTERPRETATION: _____

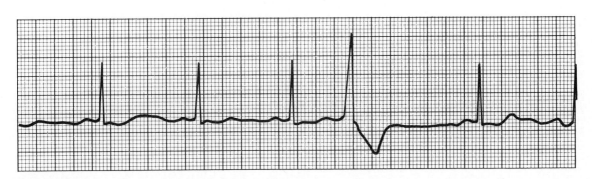

Figure 3–144

228. RATE: _____   RHYTHM: _____
P WAVES: _____   P-R INTERVALS: _____
QRS: _____   INTERPRETATION: _____

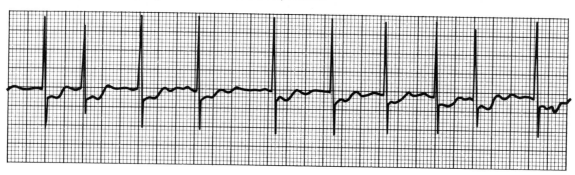

Figure 3–145

229. RATE: _____   RHYTHM: _____

P WAVES: _____   P-R INTERVALS: _____

QRS: _____   INTERPRETATION: _____

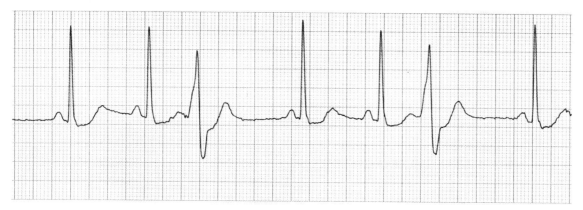

Figure 3–146

230. RATE: _____   RHYTHM: _____

P WAVES: _____   P-R INTERVALS: _____

QRS: _____   INTERPRETATION: _____

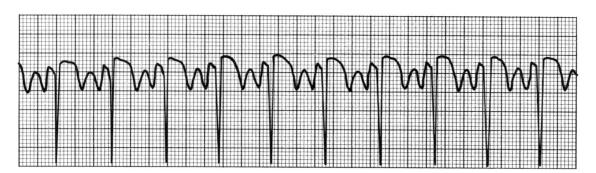

Figure 3–147

231. RATE: _____   RHYTHM: _____

P WAVES: _____   P-R INTERVALS: _____

QRS: _____   INTERPRETATION: _____

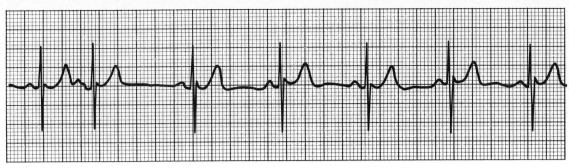

Figure 3-148

232. RATE: _____ RHYTHM: _____

P WAVES: _____ P-R INTERVALS: _____

QRS: _____ INTERPRETATION: _____

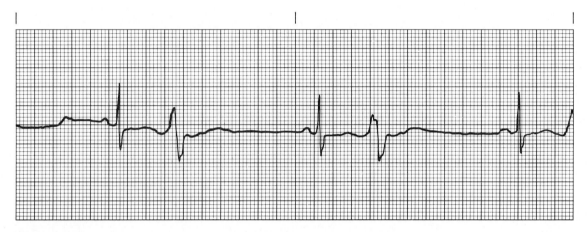

Figure 3-149

233. RATE: _____ RHYTHM: _____

P WAVES: _____ P-R INTERVALS: _____

QRS: _____ INTERPRETATION: _____

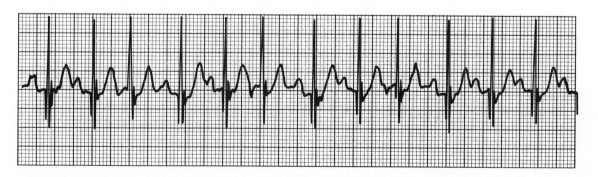

Figure 3-150

234. RATE: _____ RHYTHM: _____

P WAVES: _____ P-R INTERVALS: _____

QRS: _____ INTERPRETATION: _____

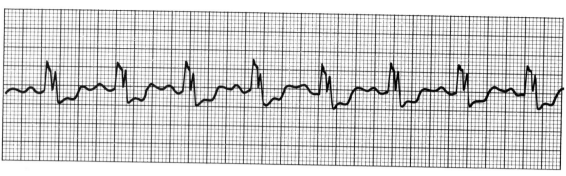

Figure 3–151

235. RATE: _____   RHYTHM: _____

　　　 P WAVES: _____   P-R INTERVALS: _____

　　　 QRS: _____   INTERPRETATION: _____

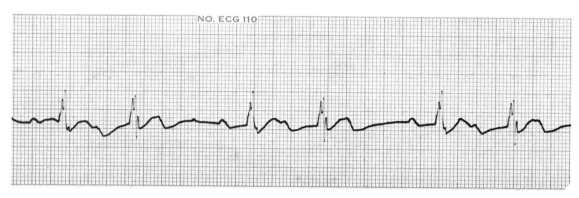

Figure 3–152

236. RATE: _____   RHYTHM: _____

　　　 P WAVES: _____   P-R INTERVALS: _____

　　　 QRS: _____   INTERPRETATION: _____

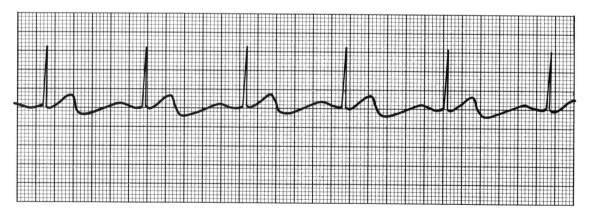

Figure 3–153

237. RATE: _____   RHYTHM: _____

　　　 P WAVES: _____   P-R INTERVALS: _____

　　　 QRS: _____   INTERPRETATION: _____

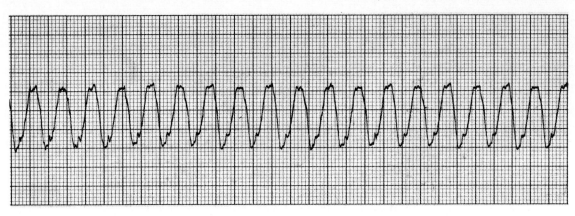

Figure 3–154

238. RATE: _____ RHYTHM: _____

P WAVES: _____ P-R INTERVALS: _____

QRS: _____ INTERPRETATION: _____

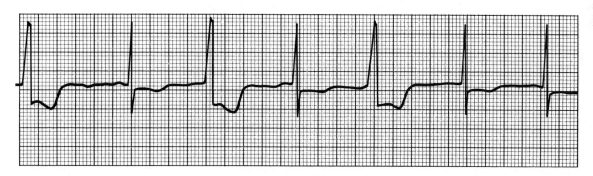

Figure 3–155

239. RATE: _____ RHYTHM: _____

P WAVES: _____ P-R INTERVALS: _____

QRS: _____ INTERPRETATION: _____

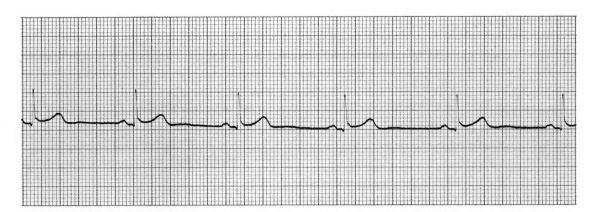

Figure 3–156

240. RATE: _____ RHYTHM: _____

P WAVES: _____ P-R INTERVALS: _____

QRS: _____ INTERPRETATION: _____

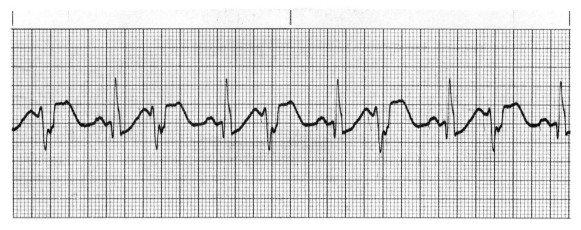

Figure 3–157

241. RATE: _____   RHYTHM: _____

P WAVES: _____   P-R INTERVALS: _____

QRS: _____   INTERPRETATION: _____

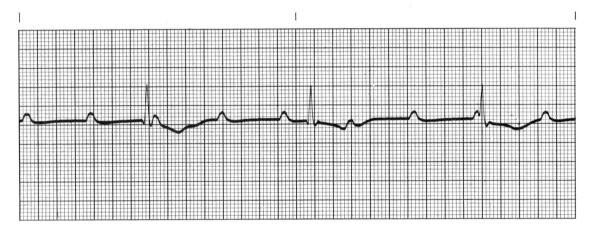

Figure 3–158

242. RATE: _____   RHYTHM: _____

P WAVES: _____   P-R INTERVALS: _____

QRS: _____   INTERPRETATION: _____

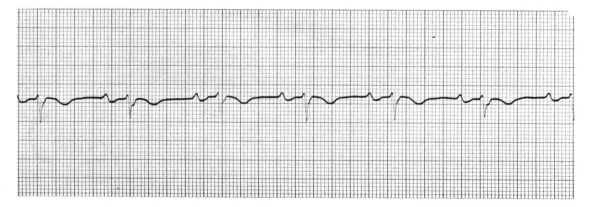

Figure 3–159

243. RATE: _____   RHYTHM: _____

P WAVES: _____   P-R INTERVALS: _____

QRS: _____   INTERPRETATION: _____

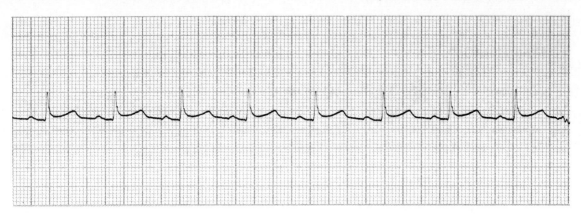

Figure 3–160

244. RATE: _____ RHYTHM: _____

   P WAVES: _____ P-R INTERVALS: _____

   QRS: _____ INTERPRETATION: _____

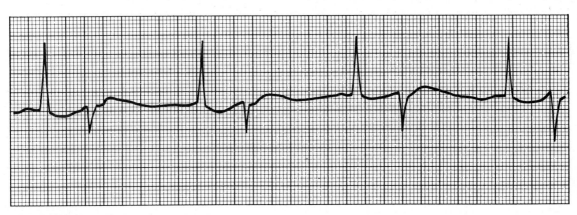

Figure 3–161

245. RATE: _____ RHYTHM: _____

   P WAVES: _____ P-R INTERVALS: _____

   QRS: _____ INTERPRETATION: _____

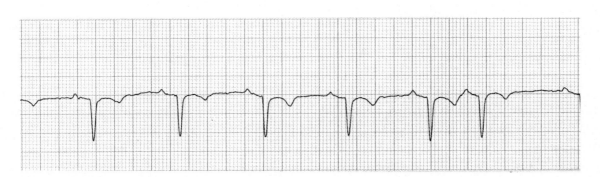

Figure 3–162

246. RATE: _____ RHYTHM: _____

   P WAVES: _____ P-R INTERVALS: _____

   QRS: _____ INTERPRETATION: _____

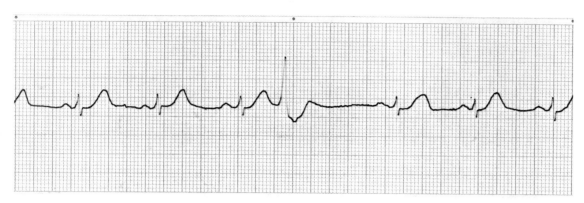

Figure 3–163

247. RATE: _____ RHYTHM: _____

  P WAVES: _____ P-R INTERVALS: _____

  QRS: _____ INTERPRETATION: _____

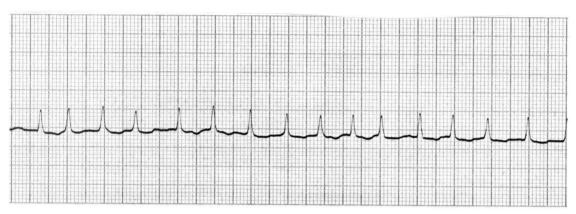

Figure 3–164

248. RATE: _____ RHYTHM: _____

  P WAVES: _____ P-R INTERVALS: _____

  QRS: _____ INTERPRETATION: _____

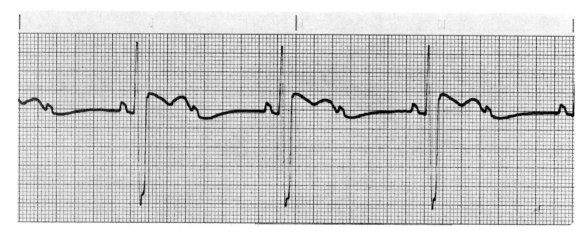

Figure 3–165

249. RATE: _____ RHYTHM: _____

  P WAVES: _____ P-R INTERVALS: _____

  QRS: _____ INTERPRETATION: _____

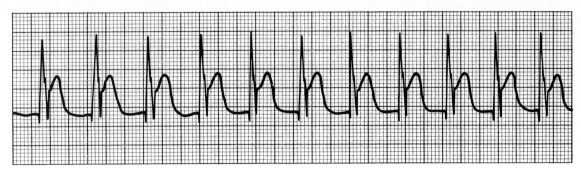

Figure 3–166

250. RATE: _____ RHYTHM: _____

    P WAVES: _____ P-R INTERVALS: _____

    QRS: _____ INTERPRETATION: _____

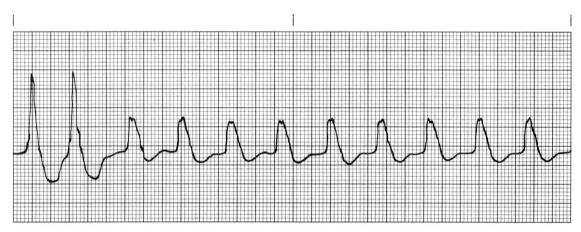

Figure 3–167

251. RATE: _____ RHYTHM: _____

    P WAVES: _____ P-R INTERVALS: _____

    QRS: _____ INTERPRETATION: _____

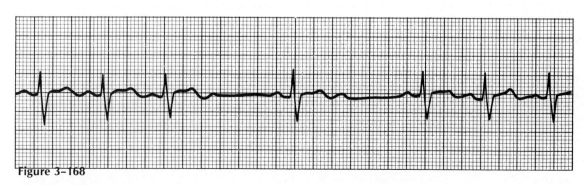

Figure 3–168

252. RATE: _____ RHYTHM: _____

    P WAVES: _____ P-R INTERVALS: _____

    QRS: _____ INTERPRETATION: _____

ANSWER KEY

1. TRUE

2. FALSE: The pulse represents the mechanical activity (contraction) of the heart; the ECG pattern represents the heart's electrical activity.

3. TRUE

4. FALSE: If individual cardiac muscle cells depolarized and contracted in an uncoordinated manner, the atria and ventricles would quiver rather than fill and empty effectively with each beat.

5. a. pacemaker cells: initiate cardiac electrical impulse
b. cardiac conduction system: transmits cardiac electrical impulse
c. automaticity: ability to generate a spontaneous electrical impulse

6. The conduction system of the heart (Figure 3–169).

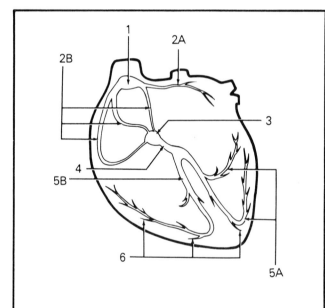

ELECTRICAL CONDUCTION THROUGH THE HEART

1.   Sinoatrial (SA) node
2A.   Interatrial pathway
2B.   Internodal pathways
3.   Atrioventricular (AV) junction
4.   Bundle of His
5A.   Left bundle branches (2 divisions)
5B.   Right bundle branch
6.   Purkinje fibers

Figure 3–169

7. FALSE: Since pacemaker cells possess the property of automaticity, they can depolarize spontaneously.

8. TRUE: See Figure 3–170.

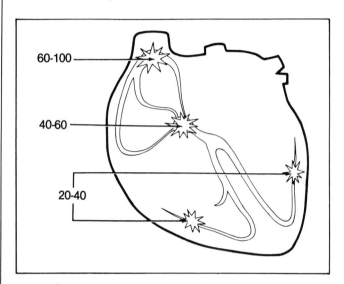

Figure 3–170

9. TRUE

10. TRUE: If the SA node fails to initiate an impulse, a lower pacemaker site will initiate the impulse. This is referred to as an "escape mechanism" (see Figure 3–171).

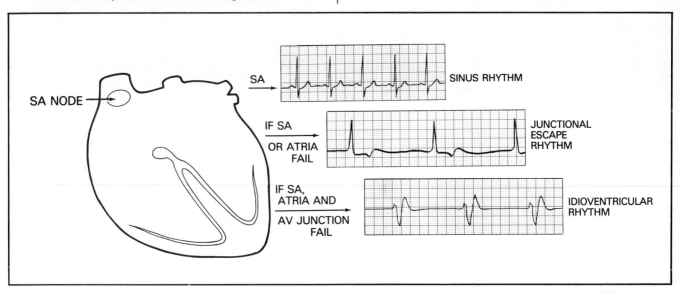

Figure 3–171

11. a. SA node: normal pacemaker of the heart; rate of automaticity between 60 and 100 per minute; b. AV junction: rate of automaticity between 40 and 60 per minute; a potential escape pacemaker (pacemaker only when higher pacemaker fails or if its own rate of automaticity exceeds that of higher pacemaker); c. ventricular conduction system: rate of automaticity is less than 40 per minute; potential escape pacemaker; initiates a rhythm if the impulse does not reach the ventricles within 1.5 seconds.

12. b: The impulse travels from the SA node to the atrial internodal pathways (Figure 3–172)

13. c (Figure 3–172)

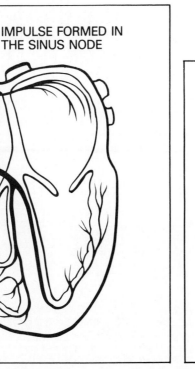

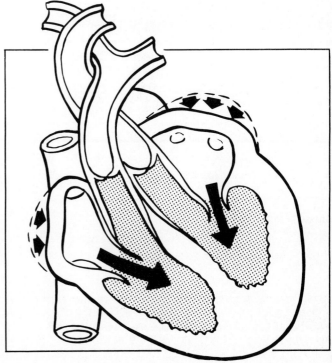

Figure 3–172

14. a: A slight delay of conduction normally occurs at the AV junction (Figure 3–173).

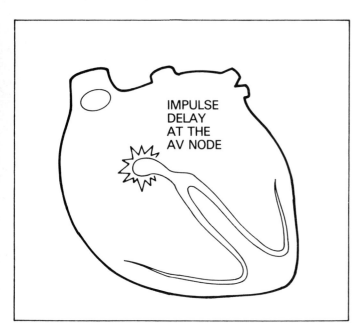

Figure 3–173

15. d: Depolarization (stimulation) of the bundle of His, left and right bundle branches, and the Purkinje fibers results in ventricular contraction (Figure 3–174).

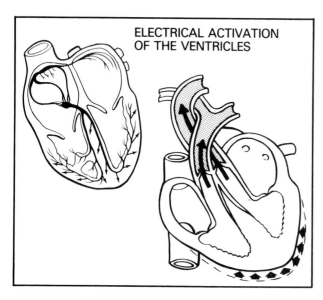

Figure 3–174

16. The major direction of the depolarization wave through the heart is from the SA node downward toward the left ventricular apex (Figure 3–175).

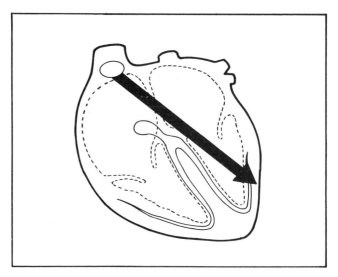

Figure 3–175

17. The relationship between cardiac electrical events and ECG waveforms and intervals is shown in Figure 3–176.

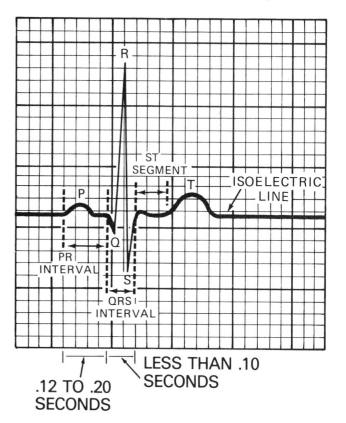

Figure 3–176

Figure 3–177 demonstrates generation of these ECG characteristics in more detail.

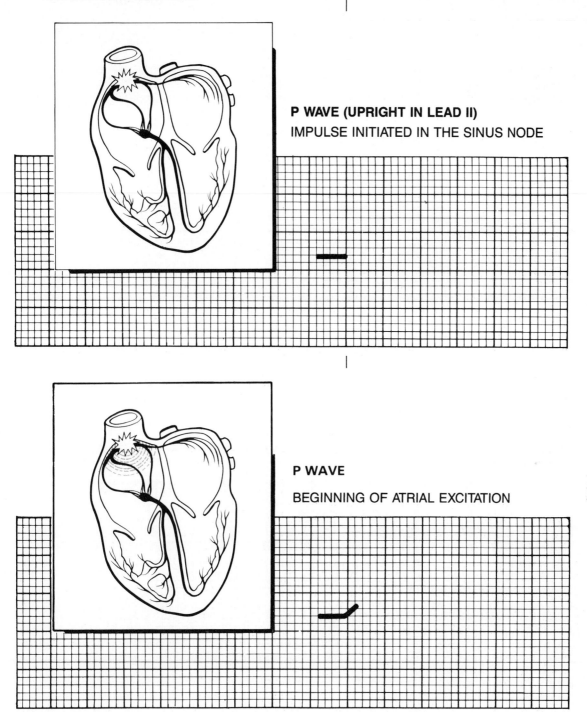

P WAVE (UPRIGHT IN LEAD II)
IMPULSE INITIATED IN THE SINUS NODE

P WAVE

BEGINNING OF ATRIAL EXCITATION

Figure 3–177

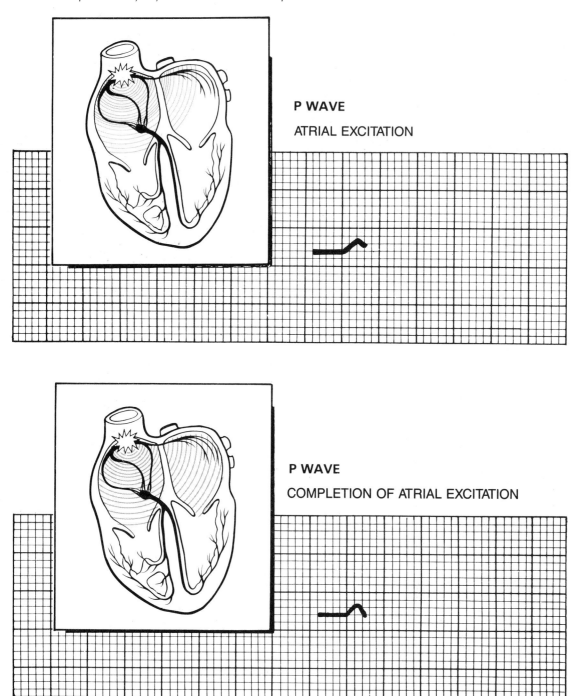

P WAVE

ATRIAL EXCITATION

P WAVE

COMPLETION OF ATRIAL EXCITATION

Figure 3–177 (continued)

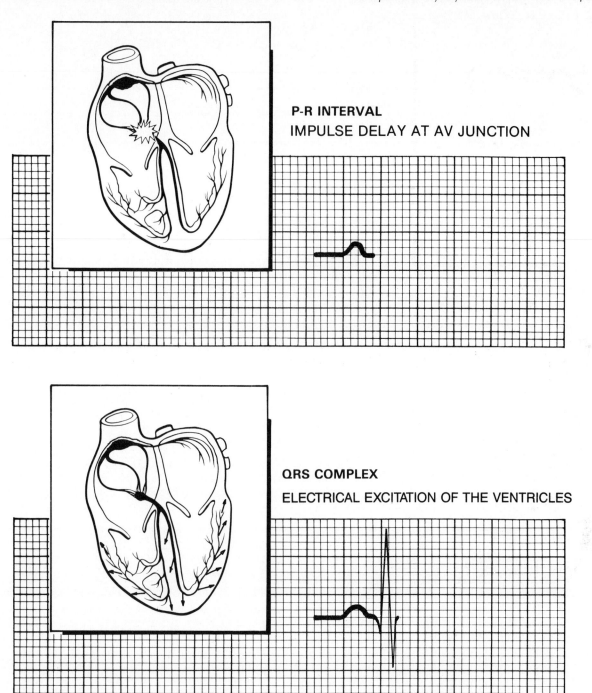

P-R INTERVAL
IMPULSE DELAY AT AV JUNCTION

QRS COMPLEX
ELECTRICAL EXCITATION OF THE VENTRICLES

Figure 3–177 (continued)

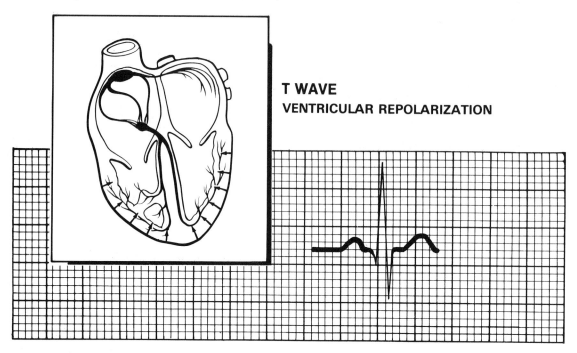

T WAVE

VENTRICULAR REPOLARIZATION

Figure 3–177 (continued)

18. ECG graph paper with time standards (see Figures 3–178 and 3–179).

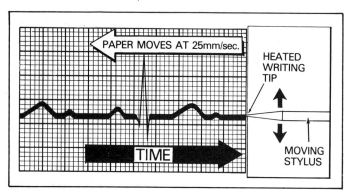

PAPER MOVES AT 25mm/sec.

HEATED WRITING TIP

TIME

MOVING STYLUS

Figure 3–178

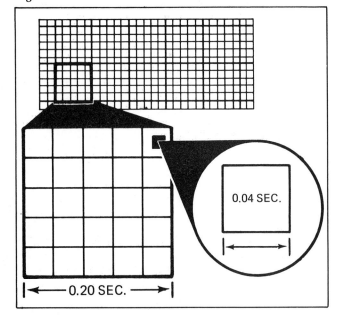

0.04 SEC.

0.20 SEC.

Figure 3–179

19. Interval A in Figure 3–180 represents 3 seconds and interval B represents 6 seconds.

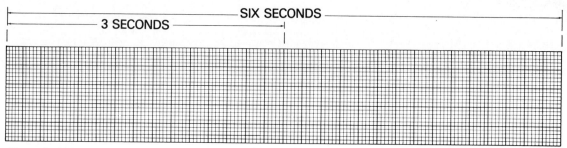

Figure 3–180

20. b: Since 6 seconds times 10 equals 60 seconds or 1 minute.

21. The normal limits for the P-R interval = 0.12 to 0.20 second. The normal limits for the QRS interval = 0.04 to 0.10 second.

22. Electrode locations for standard lead II are shown in Figure 3–181.

POSITION OF ELECTRODES: LEAD II POSITION

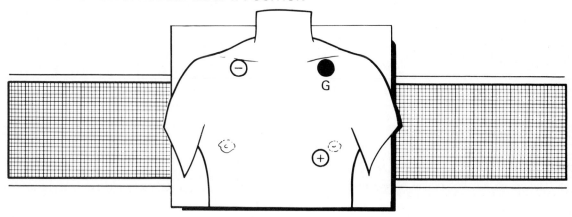

Figure 3–181

23. TRUE

24. FALSE: The SA node normally initiates atrial depolarization.

25. TRUE

26. TRUE: The pacemaking site may be variable (wandering).

27. FALSE: A negative P wave in lead II suggests that the impulse originated from the AV junction.

28. a: originated in the region of the AV junction
    b: originated in more than one location in the atria
    c: originated in the SA node

29. FALSE: This delay in impulse transmission allows the ventricles to fully fill before they contract.

30. TRUE

31. TRUE

32. a: originated in the SA node, but was abnormally delayed at the AV junction
    b: originated in the region of the AV junction
    c: originated in the SA node and has traveled through the AV junction within a normal period of time

33. c

34. a

35. a: originated from the SA node, but its conduction through the ventricles has been delayed
    b: originated in the ventricles
    c: traveled normally through the ventricles

36. d

37. b

38. d

39. e

40. c

41. d

42. a

43. a: bradycardia
b: normal rate
c: tachycardia

44. FALSE: Slow heart rates are associated with slowed conduction.

45. TRUE

46. TRUE

47. TRUE

48. FALSE: Rapid heart rates increase myocardial oxygen consumption; this effect can be especially detrimental to persons who already have diminished myocardial perfusion.

49. FALSE: Severe tachycardia usually diminishes perfusion to all of these body systems.

50. b

51. SINUS RHYTHM RATE: between 60 and 100 per minute; ATRIAL vs. VENT RATES: same; P-P: regular (constant); R-R: regular (constant); RHYTHM: essentially regular; P WAVES: precede each QRS; normal configuration; P-R: within normal limits (0.12–0.20 second); QRS: within normal limits (less than 0.10 second) (* unless an intraventricular conduction defect prolongs the QRS); PACEMAKER: SA node

52. SINUS BRADYCARDIA RATE: less than 60 per minute; ATRIAL vs. VENT RATES: same; P-P: regular; R-R: regular; RHYTHM: essentially regular; P WAVES: precede each QRS; normal configuration; P-R: within normal limits; tend to be at upper limits of normal with slower rates; QRS: within normal limits*; PACEMAKER: SA node

53. SINUS TACHYCARDIA RATE: over 100 per minute; usually 100 to 160; ATRIAL vs. VENT RATES: same; P-P: regular; R-R: regular; RHYTHM: essentially regular; P WAVES: precede each QRS; normal configuration; P-R: within normal limits; tend to be at lower limits of normal with faster rates; QRS: within normal limits*; PACEMAKER: SA node

54. WANDERING ATRIAL PACEMAKER RATE: between 60 and 100 per minute; ATRIAL vs. VENT RATES: same; P-P: generally regular, but may vary slightly as pacemaking site shifts; R-R; generally regular, but may vary slightly as pacemaking site shifts; RHYTHM: essentially regular; P WAVES: precede each QRS, but vary in configuration; P-R: within normal limits; may vary slightly; QRS: within normal limits*; PACEMAKER: more than one focus in the atria

55. ATRIAL TACHYCARDIA RATE: usually 160 to 220 per minute; ATRIAL vs. VENT RATES: same when all impulses are conducted (unless physiologic block at AV junction produces block); P-P: same; R-R: same; RHYTHM: regular; when this rhythm is paroxysmal (PAT), the rhythm is often precisely regular rather than just essentially regular; P WAVES: differ from sinus P waves; precede each QRS, but are often obscured in T wave of preceding cycle; P-R: when identifiable, are often at lower normal limits; may be prolonged in patients sensitive to rapid heart rates; often not identifiable if unable to see P waves clearly; QRS: within normal limits*; PACEMAKER: atrium, may be one or many foci

56. ATRIAL FLUTTER RATE: ventricular rate depends on how many atrial impulses are conducted to the ventricles; atrial rates are typically 300 per minute, but may range between 220 and 350 per minute; ATRIAL vs. VENT RATES: physiologic block at the AV junction normally prevents 1:1 conduction so that the atrial rate exceeds the ventricular rate; P-P: unable to determine since P waves are replaced by flutter waves; R-R: regular only if atrial impulses are conducted to ventricles at a constant ratio; otherwise, vary as conduction ratio varies; conduction ratios may range 5:1, 4:1, 3:1, etc.; RHYTHM: regular when conduction ratio constant; P WAVES: replaced by sawtooth flutter (F) waves; P-R: unable to determine (no P waves; QRS: within normal limits*; flutter waves may distort and appear to widen QRS; PACEMAKER: atrium

57. ATRIAL FIBRILLATION RATE: atrial rate is usually over 300 per minute, ranging 400 to 700 per minute, but typically cannot see atrial activity well enough to calculate rate; ventricular rate in untreated patients usually is between 160 and 180 per minute; ATRIAL vs. VENT RATES: atrial rate exceeds ventricular rate due to normal (physiologic, not pathologic) block at AV junction; ventricular rate depends on how many atrial impulses reach ventricles; P-P: unable to determine since P waves not readily identifiable; R-R: irregularly (totally) irregular; RHYTHM: irregularly irregular; P WAVES: not recognizable as P waves; replaced by fine undulations of baseline (fibrillatory waves); P-R: unable to determine without identifiable P waves; QRS: generally are within normal limits*; some atrial impulses may reach ventricles before they have fully repolarized, causing delayed ventricular conduction (Ashman's phenomenon); PACEMAKER: multiple areas in the atria

58. PREMATURE ATRIAL CONTRACTIONS (PACs) RATE: add PACs to underlying rate; ATRIAL vs. VENT RATES: most often are the same, but a PAC may be so premature that it is conducted with delay through the ventricles (PAC with aberrancy) or may not be able to be conducted at all (nonconducted PAC); in the latter case, the atrial rate would transiently exceed the ventricular rate; P-P: shortened whenever a PAC occurs; R-R: irregular (shortened) whenever a PAC occurs; RHYTHM: disrupted by the PAC; P WAVES: differ in morphology from the sinus P waves; the earlier the PAC occurs, the more likely it is to be hidden in the preceding T wave; P-R: usually normal; may be shortened or prolonged, depending on readiness of the AV junction to conduct the PAC; QRS: intervals usually normal, but may be prolonged if aberrancy occurs; PACEMAKER: PAC originates from the atrium, but underlying rhythm can originate from any location, usually the SA node

59. PREMATURE JUNCTIONAL CONTRACTIONS (PJCs) RATE: add PJC to underlying rate; ATRIAL vs. VENT RATES: often are same, but PJC may be so premature that it does not conduct (nonconducted PJC); latter could cause atrial rate to transiently exceed ventricular rate; P-P: when P wave of PJC precedes QRS complex, P-P is shortened; if P wave follows its QRS, P-P will be prolonged; R-R: irregular (shortened) when PJC occurs; RHYTHM: disrupted whenever PJC occurs; P WAVES: is a negative (inverted) deflection in leads where it is normally positive (leads II, III, avF); may precede, coincide with, or follow the QRS; P-R: less than 0.12 if P precedes QRS; if P follows QRS, P-R is converted to an R-P interval; QRS: within normal limits*; normal configuration; PACEMAKER: PJC originates in AV junction; underlying rhythm can be of any origin

60. PREMATURE VENTRICULAR CONTRACTIONS (PVCs) RATE: rate of underlying rhythm plus PVCs if latter produce palpable pulses; ATRIAL vs. VENT RATES: often are virtually the same; as PVCs become more frequent, ventricular rate may exceed atrial rate; P-P: may or may not be affected by PVC; sinus rhythm may persist despite PVCs; R-R: irregular (shortened) by PVC; RHYTHM: disrupted whenever PVC occurs; P WAVES: sinus P waves are often obscured by PVC; if P wave is conducted retrograde from ventricles, it will follow QRS of PVC; P-R: may not be able to locate P waves to determine; QRS: is greater than 0.12 second in duration, bizarre in configuration with ST segment and T wave oriented opposite to QRS. QRS complexes of PVCs may all resemble one another and have a constant coupling interval with the preceding QRS (unifocal, uniform PVCs) or may differ in their morphology and coupling intervals (multiform, multifocal PVCs); the former probably arise from a single ventricular site, whereas the latter likely arise from multiple ventricular foci. PACEMAKER: ventricles

61. JUNCTIONAL ESCAPE RHYTHM RATE: 40 to 60 per minute; ATRIAL vs. VENT RATES: usually the same; P-P: usually regular when P waves are visible; vary if SA node functions intermittently; R-R: regular; RHYTHM: regular; P WAVES: when visible, are negative deflections in leads where they are normally positive (leads II, III, avF); may precede, coincide with or follow the QRS; P-R: when negative P precedes QRS; P-R: when negative P precedes QRS, P-R usually less than 0.12 second; QRS: within normal limits*; PACEMAKER: AV junction due to failure (default) of SA node

62. ACCELERATED JUNCTIONAL RHYTHM RATE: 60 to 100 per minute (accelerated junctional rhythm); over 100 per minute (junctional tachycardia); ATRIAL vs. VENT RATES: usually the same; P-P: usually regular when P waves are visible; vary if SA node functions intermittently; R-R: regular; RHYTHM: regular; P WAVES: when visible, are negative deflections in leads where they are normally positive (leads II, III, avF); may precede, coincide with or follow QRS; P-R: when negative P precedes QRS, P-R is usually less than 0.12 second; QRS: within normal limits*; normal configuration; PACEMAKER: AV junction due to increased automaticity at this site

63. VENTRICULAR TACHYCARDIA RATE: ventricular rate usually over 100, but less than 220 per minute; ATRIAL vs. VENT RATES: ventricular rate typically faster than the coexisting atrial (sinus) rate; P-P: usually not able to determine because P waves are obscured by QRS complexes; R-R: usually regular; RHYTHM: regular; P WAVES: sinus P waves often obscured; may be retrograde from PVC; if visible and of SA origin, are typically dissociated from the QRS complexes; P-R: not able to calculate usually; QRS: wide (over 0.12 second), bizarre configuration with ST segment and T wave opposite in polarity to QRS; PACEMAKER: ventricles

64. VENTRICULAR FIBRILLATION RATE: usually over 300 per minute; lack of identifiable waveforms may preclude ability to calculate rates; ATRIAL vs. VENT RATES: (see above); P-P: unable to identify P waves; R-R: unable to distinguish R waves; RHYTHM: irregularly irregular; P WAVES: unable to identify; P-R: unable to calculate; QRS: unable to distinguish waveforms; PACEMAKER: multiple areas in ventricles

65. IDIOVENTRICULAR RHYTHM RATE: usually 20 to 40 per minute; ATRIAL vs. VENT RATES: no atrial rhythm; P-P: no P waves; R-R: often quite regular; RHYTHM: regular; P WAVES: absent; P-R: does not apply, no P waves; QRS: wide (over 0.12 second), bizarre with an ST segment and T wave oriented in opposite polarity to QRS; PACEMAKER: ventricles as escape rhythm

66. FIRST-DEGREE AV BLOCK RATE: usually 60 to 100 per minute, but can be associated with a bradycardia or tachycardia; ATRIAL vs. VENT RATES: same; P-P: regular; R-R: regular; RHYTHM: regular; P WAVES: precede each QRS; normal configuration; P-R: greater than 0.20 second, but constant; QRS: within normal limits*; PACEMAKER: usually the SA node

67. SECOND-DEGREE AV BLOCK, MOBITZ I (WENCKEBACH) RATE: may be 60 to 100, but often underlying rate less than 60 per minute; ATRIAL vs. VENT RATES: atrial rate exceeds ventricular rate; P-P: regular; R-R: shorten progressively; groups of R waves apparent; RHYTHM: atrial rhythm is regular, but ventricular rhythm is irregular because of dropped QRS complexes; P WAVES: normal configuration, but last P in each group is not followed by a QRS; are more numerous than QRS complexes; P-R: progressively lengthens until one P wave is not followed by a QRS complex, producing a conduction pattern such as 5:4, 4:3, 3:2, etc.; QRS: within normal limits*; PACEMAKER: usually SA node

68. SECOND-DEGREE AV BLOCK, MOBITZ II RATE: may be 60 to 100; often associated with rate less than 60 per minute; ATRIAL vs. VENT RATES: atrial rate exceeds ventricular rate; may be 2, 3, 4 or more times as fast as the ventricular rate; P-P: regular; R-R: depends on AV conduction ratio; regular only when conduction ratio remains constant; RHYTHM: regular only when conduction ratio remains constant; pauses occur when beats are blocked by the AV junction; P WAVES: normal in configuration; more numerous than QRS complexes; P-R: normal and constant for all conducted beats; may be associated with first-degree AV block; QRS: may be within normal limits*; often associated with prolonged QRS; PACEMAKER: usually SA node

69. THIRD-DEGREE (COMPLETE) AV BLOCK RATE: atrial rate will be 60 to 100 if of sinus origin; ventricular rate varies with site of escape rhythm: if AV junction, rate will be 40 to 60 per minute; if ventricular, rate will be 20 to 40 per minute; ATRIAL vs. VENT RATES: if P waves are visible, atrial rate exceeds ventricular rate; P-P: usually regular when P waves present; R-R: usually regular; RHYTHM: atrial and ventricular rhythms are independent and unrelated, but each is regular; P WAVES: when present, are normal in configuration and more numerous and unrelated to the QRS complexes; P-R: totally irregular due to independence of atrial and ventricular rhythms; QRS: depends on site of escape rhythm: if originating from AV junction, QRS will be normal in duration and configuration; if originating from ventricles, QRS will be prolonged and bizarre; PACEMAKER: atrial pacemaker most commonly in SA node; ventricular pacemaker may be located in AV junction or ventricles.

70. TRUE

71. TRUE

72. FALSE: (normal) sinus rhythm

73. FALSE: In sinus bradycardia, there is only one P wave for each QRS.

74. TRUE

75. TRUE: especially when the stroke volume is low

76. FALSE: Sinus tachycardia is usually due to sympathetic nervous system stimulation.

77. FALSE: Atrial rhythms originate somewhere in the atria.

78. TRUE: either by default of the SA node or by increased atrial automaticity

79. FALSE: Atrial rhythms have P waves different from sinus P waves.

TABLE 3–1—ANSWERS

	Rate	Regularity	P Waves	QRS Complexes	Ratio of Atrial to Ventricular	P-R Interval	P to P Interval (regularity)	R to R Interval (regularity)	Clinical Significance of Rhythm
Sinus Rhythm	60 to 100	Essentially regular	Normal and upright	<0.12	1:1	0.12 to 0.20	Regular	Regular	Normal
Sinus Arrhythmia	60 to 100	Irregular	Normal	<0.12	1:1	0.12 to 0.20	Slightly irregular	Slightly irregular	Generally none
Sinus Bradycardia	<60	Essentially regular	Normal	<0.12	1:1	0.12 to 0.20	Regular	Regular	Only treat if rhythm is accompanied by ↓ cardiac output
Sinus Tachycardia	100 to 160	Essentially regular	Normal	<0.12	1:1	0.12 to 0.20	Regular	Regular	Increases cardiac work and oxygen needs
Atrial Flutter	Atrial 250 to 350, ventricular variable	Regular if conduction ratio is constant	F waves sawtooth	<0.12	Variable (4:1, 3:1, 2:1)	No P waves to determine	No P waves to determine	Variable depends on conduction ratio	Depends on resulting ventricular rate
Atrial Fibrillation	Atrial >350, ventricular variable	Irregularly irregular	f waves	<0.12	Unable to calculate	No P waves to calculate	NA	Totally irregular	Depends on resulting ventricular rate
Atrial Tachycardia	Atrial 160 to 220, ventricular variable	Regular	Differs from sinus P waves	<0.12	May be 1:1, may vary	0.12 to 0.20	Regular	Regular if conduction is constant	Depends on resulting ventricular rate

TABLE 3–2—ANSWERS

	Rate	Regularity	P Waves	QRS Complexes	Ratio of Atrial to Ventricular	P-R Interval	P to P Interval (regularity)	R to R Interval (regularity)	Clinical Significance of Rhythm
Wandering Atrial Pacemaker	Variable, usually 60 to 100	Essentially regular	Morphology differs	<0.12	1:1	0.12 to 0.20	May vary slightly	May vary slightly	Atria are electrically unstable
Junctional Escape Rhythm	40 to 60	Regular	May precede, coincide with or follow QRS and may have a negative deflection	<0.12	1:1 P waves may not be visible	<0.12 usually	Regular	Regular	Failure of SA node pacemaker
Accelerated Junctional Rhythm	60 to 100	Regular		<0.12	1:1 P waves may not be visible	<0.12 usually	Regular	Regular	Enhanced automaticity of AV junction
Junctional Tachycardia	> 100	Regular		<0.12	1:1	<0.12 usually	Regular	Regular	Enhanced automaticity of the AV junction, ↑ myocardial oxygen consumption
First-degree AV Block	Usually 60 to 100	Regular	Normal	<0.12	1:1	>0.20	Regular	Regular	Conduction delay at AV junction
Mobitz I, Wenckebach	Usually 60 to 100	Irregular grouped beating	Normal	<0.12	Atrial > ventricular (5:4, 4:3, 3:2), can vary	Progressively lengthens	Regular	Progressively shortens	Rarely progresses to 3rd-degree block, progressive loss of conduction at AV junction
Mobitz II, Second-Degree AV Block	Usually 60 to 100, may be slow	Irregular skipped beats	Normal	Often are >0.12	Atrial > ventricular (5:1, 4:1, 3:1, 2:1, etc.), can vary	Constant in conducted beats 0.12 to 0.20	Regular	Depends on conduction ratio	Often progresses to 3rd-degree AV block, often associated with very slow bradycardia

TABLE 3-3—ANSWERS

	Rate	Regularity	P Waves	QRS Complexes	Ratio of Atrial to Ventricular	P-R Interval	P to P Interval (regularity)	R to R Interval (regularity)	Clinical Significance of Rhythm
Complete AV Block	Almost always <60, often <40	Usually regular	Normal	<0.12 if junctional escape, >0.12 if ventricular	Atrial rate is greater than ventricular rate	Totally variable	Regular	Regular	May result in ↓ cardiac output may lead to asystole
Ventricular Tachycardia	>100	Usually regular	Are usually buried in QRS	>0.12	NA	NA	Regular	Regular	May result in ↓ cardiac output, may lead to ventricular fibrillation
Ventricular Fibrillation	Unable to measure	Chaotic	Not recognizable	None recognizable	NA	NA	NA	NA	Lethal; no cardiac output
Idioventricular Rhythm	Usually <40	Usually regular	Usually none	>0.12	NA	NA	NA	Usually regular	Heart rate not sufficient to maintain life
Agonal Rhythm	Usually <20	Usually totally irregular	Usually none	>0.12	NA	NA	NA	Irregular	Represents dying heart, almost no cardiac output
Asystole	0	NA	None	None	NA	NA	NA	NA	No cardiac output

TABLE 3-4—ANSWERS

	Site of Origin	P Wave	QRS Complexes	T Wave	Effect on R-R Interval	Compensatory Pause
Premature Atrial Contraction	Atrium	Differs from sinus P wave; may be hidden in T wave of preceding beat	Normal in configuration, <0.12	Normal	Shortens	May be followed by a noncompensatory pause
Premature Junctional Contraction	AV junction	May precede, coincide with, or follow QRS complexes and may have a negative deflection	Normal in configuration, <0.12	Normal	Shortens	May be followed by a noncompensatory pause
Premature Ventricular Contraction	Ventricles	Usually buried in the QRS complex	Wide and bizarre, >0.12	Opposite deflection to QRS	Shortens	Often followed by a full compensatory pause

80. TRUE

81. FALSE: The P-R interval may vary from one beat to the next.

82. TRUE

83. TRUE: Atrial tachycardia may be unifocal or multifocal.

84. TRUE

85. FALSE: People with poor cardiac reserve are susceptible to hemodynamic compromise.

86. TRUE

87. FALSE: Unless ventricular conduction is otherwise impaired, the QRS complexes of atrial tachycardia will be less than 0.12 second and normal in configuration.

88. FALSE: Sawtooth waveforms characterize atrial flutter.

89. FALSE: The strip shows a constant AV conduction ratio.

90. TRUE: This is atrial fibrillation.

91. FALSE: In atrial fibrillation, some of the impulses are conducted intermittently to the ventricles; this is one reason why the R-R intervals are so irregular.

92. TRUE

93. FALSE: Retrograde atrial conduction is a normal phenomenon for rhythms that originate below the atria; it commonly occurs with junctional rhythms and with some ventricular rhythms.

94. TRUE

95. TRUE

96. TRUE

97. FALSE: You would anticipate seeing a junctional escape rhythm at a rate of 40 to 60 per minute rather than a junctional tachycardia at over 100 per minute.

98. TRUE

99. FALSE: In both of these junctional rhythms, P waves may be present and QRS complexes are normal.

100. TRUE

101. FALSE: First-degree AV block has delayed, but 1:1 conduction.

102. FALSE: This is first-degree AV block since the P-R interval is greater than 0.20 second with a normal QRS and 1:1 AV conduction.

103. FALSE: With Wenckebach there will be a QRS complex following most P waves. Conduction progressively prolongs until a QRS is dropped; these dropped QRS complexes produce the characteristic "group beating."

104. TRUE

105. TRUE

106. TRUE

107. FALSE: The ECG shows second-degree AV block, Mobitz II, with 2:1 AV conduction.

108. TRUE

109. TRUE

110. FALSE: The AV conduction ratio may be constant or variable.

111. TRUE

112. TRUE: Each will be regular, but the two rhythms are unrelated to (dissociated from) one another.

113. FALSE: In complete AV block the P-R interval is totally inconsistent because the atrial and ventricular rhythms are dissociated.

114. TRUE: Either site may serve as the escape pacemaker.

115. FALSE: Third-degree AV block represents a total and complete block at the AV junction.

116. TRUE

117. TRUE

118. FALSE: Ventricular escape rhythms usually have a heart rate of 20 to 40 beats per minute.

119. TRUE

120. TRUE

121. TRUE

122. FALSE: A PVC that falls on the "vulnerable period" of the T wave may trigger lethal dysrhythmias such as ventricular tachycardia or fibrillation.

123. TRUE

124. FALSE: When PVCs alternate with normal beats, it is called ventricular bigeminy; ventricular trigeminy exists when PVCs occur after every two normal beats.

125. TRUE

126. TRUE

127. FALSE: Ventricular tachycardia usually has a rate over 100 per minute.

128. FALSE: In ventricular tachycardia, QRS complexes are greater than 0.12 second in duration and are not usually preceded by a P wave.

129. FALSE: Ventricular fibrillation always results in hemodynamic compromise.

130. TRUE: because the heart rate is only 20 to 40 beats per minute

131. TRUE

132. TRUE

133. Dysrhythmias with more P waves than QRS complexes: second-degree AV block, Mobitz I (Wenckebach), second-degree AV block, Mobitz II, third-degree AV block *Note:* Atrial tachycardia may be associated with physiologic block and result in an atrial rate faster than the ventricular rate.

134. Dysrhythmias that could result in an irregular R-R (ventricular) rhythm: ALWAYS DO: second-degree AV block, Mobitz I (Wenckebach); atrial fibrillation; PACs; PJCs; PVCs. DO IF CONDUCTION RATIO VARIES: atrial tachycardia; second-degree AV block, Mobitz II; atrial flutter

135. a. P-R 0.12 to 0.20 second: sinus rhythm; sinus bradycardia; sinus tachycardia; atrial tachycardia; 2nd-degree AV block, Mobitz II (in all conducted beats)
   b. less than 0.12 second: junctional escape rhythm; accelerated junctional rhythm
   c. over 0.20 second: 1st-degree AV block
   d. progressively lengthens: 2nd-degree AV block Mobitz I (Wenckebach)
   e. completely inconsistent: 3rd-degree AV block

136. Rate: 104/minute; Rhythm: regular; P waves: uniform positive deflections precede each QRS complex; P-P intervals are regular; P-R: 0.26 second; QRS: 0.06 second; Interpretation: sinus tachycardia with 1st-degree AV block

137. Rate: 86/minute; Rhythm: regular; P waves: uniform positive deflections precede each QRS complex; P-P intervals are regular; P-R: 0.16 second; QRS: 0.08 second; Interpretation: (normal) sinus rhythm

138. Rate: approximately 80/minute; Rhythm: regularly irregular; P waves: uniform positive deflections precede each QRS complex in underlying rhythm; P wave morphology differs in premature beats; P-P intervals are irregular due to premature P waves; P-R: 0.12 second; QRS: 0.06 second; Interpretation: sinus rhythm with frequent PACs (atrial bigeminy)

139. Rate: 100/minute; Rhythm: regular; P waves: not observable; consider changing lead to distinguish whether notching on terminal portion of S wave is a retrograde P wave; P-R: not observable; QRS: 0.09 second; Interpretation: accelerated junctional rhythm

140. Rate: ventricular is 120/minute; cannot distinguish atrial rate; Rhythm: irregularly irregular; P waves: absent; fibrillatory waves present; P-R: none; QRS: 0.06 second; Interpretation: atrial fibrillation with a rapid ventricular response

141. Rate: 78/minute; Rhythm: irregular due to premature beats; P waves: uniform positive deflections precede each QRS complex in underlying rhythm (complexes 2,4,6,8); P waves in premature beats are negative deflections; P-P intervals are irregular due to premature beats; P-R: 0.12 second;

QRS: 0.06 second; Interpretation: sinus rhythm with 3 PJCs (junctional bigeminy)

142. Rate: 120/minute; Rhythm: regular; P waves: uniform positive deflections precede each QRS complex; P-P intervals are regular; P-R: 0.16 second; QRS: 0.06 second; Interpretation: sinus tachycardia

143. Rate: approximately 70/minute; Rhythm: regularly irregular; P waves: uniform positive deflections that precede some, but not all QRS complexes; P-P intervals are regular; P-R: lengthens progressively until a QRS complex is dropped; QRS: 0.08 second; Interpretation: 2nd-degree AV block, Mobitz I (Wenckebach)

144. Rate: 90/minute; Rhythm: irregular due to premature beats; underlying rhythm is regular; P waves: uniform positive deflections precede each QRS complex in underlying rhythm; P waves do not precede premature beats; P-P intervals are irregular because of premature beats; P-R: 0.12 second; QRS: 0.08 second in underlying rhythm; 0.14 second in premature beats; Interpretation: sinus rhythm with uniform (unifocal) PVCs (ventricular quadrigeminy)

145. Rate: 40/minute; Rhythm: regular; P waves: none; P-R: none; QRS: 0.20 second; wide and bizarre complexes with S-T and T oriented opposite to QRS deflection; Interpretation: idioventricular rhythm

146. Rate: 60/minute; Rhythm: occasionally irregular; P waves: uniform positive deflections precede each QRS complex, except in the premature complex (4th) where P wave morphology differs; P-P intervals are irregular due to premature beat; P-R: 0.18 second; QRS: 0.08 second; Interpretation: sinus rhythm with a PAC

147. Rate: 250/minute; Rhythm: regular; P waves: not readily identifiable; may follow QRS complexes; P-R: none; QRS: 0.28 second; Interpretation: (sustained) ventricular tachycardia

148. Rate: ventricular is 100/minute; atrial is 400/minute; Rhythm: regular; P waves: absent; sawtooth flutter waves present; P-R: not measurable; QRS: 0.08 second; Interpretation: atrial flutter with 4 to 1 AV conduction

149. Rate: 90/minute (ventricular); Rhythm: irregularly irregular; P waves: absent; fibrillatory waves present; P-R: not measurable; QRS: 0.08 second; Interpretation: atrial fibrillation with controlled ventricular response

150. Rate: approximately 220/minute; Rhythm: regular; P waves: not discernable; P-R: not observable; QRS: 0.06 second; Interpretation: supraventricular tachycardia (probably atrial tachycardia)

151. Rate: 92/minute; Rhythm: regular; P waves: uniform positive deflections precede each QRS complex; P-P intervals are regular; P-R: 0.28 second; QRS: 0.10 second; Interpretation: sinus rhythm with 1st-degree AV block

152. Rate: atrial is 84/minute; ventricular is 50/minute; Rhythm: regular; P waves: uniform positive deflections; are more numerous than QRS complexes; P-P intervals are regular; P-R: intervals vary widely; there is no association between P waves and QRS complexes; P waves appear to "march through" the QRS complexes; QRS: 0.06 second; Interpretation: 3rd-degree (complete) AV block with junctional escape rhythm

153. Rate: 64/minute; Rhythm: occasionally irregular; P waves: uniform positive deflections precede each QRS complex; shape of P wave changes in premature beats (beats 7 and 8); P-P intervals are irregular due to premature beats; P-R: 0.16 second; QRS: 0.08 second; Interpretation: sinus rhythm with two consecutive PACs

154. Rate: 76/minute; Rhythm: regular; P waves: uniform negative deflections precede each QRS complex; P-P intervals are regular; P-R: 0.12 second; QRS: 0.08 second; Interpretation: accelerated junctional rhythm

155. Rate: approximately 90/minute; Rhythm: irregularly irregular; P waves: absent; fibrillatory waves present; P-R: none; QRS: 0.10 second; Interpretation: atrial fibrillation with controlled ventricular response

156. Rate: 47/minute; Rhythm: regular; P waves: none; P-R: none; QRS: 0.16 second; Interpretation: idioventricular rhythm

157. Rate: 80/minute; Rhythm: underlying rhythm is regular; premature beat causes irregularity; P waves: uniform positive deflections precede each QRS complex in underlying rhythm; no P wave precedes premature beat; P-P intervals are irregular because of premature beat; P-R: 0.18 second; QRS: 0.08 second; Interpretation: sinus rhythm with a PVC

158. Rate: 110/minute; Rhythm: irregular; P waves: uniform positive deflections precede each QRS complex in underlying rhythm; no P waves precede premature beats; P-P intervals are irregular due to premature beats; P-R: 0.16 second; QRS: 0.10 second in underlying rhythm; 0.14 second in premature beats; Interpretation: sinus tachycardia with a four-beat run of ventricular tachycardia and a PVC

159. Rate: 46/minute; Rhythm: regular; P waves: uniform positive deflections precede each QRS complex; P-P intervals are regular; P-R: 0.14 second; QRS: 0.09 second; Interpretation: sinus bradycardia

160. Rate: 64/minute; Rhythm: regular; P waves: uniform positive deflections precede each QRS complex; P-P intervals are regular; P-R: 0.12 second; QRS: 0.06 second; Interpretation: sinus rhythm

161. Rate: 118/minute; Rhythm: regular; P waves: uniform positive deflections precede each QRS complex; P-P intervals are regular; P-R: 0.16 second; QRS: 0.14 second; Interpretation: sinus tachycardia with an intraventricular conduction defect

162. Rate: atrial is 70/minute; ventricular is 35/minute; Rhythm: regular; P waves: uniform positive deflections precede every other QRS complex; P-P intervals are regular; P-R: 0.22 second and constant in all conducted beats; QRS: 0.10 second; Interpretation: 2nd-degree AV block, Mobitz II with 2 to 1 AV conduction

163. Rate: 60/minute; Rhythm: regularly irregular; P waves: uniform positive deflections precede each QRS complex in underlying rhythm; no P waves precede premature beats; P-R: 0.20 second in underlying rhythm; QRS: 0.12 second in underlying rhythm; 0.14 second in premature beats; Interpre-

tation: sinus rhythm with frequent uniform/unifocal PVCs (ventricular bigeminy) and underlying intraventricular conduction defect

164. Rate: approximately 180/minute (ventricular); Rhythm: regular; P waves: not readily identifiable; waveform between QRS complexes could represent T wave, P wave, merged T and P waves, or atrial flutter wave; need to slow ventricular rate to determine origin and nature of waveform; intervals are regular; P-R: not measurable with certainty; QRS: 0.06 second; Interpretation: supraventricular tachycardia, possibly atrial flutter with 2 to 1 AV conduction

165. Rate: atrial is 76/minute; ventricular is 30/minute; Rhythm: regular; P waves: uniform positive deflections; more numerous than QRS complexes; P-P intervals are regular; P-R: intervals vary widely, suggesting a lack of association between P waves and QRS complexes; some P waves distort terminal portion of QRS (2nd and 4th complexes); QRS: 0.12 second; Interpretation: 3rd-degree (complete) AV block

166. Rate: 120/minute; Rhythm: regular; P waves: none; P-R: none; QRS: 0.18 second; Interpretation: sustained ventricular tachycardia

167. Rate: 47/minute; Rhythm: regular; P waves: uniform positive deflections precede each QRS complex; P-P intervals are regular; P-R: 0.30 second; QRS: 0.10 second; Interpretation: sinus bradycardia with 1st-degree AV block

168. Rate: 70/minute; Rhythm: slightly irregular; P waves: positive deflections, but morphology changes; each is followed by a QRS complex; P-P intervals vary slightly; P-R: varies somewhat from 0.10 to 0.16 second; QRS: 0.08 second; Interpretation: wandering atrial pacemaker

169. Rate: atrial 360/minute; ventricular 120/minute; Rhythm: regular; P waves: absent; flutter waves present; P-R: not measurable; QRS: 0.10 second; Interpretation: atrial flutter with 3 to 1 AV conduction

170. Rate: approximately 65/minute; Rhythm: irregularly irregular; P waves: absent; fibrillatory waves present; P-R: not measurable; QRS: 0.06 second; Interpretation: atrial fibrillation with a controlled ventricular response

171. Rate: atrial is 80/minute; ventricular is 40/minute; Rhythm: regular; P waves: uniform deflections; every other is followed by a QRS complex; P-R: 0.26 second and constant in conducted beats; QRS: 0.12 second; Interpretation: 2nd-degree AV block, Mobitz II, with 2 to 1 AV conduction

172. Rate: approximately 40/minute (ventricular); Rhythm: irregularly irregular; P waves: absent; fibrillatory waves are present; P-R: none; QRS: 0.10 second; Interpretation: atrial fibrillation with an extremely slow ventricular response

173. Rate: approximately 90/minute (ventricular); Rhythm: irregularly irregular; P waves: absent; fibrillatory waves are present; P-R: none; QRS: 0.08 second; Interpretation: atrial fibrillation with a controlled ventricular response

174. Rate: 150/minute (ventricular); Rhythm: regular; P waves: absent; P-R: none; QRS: 0.14 second; Interpretation: ventricular tachycardia

175. Rate: atrial is 90/minute; ventricular is 30/minute; Rhythm: regular; P waves: uniform positive deflections precede every third QRS complex; P-P intervals are regular; P-R: 0.14 second and constant in all conducted beats; QRS: 0.12 second; Interpretation: 2nd-degree AV block, Mobitz II, with 3 to 1 AV conduction

176. Rate: 68/minute; Rhythm: irregular; P waves: positive deflections precede each QRS complex in the underlying rhythm; P wave morphology changes with the premature beats (complexes 1, 6); P-P intervals are irregular due to the premature beats; P-R: 0.16 second in underlying rhythm; 0.08 second in premature beats; QRS: 0.06 second; Interpretation: sinus rhythm with 2 PACs

177. Rate: 142/minute; Rhythm: regular; P waves: uniform positive deflections precede each QRS complex; P-P intervals are regular; P-R: 0.14 second; QRS: 0.10 second; Interpretation: sinus tachycardia

178. Rate: 84/minute; Rhythm: irregular only when premature beat occurs; P waves: uniform positive deflections precede each QRS complex in the underlying rhythm; no P wave precedes the premature QRS complex; P-P intervals are regular, except with the premature beat; P-R: 0.16 second; QRS: 0.06 second in underlying rhythm; 0.14 second in premature beat; Interpretation: sinus rhythm with one PVC

179. Rate: 96/minute; Rhythm: regular, except with premature beat; P waves: uniform positive deflections precede each QRS complex in the underlying rhythm; no P wave precedes the premature complex; P-R intervals are regular, except with the premature beat; P-R: 0.18 second; QRS: 0.10 second; Interpretation: sinus rhythm with a PJC

180. Rate: atrial is 280/minute; ventricular is 70/minute; Rhythm: regular; P waves: none; flutter waves present; P-R: not measurable; QRS: 0.06 second; Interpretation: atrial flutter with constant 4 to 1 AV conduction

181. Rate: 120/minute; Rhythm: regular; P waves: uniform positive deflections precede each QRS complex; P-P intervals are regular; P-R: 0.22 second; QRS: 0.06 second; Interpretation: sinus tachycardia with 1st-degree AV block

182. Rate: approximate atrial rate of 280/minute and ventricular rate of 80/minute; Rhythm: irregular; P waves: absent; flutter waves present; P-R: not measurable; QRS: 0.08 second; Interpretation: atrial flutter with variable (4:1 and 2:1) AV conduction

183. Rate: initially ventricular rate only about 30/minute; ventricular rate then increases abruptly to about 150/minute; Rhythm: initially irregular; regular when rate increases; P waves: uniform positive deflections precede the two sinus beats; no P waves precede the premature complexes; P-P intervals are irregular because of the premature beats; P-R: 0.16 second in sinus beats; QRS: 0.06 second in underlying rhythm and 0.14 in ventricular beats; Interpretation: sinus bradycardia with ventricular bigeminy followed by sustained ventricular tachycardia

184. Rate: 43/minute; Rhythm: regular; P waves: none; P-R: none; QRS: 0.10 second; Interpretation: junctional (escape) rhythm

185. Rate: approximately 56/minute in underlying rhythm and 110/minute with premature beats; Rhythm: regularly ir-

regular; P waves: uniform positive deflections precede each QRS complex in underlying rhythm; no P waves precede the premature beats; P-R: 0.12 second; QRS: 0.08 second in underlying rhythm and 0.14 second with premature beats; Interpretation: sinus bradycardia with ventricular bigeminy

186. Rate: atrial 84/minute; ventricular is 40/minute; Rhythm: regular, but independent atrial and ventricular rhythms; P waves: uniform positive deflections; are more numerous than QRS complexes; P-P intervals are regular; P-R: intervals vary widely, suggesting a lack of association between P waves and QRS complexes; QRS: 0.16 second; Interpretation: 3rd-degree (complete) AV block with a ventricular escape rhythm

187. Rate: 70/minute; Rhythm: regular, except when premature beats occur; P waves: uniform positive deflections precede each QRS complex, except in premature beats; P-P intervals are irregular because of premature beats; P-R: 0.16 second; QRS: 0.08 second; Interpretation: sinus rhythm with two consecutive PJCs

188. Rate: approximately 120/minute (ventricular); Rhythm: irregularly irregular; P waves: absent; fibrillatory waves present; P-R: none; QRS: 0.06 second; Interpretation: atrial fibrillation with a rapid ventricular response

189. Rate: atrial is 90/minute and ventricular is 60/minute; Rhythm: regularly irregular; P waves: uniform positive deflections precede some, but not all, QRS complexes; P-P intervals are regular; P-R: lengthens progressively until a QRS complex is dropped; QRS: 0.18 second; Interpretation: 2nd-degree AV block, Mobitz I (Wenckebach), with 2:1 and 3:2 AV conduction in an intraventricular conduction defect

190. Rate: 110/minute; Rhythm: regular; P waves: upright; P-R: beyond 0.20; QRS: 0.06 second; Interpretation: sinus tachycardia with 1st-degree AV block

191. Rate: 44/minute; Rhythm: regular; P waves: uniform negative deflections precede each QRS complex; P-P intervals are regular; P-R: 0.12 second; QRS: 0.07 second; Interpretation: junctional (escape) rhythm

192. Rate: 64/minute; Rhythm: regular; P waves: uniform positive deflections precede each QRS complex; P-P intervals are regular; P-R: 0.20 second; QRS: 0.10 second; Interpretation: (normal) sinus rhythm

193. Rate: the rate is 60/minute initially, then increases to 150/minute; Rhythm: regular; P waves: uniform positive deflections precede each QRS complex before and after the run of tachycardia; the P wave preceding the tachycardia (4th complex) differs and is likely of atrial origin; P waves are not visible during the tachycardia and may be merged into the T waves; P-P intervals are irregular; P-R: 0.18 second in underlying rhythm; QRS: 0.06 second; Interpretation: sinus rhythm with a run of paroxysmal atrial tachycardia

194. Rate: 75/minute; Rhythm: regular; P waves: none; P-R: none; QRS: 0.06 second; Interpretation: accelerated junctional rhythm

195. Rate: 62/minute; Rhythm: regular, except when premature beats occur; P waves: uniform positive deflections precede each QRS complex of the underlying rhythm; P waves do not precede the premature beats; P-P intervals are irregular because of the premature beats; P-R: 0.16 second; QRS:

0.06 second in underlying rhythm; 0.16 second in premature beats; Interpretation: sinus rhythm with two consecutive PVCs

196. Rate: 52/minute; Rhythm: regular; P waves: uniform positive deflections precede each QRS complex; P-P intervals are regular; P-R: 0.18 second; QRS: 0.08 second; Interpretation: sinus bradycardia

197. Rate: atrial rate is 72/minute; ventricular rate is 50/minute; Rhythm: regular, but independent atrial and ventricular rhythms; P waves: uniform positive deflections that are more numerous than QRS complexes; P-P intervals are regular; P-R: intervals vary widely, suggesting a lack of association between P waves and QRS complexes; QRS: 0.08 second; Interpretation: 3rd-degree (complete) AV block

198. Rate: approximately 100/minute (ventricular); Rhythm: irregularly irregular; P waves: absent; fibrillatory waves present; P-R: none; QRS: 0.08 second; Interpretation: atrial fibrillation with a controlled ventricular response

199. Rate: atrial rate is 110/minute; ventricular is 55/minute; Rhythm: regular; P waves: uniform positive deflections precede each QRS complex, but only every other P wave is followed by a QRS complex; P-P intervals are regular; P-R: 0.14 second and constant in conducted beats; QRS: 0.12 second; Interpretation: 2nd-degree AV block, Mobitz II, with 2 to 1 AV conduction

200. Rate: approximately 75/minute atrial and 60/minute ventricular; Rhythm: regularly irregular; P waves: uniform positive deflections not all followed by a QRS complex; P-P intervals are regular; P-R: lengthens progressively until a QRS complex is dropped; QRS: 0.06 second; Interpretation: 2nd-degree AV block, Mobitz I (Wenckebach), with 4 to 3 AV conduction

201. Rate: approximately 75/minute; Rhythm: regularly irregular; P waves: uniform positive deflections precede each QRS complex in the underlying rhythm; P waves do not precede the premature impulses; P-R: 0.20 second; QRS: 0.08 second in sinus beats; 0.18 second in premature beats; Interpretation: sinus rhythm with frequent uniform (unifocal) PVCs (ventricular bigeminy)

202. Rate: ventricular rate is about 45/minute; Rhythm: regularly irregular; P waves: absent; fibrillatory waves appear to be present (also artifact); P-R: none; QRS: 0.08 second; Interpretation: atrial fibrillation with a slow ventricular response

203. Rate: 96/minute; Rhythm: regular; P waves: uniform positive deflections precede each QRS complex; P-P intervals are regular; P-R: 0.24 second; QRS: 0.08 second; Interpretation: sinus rhythm with 1st-degree AV block

204. Rate: 60/minute; Rhythm: irregular; P waves: positive deflections precede each QRS complex; P waves preceding premature beats (complexes 2, 4) differ from sinus P waves and are likely of atrial origin; pacemaking site may be unstable because P waves in beats 1 and 6 also differ from sinus P waves; P-P intervals are irregular due to the premature beats; P-R: 0.12 second in underlying rhythm and 0.14 second in premature beats; QRS: 0.06 second; Interpretation: sinus rhythm with 2 PACs; rule out wandering atrial pacemaker

205. Rate: 100/minute; Rhythm: regular; P waves: none observable; P-R: none; QRS: 0.16 second; Interpretation: (sustained) ventricular tachycardia

206. Rate: atrial is 90/minute and ventricular is 45/minute; Rhythm: regular; P waves: uniform positive deflections precede every other QRS complex; P-P intervals are regular; P-R: 0.24 second and constant in conducted beats; QRS: 0.10 second; Interpretation: 2nd-degree AV block, Mobitz II, with 2 to 1 AV conduction; 1st-degree AV block

207. Rate: approximately 90/minute in underlying rhythm and 200/minute in run of tachycardia; Rhythm: irregular; P waves: uniform positive deflections precede each narrow QRS complex; P waves do not precede the premature beats; P-R: 0.16 second; QRS: 0.08 second in sinus beats and 0.16 second in premature beats; Interpretation: sinus rhythm with two runs of ventricular tachycardia

208. Rate: atrial rate is 58/minute and ventricular rate is 50/minute; Rhythm: irregular; P waves: uniform positive deflections; not all are followed by a QRS complex; P-P intervals are regular; P-R: lengthens progressively until a QRS complex is dropped; QRS: 0.08 second; Interpretation: 2nd-degree AV block, Mobitz I (Wenckebach)

209. Rate: 120/minute; Rhythm: regular; P waves: uniform positive deflections precede each QRS complex; P-P intervals are regular; P-R: 0.22 second; QRS: 0.08 second; Interpretation: sinus tachycardia with 1st-degree AV block

210. Rate: 56/minute; Rhythm: regular; P waves: uniform positive deflections precede each QRS complex; P-P intervals are regular; P-R: 0.28 second; QRS: 0.08 second; Interpretation: sinus bradycardia with 1st-degree AV block

211. Rate: atrial rate is 33/minute; ventricular is 16/minute; Rhythm: regular; P waves: uniform positive deflections; not all followed by a QRS complex; P-P intervals are regular; P-R: variable; QRS: 0.08 second; Interpretation: 3rd-degree (complete) AV block with junctional escape rhythm

212. Rate: 84/minute; Rhythm: regular, except when premature beats occur; P waves: uniform positive deflections precede each QRS complex in all but premature beats; P-P intervals are irregular because of premature beats; P-R: 0.20 second; QRS: 0.10 second in underlying rhythm and 0.23 second in premature beats; Interpretation: sinus rhythm with two PVCs

213. Rate: atrial is 300/minute; ventricular is 130/minute; Rhythm: irregular; P waves: absent; flutter waves present; P-R: none; QRS: 0.06 second; Interpretation: atrial flutter with 2:1 and 3:1 AV conduction

214. Rate: approximately 56/minute in underlying rhythm; Rhythm: regular, except for premature beat; P waves: uniform positive deflections precede each QRS complex; P-P intervals are regular, except with premature beat; P-R: 0.16 second; QRS: 0.09 second; Interpretation: sinus bradycardia with one PAC

215. Rate: 72/minute; Rhythm: regular, except for the premature beat; P waves: uniform positive deflections precede each QRS complex; P wave of premature beat differs in morphology from other P waves; P-P intervals are irregular; P-R: 0.16 second; QRS: 0.10 second; Interpretation: sinus rhythm with one PAC

216. Rate: atrial is 95/minute; ventricular is 35/minute; Rhythm: regular; P waves: uniform positive deflections that are more numerous than and not associated with QRS complexes; P-P intervals are regular; P-R: intervals vary widely, suggesting a lack of association between P waves and QRS complexes; QRS: 0.12 second; Interpretation: 3rd-degree (complete) AV block

217. Rate: 80/minute; Rhythm: irregular; P waves: positive deflections of somewhat variable configuration precede sinus QRS complexes; P waves preceding the premature beats appear to be negative deflections; P-P intervals are irregular; P-R: 0.12 second in underlying rhythm and 0.10 second in premature beats; QRS: 0.08 second; Interpretation: sinus rhythm with 2 PJCs

218. Rate: approximately 100/minute (ventricular); Rhythm: irregularly irregular; P waves: absent; fibrillatory waves present; P-R: none; QRS: 0.08 second; Interpretation: atrial fibrillation with a rapid ventricular response

219. Rate: 84/minute; Rhythm: regular; P waves: uniform positive deflections precede each QRS complex; P-P intervals are regular; P-R: 0.26 second; QRS: 0.12 second; Interpretation: sinus rhythm with 1st-degree AV block

220. Rate: approximately 80/minute (ventricular); Rhythm: irregularly irregular; P waves: absent; fibrillatory waves present; P-R: none; QRS: 0.08 second; Interpretation: atrial fibrillation with a controlled ventricular response

221. Rate: approximately 90/minute; Rhythm: regularly irregular; P waves: uniform positive deflections precede each QRS complex of the underlying rhythm; P waves do not precede the premature beats; P-R: 0.14 second; QRS: 0.08 second in underlying rhythm and 0.14 second in premature beats; Interpretation: sinus rhythm with frequent PVCs (ventricular bigeminy)

222. Rate: 118/minute; Rhythm: regular; P waves: uniform positive deflections precede each QRS complex; P-P intervals are regular; P-R: 0.14 second; QRS: 0.06 second; Interpretation: sinus tachycardia

223. Rate: atrial rate is 54/minute; ventricular is 30/minute; Rhythm: irregular; P waves: uniform positive deflections; not all are followed by a QRS complex; P-P intervals are regular; P-R: 0.20 second and constant in conducted beats; QRS: 0.12 second; Interpretation: intermittent 2nd-degree AV block, Mobitz II, with 2 to 1 AV conduction

224. Rate: 70/minute in underlying rhythm; Rhythm: regular, except when premature beat occurs; P waves: uniform positive deflections precede each QRS complex, except with premature beat; P-P intervals are irregular; P-R: 0.18 second; QRS: 0.12 second in underlying rhythm; 0.18 second and 0.21 second in premature beat; Interpretation: sinus rhythm with a PVC

225. Rate: 40/minute; Rhythm: regular; P waves: uniform positive deflections precede each QRS complex; P-P intervals are regular; P-R: 0.14 second; QRS: 0.10 second; Interpretation: sinus bradycardia

226. Rate: 46/minute; Rhythm: regular; P waves: none; P-R: none; QRS: 0.08 second; Interpretation: junctional (escape) rhythm

227. Rate: approximately 160/minute; Rhythm: irregular; P waves: none observable; P-R: none; QRS: 0.10 second in narrow QRS complexes; 0.20 second in wide QRS complexes; Interpretation: junctional rhythm with ventricular tachycardia

228. Rate: 60/minute; Rhythm: regular, except for premature beats; P waves: uniform positive deflections precede each QRS complex, except in the premature beats; P-R: 0.18 second; QRS: 0.10 second in underlying rhythm; 0.18 second in premature beat; Interpretation: sinus rhythm with one PVC

229. Rate: approximately 100/minute; Rhythm: irregularly irregular; P waves: absent; fibrillatory waves present; P-R: none; QRS: 0.06 second; Interpretation: atrial fibrillation with a rapid ventricular response

230. Rate: about 70/minute; Rhythm: irregular; P waves: uniform positive deflections precede each QRS complex, except in premature beats; P-R: 0.18 second; QRS: 0.10 second in underlying rhythm and 0.20 second in premature beats; Interpretation: sinus rhythm with frequent uniform (unifocal) PVCs (ventricular trigeminy)

231. Rate: atrial rate is approximately 300/minute; ventricular is 100/minute; Rhythm: regular; P waves: absent; flutter waves present; P-R: none; QRS: 0.06 second; Interpretation: atrial flutter with 3 to 1 AV conduction

232. Rate: 67/minute; Rhythm: regular, except for premature beat; P waves: uniform positive deflections precede each QRS complex; the P wave of the premature beat differs in morphology from the sinus P waves; P-P intervals are regular, except for the premature beat; P-R: 0.12 second; QRS: 0.06 second; Interpretation: sinus rhythm with one PAC

233. Rate: approximately 55/minute; Rhythm: regularly irregular; P waves: uniform positive deflections precede each sinus QRS complex; P waves do not precede the premature beat; P-R: 0.18 second; QRS: 0.08 second in underlying rhythm; 0.20 second in premature beat; Interpretation: sinus bradycardia alternating with PVCs (ventricular bigeminy)

234. Rate: 135/minute; Rhythm: irregular; P waves: uniform positive deflections precede each QRS complex; P waves preceding the premature beats are negative deflections; P-P intervals are irregular; P-R: 0.18 second in underlying rhythm; 0.10 in premature beats; QRS: 0.08 second; Interpretation: sinus tachycardia with frequent PJCs (junctional trigeminy)

235. Rate: 80/minute; Rhythm: regular; P waves: uniform positive deflections precede each QRS complex; P-P intervals are regular; P-R: 0.20 second; QRS: 0.16 second; Interpretation: sinus rhythm with an intraventricular conduction defect

236. Rate: atrial rate is 90/minute; ventricular rate is 60/minute; Rhythm: regularly irregular; P waves: uniform deflections; not all are followed by a QRS complex; P-P intervals are regular; P-R: lengthens progressively until a QRS complex is dropped; shortest; P-R is 0.32 second; QRS: 0.14 second; Interpretation: 2nd-degree AV block, Mobitz I (Wenckebach), with 3:2 AV conduction.

237. Rate: 55/minute; Rhythm: regular; P waves: uniform positive deflections precede each QRS complex; P-P intervals are regular; P-R: 0.32 second; QRS: 0.07 second; Interpretation: sinus bradycardia with 1st-degree AV block

238. Rate: 210/minute; Rhythm: regular; P waves: none readily apparent; P-R: none; QRS: 0.24 second; Interpretation: ventricular tachycardia

239. Rate: approximately 66/minute; Rhythm: irregular; P waves: positive deflections that vary somewhat in configuration; precede each QRS complex, except for premature beats; P-R: 0.13 second; QRS: 0.08 second in sinus beats; 0.12 second in premature beats; Interpretation: run of ventricular bigeminy followed by sinus rhythm

240. Rate: 56/minute; Rhythm: regular; P waves: uniform positive deflections precede each QRS complex; P-P intervals are regular; P-R: 0.16 second; QRS: 0.06 second; Interpretation: sinus bradycardia

241. Rate: about 100/minute; Rhythm: regularly irregular; P waves: uniform positive deflections precede each QRS complex, except for the premature beats; P-R: 0.18 second; QRS: 0.12 second in sinus beats; 0.16 in premature beats; Interpretation: sinus rhythm alternating with PVCs (ventricular bigeminy)

242. Rate: atrial rate is 90/minute; ventricular rate is 35/minute; Rhythm: essentially regular; P waves: uniform positive deflections that are more numerous than QRS complexes; P-P intervals are regular; P-R: intervals vary; there is no association between P waves and QRS complexes; QRS: 0.11 second; Interpretation: 3rd-degree (complete) AV block with junctional escape rhythm

243. Rate: 65/minute; Rhythm: regular; P waves: uniform positive deflections precede each QRS complex; P-P intervals are regular; P-R: 0.25 second; QRS: 0.10 second; Interpretation: sinus rhythm with 1st-degree AV block

244. Rate: 85/minute; Rhythm: regular; P waves: uniform positive deflections precede each QRS complex; P-R: 0.20 second; QRS: 0.08 second; Interpretation: sinus rhythm

245. Rate: approximately 80/minute; Rhythm: regularly irregular; P waves: uniform positive deflections precede each sinus QRS complex; P waves do not precede the premature beats; P-R: 0.16 second; QRS: 0.10 second in underlying rhythm; 0.16 second in premature beats; Interpretation: sinus rhythm alternating with PVCs (ventricular bigeminy)

246. Rate: 70/minute; Rhythm: regular, except for premature beat; P waves: uniform positive deflections precede each QRS complex; P-P intervals are irregular only with the premature beat; P-R: 0.20 second; QRS: 0.06 second; Interpretation: sinus rhythm with one PAC

247. Rate: 72/minute; Rhythm: regular, except for premature beat; P waves: uniform positive deflections precede each QRS complex, except with premature beat; P-P intervals are irregular; P-R: 0.18 second; QRS: 0.08 second in underlying rhythm; 0.12 second in premature beat; Interpretation: sinus rhythm with one PVC

248. Rate: approximately 150/minute; Rhythm: irregularly irregular; P waves: none observable; P-R: none; QRS: 0.06 second; Interpretation: (fine) atrial fibrillation with a rapid ventricular response

249. Rate: atrial is 76/minute; ventricular is 38/minute; Rhythm: regular; P waves: uniform positive deflections precede every other QRS complex; P-P intervals are regular; P-R: 0.16 second and constant in all conducted beats; QRS: 0.14 second; Interpretation: 2nd-degree AV block, Mobitz II, with 2:1 AV conduction

250. Rate: 110/minute; Rhythm: regular; P waves: none observable; P-R: none; QRS: 0.08 second; Interpretation: junctional tachycardia

251. Rate: 110/minute; Rhythm: regular; P waves: none observable; P-R: none; QRS: 0.24 second; Interpretation: ventricular tachycardia

252. Rate: 86/minute; Rhythm: irregular; P waves: uniform positive deflections precede some, but not all, QRS complexes; P-P intervals are regular; P-R: 0.16 second; QRS: 0.12 second; Interpretation: sinus rhythm with intermittent 2nd-degree AV block, Mobitz II, with 2:1 AV conduction

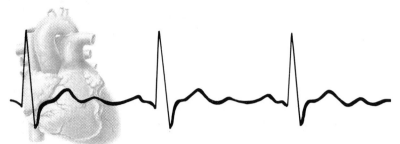

Chapter 4

Cardiovascular Pharmacology

OBJECTIVES

Upon completion of this chapter, you will be able to:

- Specify the appropriate emergency use of oxygen to treat hypoxia.

- Describe the actions, indications, dosage, precautions, preparation, and administration of medications used for treatment of metabolic acidosis.

- Distinguish among the four types of cardiovascular adrenergic receptors.

- Explain the actions, indications, dosage, precautions, preparation, and administration of medications used in emergency cardiac care to enhance cardiac automaticity, conductivity, and contractility.

- Identify the actions, indications, dosage, precautions, preparation, and administration of medications used to reduce cardiac workload and enhance myocardial perfusion.

- Explain the concept of fibrillation threshold in relation to various emergency drugs.

- Relate the mechanisms of reentry and automaticity to the treatment of cardiac dysrhythmias.

- Compare the actions, indications, dosage, precautions, preparation, and administration of antidysrhythmic agents used in emergency cardiac care.

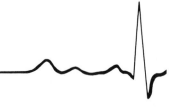

Oxygen

1. Which of the following is true about hypoxia? (More than one may be correct.)

   a. It can only be recognized as shortness of breath.
   b. It should be treated with oxygen.
   c. It is defined as a lack of oxygen in the tissues.
   d. It is often seen with shock.

2. List three factors that contribute to severe hypoxia in cardiac arrest.

   1) _____

   2) _____

   3) _____

3. List the effects of oxygen administration in the hypoxemic patient.

   1) _____

   2) _____

   3) _____

4. Identify three situations when oxygen should be administered.

   1) _____

   2) _____

   3) _____

True or False

5. T F During cardiopulmonary resuscitation (CPR), oxygen therapy should be discontinued if the patient might develop oxygen toxicity.

6. T F Oxygen administration in acute myocardial infarction may reduce or eliminate ischemic zones surrounding areas of infarction.

Sodium Bicarbonate

7. T F Acidosis affects the myocardium by decreasing the contractility and lowering the fibrillation threshold.

8. T F Sodium bicarbonate is a first-line treatment for cardiac arrest.

9. T F The most effective treatment for respiratory acidosis is sodium bicarbonate.

10. T F Sodium bicarbonate is administered before each defibrillation attempt to enhance the likelihood of successful termination of ventricular fibrillation.

11. T F Persistent ventilatory insufficiency contributes to refractory acidosis.

12. T F Cardiac muscle performance is depressed by increases in $PaCO_2$.

13. T F Respiratory compensation (hyperventilation) for metabolic acidosis can help offset intracellular acidosis.

14. T F Alveolar hyperventilation with a $PaCO_2$ in the 25- to 35-mm of Hg range may be helpful in raising the pH in metabolic acidosis.

15. List potential hazards of sodium bicarbonate administration.

   _____

   _____

   _____

   _____

   _____

16. Briefly explain how an overdose of sodium bicarbonate may result in tissue hypoxia.

   _____

   _____

   _____

   _____

   _____

   _____

17. On the prefilled syringe in Figure 4-1, shade in the area that denotes the amount of sodium bicarbonate that should be initially administered to a 150-lb cardiac arrest victim. Each syringe contains 50 mEq of $NaHCO_3$.

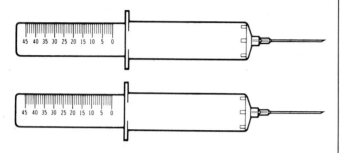

Figure 4-1

18. On the prefilled syringe in Figure 4-2, shade in the area that denotes the dosage of sodium bicarbonate that should be given to the patient approximately 10 minutes after the initial dose.

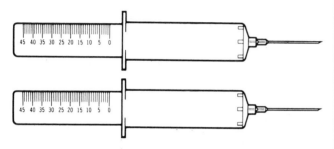

Figure 4-2

19. Explain the mechanisms of action by which medications enhance cardiac electrical or mechanical activity.

_____

_____

_____

_____

_____

_____

_____

Atropine

True or False

20. T   F   Stimulation of the parasympathetic nervous system (vagus nerve) may drastically slow the heart rate and thus deleteriously affect cardiac output.

21. T   F   Hypotension can result from a heart rate that is too slow.

22. T   F   Hemodynamically compromising bradycardia may be treated with medications that improve cardiac output by increasing the heart rate.

23. T   F   Asystole can be thought of as the "ultimate bradycardia."

24. T   F   Atropine increases the heart rate and enhances impulse conduction by stimulating the sympathetic nervous system directly.

25. T   F   Atropine should always be given when the heart rate is less than 60 beats per minute and may be valuable in high-degree AV block.

26. T   F   If hypotension is accompanied by bradycardia, atropine administration is usually the treatment of choice.

27. T   F   Atropine works by blocking the release of acetylcholine from the distal nerve ending.

28. T   F   Atropine doses of less than 0.5 mg IV may slow the heart rate.

29. T   F   Atropine may cause myocardial ischemia.

30. T   F   Atropine can be administered in an unlimited number of doses once every 5 minutes.

31. List two effects of atropine on the cardiac conduction system.

_____

_____

_____

32. Explain the rationale for using atropine in the treatment of asystole.

_____

_____

_____

33. For each of the dysrhythmias in Figures 4-3, 4-4, and 4-5, describe the changes you would expect following atropine administration and the action of atropine responsible for the change(s).

_____

_____

_____

_____

_____

_____

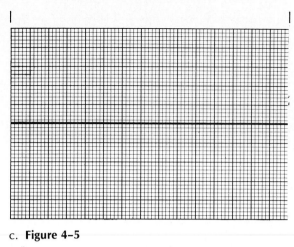

c. **Figure 4-5**

Changes _____ *Actions* _____

34. On the prefilled syringe in Figure 4-6, shade in the area that denotes the dosage range of atropine that should be initially administered to a patient with hemodynamically compromising bradycardia. Each syringe contains 10 ml (1.0 mg) of atropine.

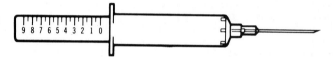

Figure 4-6

35. The initial dose of atropine did not relieve the problem and 5 minutes have passed. Shade in the area on the prefilled syringe in Figure 4-7 that indicates the dosage of atropine that should now be administered to this patient.

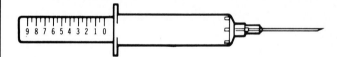

Figure 4-7

True or False

36. T   F   The appropriate initial dose of atropine for a patient in asystole is 1 mg (10 ml).

37. T   F   Atropine may be administered via endotracheal tube.

Isoproterenol

38. T   F   Isoproterenol is a virtually pure beta adrenergic receptor blocker.

39. T   F   Isoproterenol increases both preload and venous constriction and decreases both heart rate and contractility.

a. **Figure 4-3**

Changes _____ *Actions* _____

b. **Figure 4-4**

Changes _____ *Actions* _____

40. Briefly explain how to mix and administer an iso-proterenol infusion.

_____

_____

_____

_____

_____

True or False

41. T   F   Isoproterenol may increase myocardial oxygen consumption.

42. T   F   Isoproterenol increases blood pressure by increasing peripheral vascular resistance.

43. T   F   Isoproterenol increases cardiac output through its positive inotropic and chronotropic properties.

44. T   F   In a patient with a pulse, isoproterenol may be used to treat bradycardia that is refractory to atropine.

45. T   F   Isoproterenol may be used to treat ventricular asystole and electromechanical dissociation.

46. T   F   Isoproterenol is administered in a continuous IV infusion at a dosage range of 2 to 10 µg (micrograms) per minute.

47. T   F   Electrical pacing provides better control of significant bradycardia than does isoproterenol.

48. T   F   When administering isoproterenol, the desired heart rate is approximately 85 beats per minute.

49. For the dysrhythmia in Figure 4–8, describe the change(s) you would expect following isoproterenol administration and the action of isoproterenol responsible for the change(s).

_____

_____

_____

_____

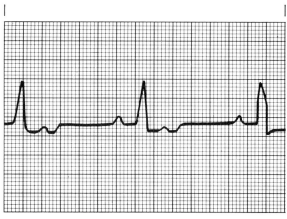

Figure 4–8

Changes _____ *Actions* _____

50. Briefly explain why it is important to decrease or discontinue isoproterenol administration if PVCs are observed.

_____

_____

_____

_____

True or False

51. T   F   Although defibrillation is the true definitive treatment for ventricular fibrillation, some medications may help improve cardiac output and subsequently increase the chances for successful resuscitation.

52. T   F   In ventricular asystole, there is a total absence of ventricular electrical and mechanical activity.

53. T   F   Electromechanical dissociation (EMD) rarely affects cardiac output.

54. T   F   In EMD, there is coordinated cardiac electrical activity, but no mechanical response (contraction).

55. T   F   Treatment of EMD is directed toward getting the heart muscle to contract effectively.

56. T   F   Epinephrine, calcium chloride, and isoproterenol are used in the treatment of EMD.

Epinephrine

True or False

57. T   F   Epinephrine decreases the pressure generated during cardiac compressions and decreases spontaneous cardiac contractions.

58. T   F   Epinephrine has both alpha and beta stimulating properties.

59. T   F   A primary beneficial effect of epinephrine in cardiac arrest is its vasoconstrictive action.

60. T   F   Epinephrine can be administered via endotracheal tube since it is rapidly absorbed across the bronchoaveolar structures.

61. T   F   Epinephrine is administered via endotracheal tube in its full 10-ml dosage (1 mg).

62. T   F   Catecholamines such as epinephrine may not be effective in stimulating the heart when the patient is acidotic.

63. T   F   In doses used during cardiac arrest, epinephrine causes coronary vasoconstriction.

64. T   F   During cardiac arrest, epinephrine can be administered every 5 minutes.

65. T   F   Epinephrine can also be used as a pressor agent via continuous infusion.

66. List the cardiac conditions that epinephrine may be used to treat.

_____

_____

_____

_____

67. Explain why epinephrine is given before sodium bicarbonate in cardiac arrest situations.

_____

_____

_____

_____

_____

_____

_____

_____

_____

_____

68. On the prefilled syringe in Figure 4–9, shade in the area that denotes the dosage range of epinephrine that should be initially administered to a cardiac arrest patient. Each syringe contains 10 ml of 1:10,000 solution (0.1 mg/ml) epinephrine.

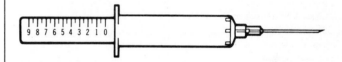

Figure 4–9

69. Now that 5 minutes have passed, shade in the area on the prefilled syringe in Figure 4–10 that indicates the dosage range of epinephrine that should now be administered to this patient.

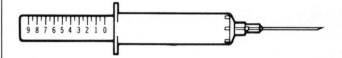

Figure 4–10

70. For each of the situations in Figures 4–11 through 4–15, describe the changes you would expect following epinephrine administration and the action of epinephrine that has contributed to that change.

_____

_____

_____

_____

_____

_____

_____

_____

_____

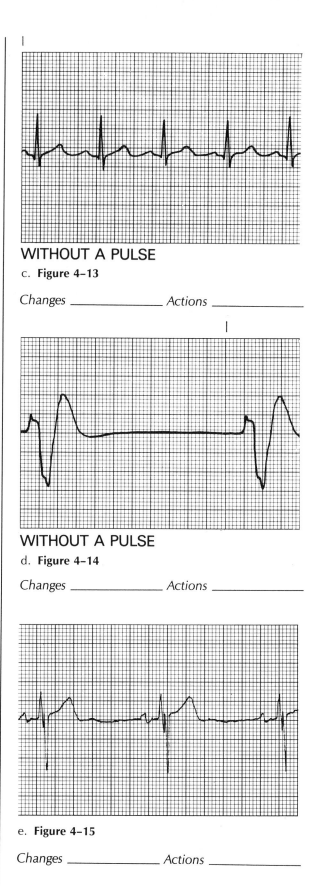

a. **Figure 4–11**

Changes _____ *Actions* _____

b. **Figure 4–12**

Changes _____ *Actions* _____

WITHOUT A PULSE

c. **Figure 4–13**

Changes _____ *Actions* _____

WITHOUT A PULSE

d. **Figure 4–14**

Changes _____ *Actions* _____

e. **Figure 4–15**

Changes _____ *Actions* _____

71. Describe how epinephrine is prepared and administered by IV infusion.

_____

_____

_____

True or False

72. T   F   Hemodynamically significant hypotension may be defined as a systolic blood pressure of less than 90 mm of Hg with accompanying signs of inadequate perfusion.

73. T   F   The danger of hypotension is that perfusion to the vital organs may be significantly decreased.

74. T   F   Hypotension can result from diminished stroke volume seen with massive myocardial infarction.

75. T   F   Inotropic agents are of little value in the treatment of hypotension due to depressed left ventricular function.

76. T   F   Inappropriate systemic vascular resistance can cause hypotension.

Norepinephrine

True or False

77. T   F   Norepinephrine has only alpha stimulating properties.

78. Place a check mark next to the statements that describe actions of norepinephrine.

_____ a. causes the venous system to constrict, thereby increasing venous return to the heart

_____ b. increases myocardial contractility

_____ c. decreases preload by decreasing end-diastolic volume

_____ d. increases the rate of spontaneous contractions by increasing automaticity

_____ e. increases arterial blood pressure by causing arterial vasoconstriction

True or False

79. T   F   Norepinephrine may be a useful drug for the treatment of hypotension related to peripheral vasodilation.

80. T   F   Norepinephrine is contraindicated in cardiogenic shock.

81. T   F   Norepinephrine is useful in cardiac arrest because it decreases myocardial oxygen consumption.

82. T   F   Norepinephrine dilates the coronary circulation directly, thereby improving myocardial perfusion.

83. T   F   Norepinephrine raises the blood pressure slightly more rapidly than other catecholamines.

84. Explain how norepinephrine may improve cardiac output when vasoconstriction is already extreme.

_____

_____

_____

85. Briefly explain how norepinephrine may enhance cardiac output further once an optimal blood pressure has been restored.

_____

_____

_____

86. Why may norepinephrine be particularly harmful in the patient with myocardial ischemia and/or infarction?

_____

_____

_____

87. What three types of monitoring should be done during norepinephrine administration?

1) _____

2) _____

3) _____

88. Which of the following items are precautions to consider when administering norepinephrine?

    1) Do not administer if patient is hypovolemic. *Answers*
    2) Causes renal and mesenteric vasoconstriction.   a. 1, 2, 3
    3) Abrupt cessation may produce hypertension.   b. 1, 2, 5
    4) May be used for a maximum of 1 to 2 hours.   c. 2, 3, 4
    5) May cause necrosis and sloughing if allowed to extravasate.   d. 2, 4, 5

89. The initial dosage for norepinephrine should be:

    a. 1 mg/kg, IV push
    b. 2 to 20 μg, IV infusion
    c. 8 to 16 μg/ml, IV infusion, titrated to effect
    d. 100 mEq, IV push
    e. 0.5 to 1.0 mg, IV push

90. Norepinephrine administration should be adjusted to maintain a systolic blood pressure at or above _____ mm of Hg.

    a. 70
    b. 80
    c. 90
    d. 100

91. On Figure 4–16, fill in the correct information for the preparation and administration of norepinephrine.

92. Describe what should be done if there is extravasation of norepinephrine.

    _____
    _____
    _____

Dopamine

93. Which of the following are properties of dopamine?

    1) alpha stimulation
    2) alpha receptor blockade   *Answers*
    3) beta receptor stimulation   a. 1, 2, 3
    4) beta receptor blockade   b. 1, 3, 5
    5) dopaminergic receptor stimulation   c. 2, 3, 5
      d. 3, 4, 5

94. Place a check mark next to the items that are actions of dopamine.

    _____ a. causes vasoconstriction and increased venous return

    _____ b. increases myocardial contractility

    _____ c. decreases preload by decreasing end-diastolic volume

    _____ d. increases automaticity

    _____ e. increases arterial blood pressure through arterial vasoconstriction

1.
DRAWING-IT-UP

2.
MIXING

3.
ADMINISTERING

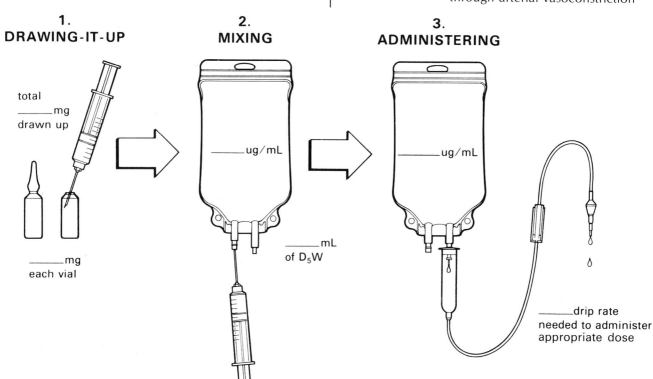

total _____ mg drawn up

_____ ug/mL

_____ ug/mL

_____ mg each vial

_____ mL of D$_5$W

_____ drip rate needed to administer appropriate dose

Figure 4–16

True or False

95. T   F   The actions of dopamine remain the same regardless of the dose administered.

96. T   F   In the emergency setting, the primary indication for dopamine is bradycardia.

97. T   F   The initial dosage for dopamine varies from 250 to 500 μg/kg/minute.

98. On Figure 4–17, fill in the correct information regarding the preparation and administration of dopamine.

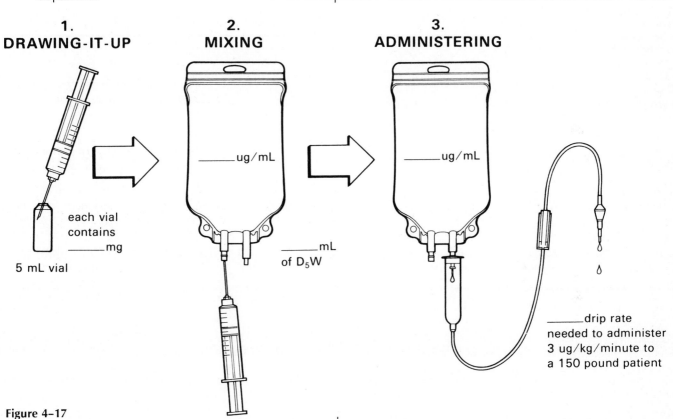

1.
DRAWING-IT-UP

each vial contains _____mg

5 mL vial

2.
MIXING

_____ug/mL

_____mL of D$_5$W

3.
ADMINISTERING

_____ug/mL

_____drip rate needed to administer 3 ug/kg/minute to a 150 pound patient

Figure 4–17

99. Briefly describe why the lowest possible dosage of dopamine is preferred.

_____

_____

_____

_____

100. Match the following dopamine dosage levels with the corresponding effects:

Dosage Level
(μg/kg/minute)

a. 1 to 2
b. 2 to 10
c. more than 10
d. more than 20

Effects

_____ dilates renal and mesenteric vessels

_____ constricts renal and mesenteric vessels

_____ beta stimulation increasing cardiac output

_____ alpha stimulation increasing peripheral resistance

101. List seven side effects of dopamine.

1) _____

2) _____

3) _____

4) _____

5) _____

6) _____

7) _____

Dobutamine

True or False

102.   T   F   Dobutamine is an alpha stimulant.

103.   T   F   Dobutamine increases cardiac output primarily by enhancing myocardial contractility.

104. Dobutamine differs from norepinephrine at usual doses, because dobutamine

a. has little effect on myocardial contractility
b. causes bradycardia
c. may induce peripheral vasodilation
d. causes systemic vasodilation

105. Dobutamine differs from isoproterenol in that dobutamine

a. has little effect on myocardial contractility
b. seldom causes tachycardia
c. produces severe systemic arterial constriction
d. increases end-diastolic volume

True or False

106.   T   F   Dobutamine can be used with sodium nitroprusside to further enhance cardiac output.

107.   T   F   The usual dosage range of dobutamine is from 2.5 to 10 μg/kg/minute.

108.   T   F   Higher doses of dobutamine may cause tachycardia and dysrhythmias.

109. On Figure 4–18, fill in the correct information regarding preparation and administration of dobutamine.

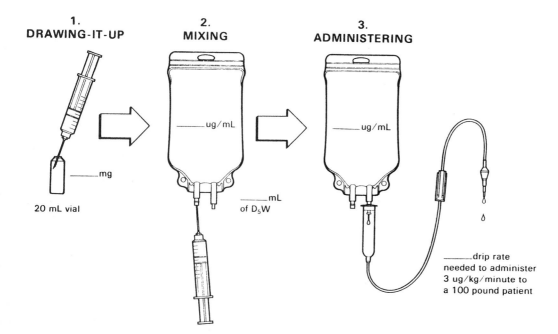

1.
DRAWING-IT-UP

2.
MIXING

3.
ADMINISTERING

_____ ug/mL

_____ ug/mL

_____ mg

20 mL vial

_____ mL
of D$_5$W

_____ drip rate
needed to administer
3 ug/kg/minute to
a 100 pound patient

Figure 4–18

110. Which of the following conditions is dobutamine used to treat?

    a. symptomatic bradycardia due to increased parasympathetic tone

    b. ventricular tachycardia

    c. refractory congestive heart failure due to depressed ventricular function

    d. electromechanical dissociation

Amrinone

True or False

111. T   F   Amrinone is a strong alpha and beta stimulant.

112. T   F   Amrinone acts similarly to dobutamine, increasing cardiac output primarily by enhancing myocardial contractility.

113. T   F   The usual dosage range of amrinone is from 2.5 to 10 μg/kg/minute.

114. T   F   Amrinone may exacerbate myocardial ischemia.

115. T   F   When afterload is increased, the myocardial workload and oxygen consumption are reduced.

116. T   F   Increases in peripheral vascular resistance will increase afterload.

Morphine Sulfate

117. Which of the following are actions of morphine sulfate?

	Answers
1) an analgesic action that reduces pain in myocardial infarction	a. 1 and 2
2) a cardioinhibitory action that slows ventricular impulse conduction	b. 1 and 3
3) a vasodilatory action that increases venous capacitance and decreases preload	c. 2 and 4
4) a vasoconstrictive action that increases afterload and myocardial workload	d. 3 and 4

118. Morphine sulfate reduces myocardial oxygen consumption by

	Answers
1) reducing left ventricular end-diastolic dimensions (preload) and wall stress	a. 1, 2, 3
2) slowing heart rate and myocardial workload	b. 1, 3, 5
3) decreasing myocardial contractility and perfusion pressures	c. 2, 3, 4
4) increasing myocardial contractility and perfusion pressures	d. 2, 4, 5
5) increasing vagal tone at the SA node	

119. Identify two indications for the administration of morphine sulfate.

1) _____

2) _____

120. T   F   The customary dosage for morphine sulfate is 2 to 5 mg IV every 5 to 30 minutes until the desired effects are achieved.

121. List the hemodynamic effects of morphine sulfate.

1) _____

2) _____

3) _____

122. Describe how morphine sulfate may assist in relieving pulmonary congestion.

_____

_____

_____

_____

123. List two side effects of morphine sulfate.

1) _____

2) _____

Nitroglycerin

124. T F Nitroglycerin dilates coronary arteries and systemic veins.

125. Briefly describe the two competing theories for how nitroglycerin relieves angina.

_____

_____

_____

_____

True or False

126. T F Nitroglycerin relieves coronary artery spasm.

127. T F Nitroglycerin is the treatment of choice for ventricular tachycardia.

128. T F Nitroglycerin may be used for reducing pain and myocardial oxygen consumption in acute myocardial infarction.

129. T F Nitroglycerin may produce maldistribution of coronary blood flow and reperfusion dysrhythmias in myocardial infarction patients.

130. T F Following nitroglycerin administration, the patient should be monitored for an excessive drop in blood pressure.

131. T F Initial administration of sublingual nitroglycerin should be at a dose of 0.3 to 0.4 mg.

132. T F Nitroglycerin can also be administered by IV.

133. List two indications for IV administration of nitroglycerin.

_____

_____

_____

134. Describe the initial IV dosage for nitroglycerin.

_____

_____

_____

_____

135. Identify the most common side effects of nitroglycerin.

1) _____

2) _____

Sodium Nitroprusside

True or False

136. T F Sodium nitroprusside constricts systemic arteries and veins.

137. T F The effects of IV sodium nitroprusside persist for about 30 minutes following cessation of its administration.

138. T F Sodium nitroprusside usually does NOT cause a reflex mediated increase in heart rate.

139. Briefly describe the effects of sodium nitroprusside on pump failure associated with myocardial infarction.

_____

_____

_____

_____

_____

140. For which of the following conditions is sodium nitroprusside the treatment of choice?

1. pump failure in MI   *Answers*
2. hypertensive crisis   a. 1, 2, 5
3. angina pectoris   b. 2 and 3 only
4. symptomatic bradycardia   c. 2, 3, 4
5. CHF refractory to   d. 3, 4, 5
   diuretics

True or False

141. T   F   Since sodium nitroprusside is a potent, rapid-acting direct peripheral vasodilator, its use is recommended when immediate reduction in peripheral arterial resistance is necessary.

142. T   F   Heart rate increases following sodium nitroprusside suggest either hypotension or inadequate left ventricular filling pressure.

143. T   F   Sodium nitroprusside may be more effective in combination with other agents than when it is utilized alone.

144. T   F   Once sodium nitroprusside is prepared, it can be refrigerated or used for several days without ill effects.

145. T   F   Sodium nitroprusside should NOT be diluted with solutions other than dextrose in water.

146. On Figure 4–19, fill in the correct information regarding the preparation and administration of sodium nitroprusside.

True or False

147. T   F   The average initial dose of sodium nitroprusside ranges from 0.5 to 8.0 μg/kg/minute.

148. T   F   Sodium nitroprusside levels may become toxic at dosages at or above 0.5 mg/kg/hour.

149. T   F   Hemodynamic monitoring during sodium nitroprusside administration is mandatory in the treatment of patients with heart failure who have ischemic heart disease.

Furosemide

150. T   F   Circulatory overload may increase cardiac preload as well as afterload.

151. T   F   Furosemide is a potent vasoconstrictor.

152. T   F   In emergency cardiac care, furosemide is the treatment of choice for acute myocardial infarction.

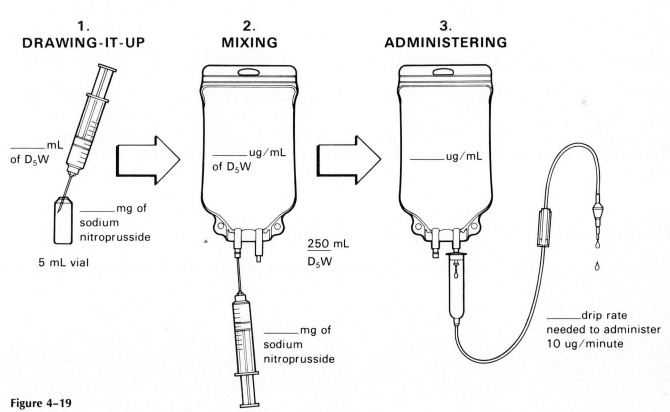

1.
DRAWING-IT-UP

_____mL of D₅W

_____mg of sodium nitroprusside

5 mL vial

2.
MIXING

_____ug/mL of D₅W

$\dfrac{250 \text{ mL}}{D_5W}$

_____mg of sodium nitroprusside

3.
ADMINISTERING

_____ug/mL

_____drip rate needed to administer 10 ug/minute

Figure 4–19

153. T   F   Furosemide works by inhibiting reabsorption of sodium in the proximal and distal tubules in the loop of Henle.

154. T   F   The onset of diuresis after IV administration of furosemide occurs after 30 minutes, peaks at 1 hour, and lasts 4 hours.

155. T   F   In addition to its diuretic effect, furosemide may reduce pulmonary edema by reducing preload through venous dilation.

156. T   F   The initial dosage for furosemide is 5.0 mg, slow IV push.

157. List six side effects of furosemide.

1) _____

2) _____

3) _____

4) _____

5) _____

6) _____

158. Describe how changes in automaticity may lead to dysrhythmias.

_____

_____

_____

_____

_____

_____

_____

_____

159. Explain the reentry mechanism in the genesis of dysrhythmias.

_____

_____

_____

_____

_____

_____

_____

_____

_____

True or False

160. T   F   A discrepancy in conduction times between normal and injured areas of the myocardium makes the heart prone to reentrant dysrhythmias.

161. T   F   Ischemic heart muscle has faster conduction than normal tissue.

162. Describe the mechanisms by which medications can control dysrhythmias due to increased automaticity and reentry.

_____

_____

_____

_____

_____

_____

_____

_____

Lidocaine

True or False

163. T   F   Lidocaine is used to treat dysrhythmias that originate from the ventricles.

164. T   F   Lidocaine enhances conduction velocity, decreases the effective refractory period, and increases the degree of dispersion of recovery in the ventricles.

165. T   F   Lidocaine is indicated for ventricular tachycardia, ventricular fibrillation, PVCs, and suspected myocardial ischemia.

166. T   F   The initial IV push dosage for lidocaine is 1 mEq/kg.

167. T   F   In doses applied clinically, lidocaine has little effect on myocardial contractility or ventricular conduction velocity.

168. For the dysrhythmias in Figures 4–20, 4–21, and 4–22, describe the changes you would expect following lidocaine administration and the action(s) of lidocaine responsible for the change(s).

_____

_____

_____

_____

_____

_____

_____

_____

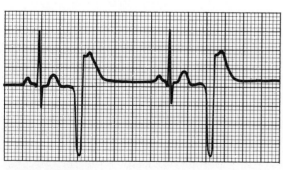

a. **Figure 4–20**

Changes _____ *Actions* _____

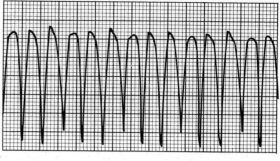

b. **Figure 4–21**

Changes _____ *Actions* _____

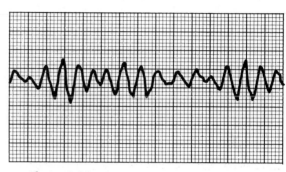

c. **Figure 4–22**

Changes _____ *Actions* _____

169. If a 10-ml syringe contains 100 mg of lidocaine, _____ mL would need to be administered to give a dose of 75 mg.

170. Calculate the correct lidocaine dosage for each of the following patient weights:

Body Weight (lb)	Lidocaine Dose
90	_____
168	_____
300	_____

171. Describe the preferred method for administering the loading and maintenance doses of lidocaine.

_____

_____

_____

_____

_____

_____

172. If 1 gm of lidocaine is added to 250 ml of D_5W and delivered with a microdrip set (60 drops/ml), the patient would receive a dose of 2 mg per minute when the infusion rate was _____ drops per minute.

173. When should prophylactic lidocaine be administered?

_____

_____

_____

_____

_____

174. Describe what action should be taken if ventricular ectopy persists following initial IV bolus and infusion administration of lidocaine.

_____

_____

_____

_____

_____

175. T   F   Signs of lidocaine toxicity include disorientation, impaired hearing, paresthesia, and muscle twitching.

176. How should seizures associated with lidocaine therapy be treated?

_____

_____

_____

True or False

177. T   F   Unless it is followed by a continuous IV infusion of lidocaine, a single 100-mg bolus of lidocaine will fall to subtherapeutic blood levels within about 45 minutes.

178. T   F   Lidocaine has different actions in acutely infarcted and normal zones of the myocardium.

179. T   F   Lidocaine suppresses reentry dysrhythmias by further depressing conduction in injured myocardium so impulses cannot conduct to adjacent normal tissue.

180. T   F   Lidocaine toxicity is usually manifested in the respiratory system.

181. T   F   When treating cardiac arrest, additional 0.5-mg/kg boluses can be given every 8 to 10 minutes after an initial 1-mg/kg bolus if necessary to a total of 3 mg/kg.

182. T   F   Since lidocaine is degraded by the liver and excreted by the kidneys, the lidocaine dosage should be reduced whenever hepatic, cardiac, or renal function is diminished.

183. T   F   In cases of heart failure or shock, lidocaine toxicity may develop after relatively short periods of time.

184. T   F   Lidocaine should never be used in the presence of cardiac conduction disturbances.

185. T   F   Lidocaine may be administered endotracheally.

186. Which of the following medications can be used to treat PVCs refractory to lidocaine?

a. atropine or isoproterenol
b. calcium chloride or sodium bicarbonate
c. procainamide or bretylium
d. morphine sulfate or furosemide

Procainamide

187. T   F   Procainamide reduces automaticity by suppressing phase 4 diastolic depolarization.

188. T   F   Procainamide slows conduction velocity and produces a bidirectional block that terminates reentry mechanisms.

189. T   F   Procainamide is indicated for persistent ventricular fibrillation.

190. T   F   Procainamide increases ion flow through myocardial membranes and subsequently increases automaticity in these cells.

191. Briefly explain how procainamide affects the action potential and speed of impulse conduction.

_____

_____

_____

_____

True or False

192. T   F   Procainamide increases threshold potential.

193. T   F   Procainamide has a secondary anticholinergic action that allows the sympathetic nervous system to accelerate impulse formation and conduction.

194. T   F   Procainamide inhibits transportation of calcium ions across the cell membrane, thereby reducing myocardial contractility.

195. List the four indicators for the termination of procainamide therapy.

1) _____

2) _____

3) _____

4) _____

196. On the syringe in Figure 4–23, shade in the correct area to indicate the maximum amount that should be administered in 5 minutes from a 10-ml vial containing 1000 mg.

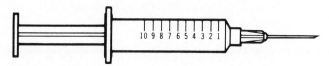

Figure 4–23

197. What infusion rate would need to be used to deliver a 2 mg/minute dose of procainamide if 1 gm is added to 250 ml of D_5W and a microdrip administration set (60 drops/ml) is attached?

_____

Bretylium (Bretylium tosylate)

True or False

198. T   F   Bretylium has postganglionic adrenergic blocking properties, antidysrhythmic effects, and a positive inotropic action.

199. T   F   The initial actions of bretylium (increased arterial pressure and heart rate) are mediated by a bretylium-provoked catecholamine release.

200. T   F   A decline in arterial pressure following bretylium administration is due to the adrenergic blocking action of bretylium.

201. T   F   The antidysrhythmic action of bretylium is due to its effect on adrenergic nerve terminals.

202. T   F   Bretylium works by prolonging the action potential throughout the entire conduction system without affecting the infarcted areas; because all areas have slower conduction, reentry is less likely.

203. T   F   Indications for bretylium therapy include ventricular fibrillation, PVCs, and ventricular tachycardia that is refractory to other treatments.

204. T   F   In ventricular fibrillation refractory to countershock and lidocaine, bretylium may be administered in a dosage of 10-mg/kg bolus repeated at 5 minute intervals up to 30 mg/kg.

205. Specify two side effects of bretylium:

1) _____

2) _____

206. T   F   Bretylium lowers the fibrillation threshold.

207. On the prefilled syringe in Figure 4–24, shade in the area that denotes the amount of bretylium that should be given to deliver 350 mg from an ampule containing 500 mg/10 ml.

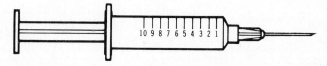

Figure 4–24

208. Calculate the correct initial and repeat dosages for each of the following patient weights:

Weight (lb)	Initial Dose	Repeat Dose
85	_____	_____
205	_____	_____
330	_____	_____

Propranolol

209. Which of the following describes the actions of propranolol?

    a. stimulates alpha receptors

    b. stimulates the parasympathetic nervous system

    c. blocks the vagus nerve

    d. blocks beta receptors

210. Briefly describe the effects of propranolol on the:

    a. SA node _____

    _____

    b. AV junction _____

    _____

    c. contractility of the heart _____

    _____

True or False

211. T   F   The effectiveness of propranolol depends on the existing degree of sympathetic stimulation.

212. T   F   When the sympathetic nervous system is functioning as a compensatory mechanism (i.e., for heart failure), use of propranolol is contraindicated as it may result in acute cardiac decompensation.

213. T   F   Propranolol can be safely used in patients who are subject to bronchospasm.

214. T   F   An appropriate IV dosage for propranolol is 1 to 3 mg repeated every 5 minutes, not to exceed a total dose of 0.1 mg/kg.

215. For which types of patients should propranolol be used with caution?

_____

_____

_____

_____

216. What two medications should be used if significant bradycardia occurs following propranolol administration?

    1) _____

    2) _____

217. T   F   If significant bronchospasm occurs following propranolol administration, isoproterenol or aminophylline should be used to provide bronchodilation.

218. Propranolol may be useful in the treatment of:

    a. atrial fibrillation with a ventricular rate > 80 per minute

    b. congestive heart failure

    c. recurrent episodes of supraventricular tachydysrhythmias

    d. third-degree AV block

    e. asystole

Verapamil

219. Which of the following are true statements about "fast response" cardiac fibers?

    1) They depend on sodium ion influx for depolarization.

    2) They are characterized by a slow-rising phase O depolarization.

    3) They are found in myocardial cells specialized for contraction.

    4) They are responsible for initiation of the cardiac impulse.

    5) They can be stimulated during their relative refractory period.

Answers

    a. 1, 2, 3

    b. 1, 2, 5

    c. 2, 3, 4

    d. 2, 4, 5

220. Which of the following are true statements about "slow response" cardiac fibers?

1) They depend on influx of calcium ions for depolarization.

Answers

2) They are characterized by a slow-rising phase O depolarization.

a. 1, 2, 5

3) They are found in tissues of the SA node and AV junction.

b. 1, 2, 4

4) They are responsible for initiation of impulses that stimulate the myocardium.

c. 2, 3, 4

5) They depend on the efflux of sodium ions for depolarization.

d. all except 5

True or False

221. T   F   Stimulation of fast-responsive fibers during their relative refractory period may result in ectopic impulses and tachydysrhythmias.

222. T   F   Verapamil eliminates abnormal slow responses by increasing the flow of ions through the cell membrane.

223. Match the following actions of verapamil with their respective effect:

Action

_____ prolongs relative refractory period of the AV junction

_____ causes vasodilation of the peripheral vascular beds and decreased blood pressure

_____ decreases peripheral resistance

_____ relaxes coronary vasculature

_____ decreases myocardial contractility

Effect

a. increases myocardial oxygen supply
b. slows AV conduction
c. decreases myocardial work and oxygen consumption
d. improves ventricular performance and cardiac output
e. counteracted by improved ventricular performance

True or False

224. T   F   Verapamil relaxes coronary and peripheral vascular smooth muscle by increasing inward movement of sodium across the cardiac cell membrane.

225. T   F   Indications for the use of verapamil include atrial fibrillation, atrial flutter, paroxysmal supraventricular tachycardias, and chronic angina.

226. T   F   Hypotension that occurs as a result of verapamil administration can be reversed by the administration of 0.5 to 1.0 gm of IV calcium chloride.

227. Specify the initial and repeat dosage ranges of verapamil for an adult.

_____

_____

_____

_____

_____

228. List three precautions for verapamil administration.

1) _____

2) _____

3) _____

229. Match the following medications with the conditions they may be used to treat. (More than one answer may be correct.)

Medication

a. atropine
b. dopamine
c. oxygen
d. sodium bicarbonate (when considered for use)
e. epinephrine
f. lidocaine
g. bretylium
h. morphine sulfate
i. verapamil
j. procainamide
k. furosemide
l. isoproterenol

Condition

_____ ventricular fibrillation

_____ acute pulmonary edema

_____ symptomatic bradycardia

_____ asystole

_____ PVCs

_____ chest pain with acute MI

_____ electromechanical dissociation

_____ metabolic acidosis

_____ hypoxia

_____ PVCs refractory to lidocaine

_____ supraventricular tachycardia, atrial fibrillation or flutter, chronic angina

_____ cardiogenic shock

230. Match the following medications with their respective effects.

Medication

a. furosemide
b. sodium nitroprusside
c. nitroglycerin
d. propranolol
e. amrinone
f. dobutamine
g. isoproterenol
h. dopamine
i. norepinephrine

Effects

_____ in low doses, dilates renal and mesenteric blood vessels

_____ a pure beta receptor stimulator

_____ dilates coronary vessels directly and relaxes peripheral blood vessels

_____ a beta receptor blocker

_____ a potent peripheral vasoconstrictor that causes mesenteric vasoconstriction

_____ a beta stimulator that seldom causes arterial constriction or tachycardia

_____ a potent diuretic

_____ a nonadrenergic cardiotonic agent

231. Match the following medications with the conditions they are used to treat. (Each medication is used only once.)

Medication

a. furosemide
b. sodium nitroprusside
c. nitroglycerin
d. propranolol
e. morphine sulfate
f. dobutamine
g. isoproterenol
h. dopamine
i. norepinephrine

Condition

_____ refractory congestive heart failure due to depressed ventricular function and contractility

_____ hemodynamically significant bradycardia that is refractory to atropine

_____ symptomatic hypotension due to cardiogenic shock or low peripheral resistance

_____ hemodynamically significant hypotension

_____ cerebral edema after cardiac arrest and acute pulmonary edema

_____ hypertensive crisis or for immediate reduction of peripheral vascular resistance

_____ angina and some cases of myocardial infarction

_____ acute myocardial infarction and acute pulmonary edema

232. Fill in the initial dosage for each of the following medications.

Medication

furosemide _____

sodium nitroprusside _____

nitroglycerin (sublingual) _____

propranolol _____

dobutamine _____

isoproterenol _____

dopamine _____

norepinephrine _____

233. For each of the medications in Table 4–1, indicate the effect it has on the clinical parameters listed. Use an up arrow (↑) to denote that the medication increases the parameter, a down arrow (↓) to denote that the medication decreases the parameter, and a horizontal line (↔) to denote that the medication has no effect on the parameter.

TABLE 4–1

	Afterload	Preload	MVO$_2$	Contractility	Heart Rate
Morphine sulfate					
Nitroglycerin					
Furosemide					
Sodium nitroprusside					
Isoproterenol					
Norepinephrine					
Dopamine					
Dobutamine					
Propranolol					

234. Mark an × to indicate which medications in Table 4–2 would be used to treat the indicated conditions.

TABLE 4–2

	Angina	Myocardial infarction	Acute pulmonary edema	Congestive heart failure	Refractory CHF	Hypertensive crisis	Cardiogenic shock	Bradycardia	Premature ventricular complexes (PVCs)	Ventricular tachycardia	Ventricular fibrillation	Rapid supraventricular tachycardia	Asystole	Electromechanical dissociation (EMD)
Atropine														
Isoproterenol														
Oxygen														
Morphine sulfate														
Nitroglycerin														
Furosemide														
Sodium nitroprusside														
Norepinephrine														
Dopamine														
Dobutamine														
Lidocaine														
Bretylium														
Procainamide														
Propranolol														
Verapamil														
Epinephrine														

ANSWER KEY

1. b, c, d

2. Factors contributing to severe hypoxia in cardiac arrest include (1) even when CPR is properly performed, cardiac output is only 25% to 30% of normal; (2) right-to-left shunting (severely desaturated blood mixing with nonshunted blood); (3) ventilation–perfusion mismatching in lungs. See Figure 4–25.

PULMONARY ARTERIOLE

BLOOD VESSEL DOES NOT PERFUSE VENTILATED ALVEOLI, OXYGEN CANNOT DIFFUSE INTO BLOOD STREAM

BRONCHIOLE

AIR

ALVEOLI PULMONARY CAPILLARIES

COLLAPSED ALVEOLI

PULMONARY VENULE

ALVEOLI ARE NOT VENTILATED, SUBSEQUENTLY THE BLOODSTREAM ISN'T OXYGENATED.

Figure 4–25

3. Figure 4–26 describes the effects of oxygen administration in the hypoxemic patient.

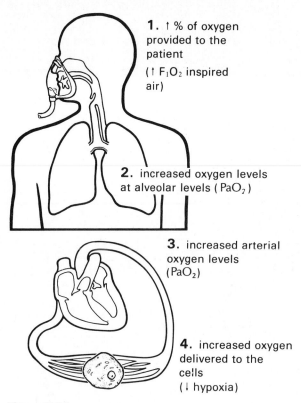

1. ↑ % of oxygen provided to the patient (↑ F_IO_2 inspired air)

2. increased oxygen levels at alveolar levels (PaO_2)

3. increased arterial oxygen levels (PaO_2)

4. increased oxygen delivered to the cells (↓ hypoxia)

Figure 4–26

4. Oxygen should be administered (1) for myocardial ischemia and/or infarction, (2) in all cases of cardiopulmonary arrest, and (3) in the presence of suspected hypoxemia of any cause.

5. FALSE: During CPR, oxygen toxicity should not be a concern; cardiac arrest always requires oxygen therapy.

6. TRUE: Oxygen administration in the acute myocardial infarction may reduce or eliminate ischemic zones surrounding the infarction.

7. TRUE: Acidosis affects the myocardium by decreasing contractility and lowering the fibrillation threshold.

8. FALSE: Sodium bicarbonate is no longer considered a first-line treatment in cardiac arrest. Sodium bicarbonate administration should be reserved until after other "more proven" treatments have been employed.

9. FALSE: The accumulation of CO_2 contributes to the formation of carbonic acid (H_2CO_3). An increase in H_2CO_3 will move the pH downward (toward acidosis) by decreasing the ratio of weak acids (H_2CO_3) to bicarbonate ($NaHCO_3$); see Figure 5–11. Improved alveolar ventilation is the most effective treatment for respiratory acidosis because this will rid the body of excess carbon dioxide (CO_2).

10. FALSE: It appears that sodium bicarbonate does not improve the ability to defibrillate or improve survival rates.

11. TRUE: Persistent ventilatory insufficiency contributes to refractory acidosis by increasing the PaCO$_2$ (and subsequently increasing the H$_2$CO$_3$) and creating hypoxemia, which will eventually result in hypoxia-induced anaerobic metabolism and metabolic acidosis. This emphasizes the critical need for maintaining a patent airway and alveolar hyperventilation, and administering 100% oxygen in the management of cardiac arrest.

12. TRUE: Carbon dioxide is freely diffusible across cellular and organ membranes (i.e., the heart and brain) and may readily contribute to intracellular acidosis. As a result, function of these organs may be depressed, particularly in ischemic myocardium.

13. TRUE: Hyperventilation will blow off CO$_2$, which may be contributing to acidosis.

14. TRUE: Although alveolar hyperventilation will not correct metabolic acidosis, it may prevent the pH from falling to more critical levels.

15. Potential hazards of NaHCO$_3$ include (1) sodium and water overload, (2) hypernatremia, (3) hyperosmolality, (4) metabolic alkalosis, (5) hypoxia secondary to a shift in the oxyhemoglobin saturation curve (oxygen release is inhibited), (6) paradoxical acidosis due to the production of carbon dioxide, (7) exacerbation of central venous acidosis, and (8) inactivation of simultaneously administered catecholamines (thus it is best to avoid mixing any medication with NaHCO$_3$).

16. Excessive amounts of NaHCO$_3$ result in alkalosis and cause a leftward displacement of the oxyhemoglobin curve, with consequent impairment in oxygen release from hemoglobin to the tissues. Hemoglobin can be thought of as an oxygen magnet that becomes stronger during alkalosis and weaker in acidosis. Unless hemoglobin releases the oxygen it carries, the tissues will become hypoxic. See Figure 4–27.

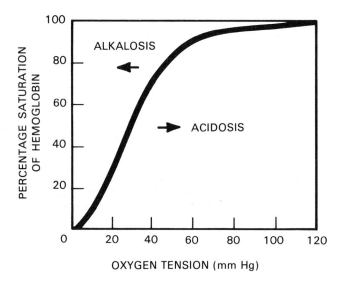

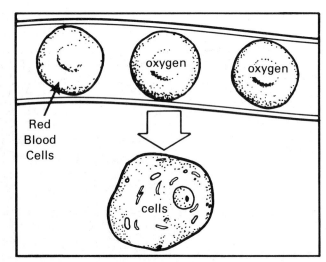

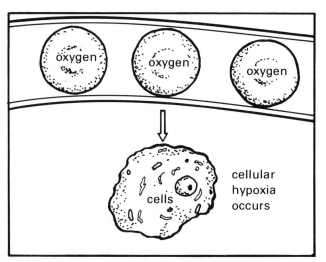

1. DURING ACIDOSIS

More oxygen is released from the hemoglobin of the red blood cells to the tissues

2. DURING ALKALOSIS

Less oxygen is released from the hemoglobin of the red blood cells to the tissues

Figure 4–27

17. When administered in cardiac arrest, the initial dosage for a 150-lb victim is shown in Figure 4–28.

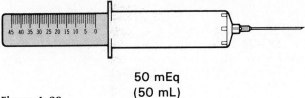

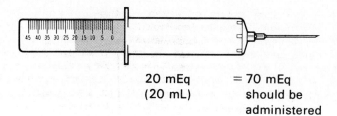

Figure 4–28

50 mEq
(50 mL)

20 mEq
(20 mL)

= 70 mEq
should be
administered

18. When administered in cardiac arrest, the amount of $NaHCO_3$ that should be administered to the 150-lb patient 10 minutes after the initial dose is shown in Figure 4–29.

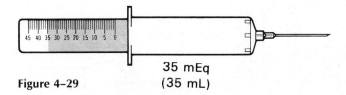

Figure 4–29

35 mEq
(35 mL)

19. Medications that enhance cardiac electrical or mechanical activity do so by accelerating the opening of channels that control ion flux into the cell. By increasing the slow inward calcium current, catecholamines increase the slope of phase 4 depolarization in the SA node and subsequently increase heart rate. Catecholamines also accelerate AV conduction by increasing the slope and amplitude of action potential in the AV junction. The increased number of calcium ions entering the cell during the plateau phase enhances myocardial contractility.

20. TRUE: The parasympathetic nervous system can be thought of as the "brake," while the sympathetic nervous system can be thought of as the "accelerator." When the parasympathetic nervous system is stimulated, the heart rate is slowed. Bradycardia may cause decreased cardiac output as the heart is not contracting at a fast enough pace per minute.

21. TRUE: Hypotension can result when the heart rate is too slow.

22. TRUE: Medications that increase the heart rate may be used to treat hemodynamically compromising bradycardia.

23. TRUE: There is no more significant bradycardia than ventricular standstill (asystole).

24. FALSE: Atropine speeds the heart rate and impulse conduction by blocking the parasympathetic nervous system (vagus nerve) at the SA node and AV junction. This action allows the heart to initiate and conduct impulses at an intrinsic rate. See Figure 4–30.

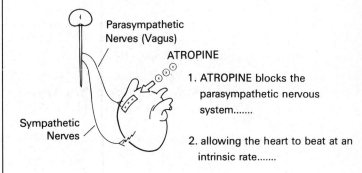

Parasympathetic
Nerves (Vagus)

ATROPINE

1. ATROPINE blocks the parasympathetic nervous system.......

Sympathetic
Nerves

2. allowing the heart to beat at an intrinsic rate.......

3. or allowing the sympathetic nervous system to accelerate the heart rate

Figure 4–30

25. FALSE: Atropine may be of value in high-degree AV block, but is only given for bradycardia that is hemodynamically significant (e.g., hypotension), impairs coronary perfusion, or is associated with frequent PVCs.

26. TRUE: In cases where hypotension is accompanied by bradycardia, the heart rate should be increased; the medication of choice for this is atropine.

27. FALSE: Atropine does not affect acetylcholine release. Atropine works by occupying acetylcholine receptor sites of the effector organs such as the heart; with atropine in its receptor sites, acetylcholine is unable to affect the heart. See Figure 4–31.

PRESYNAPTIC
NEURON

1. Under normal conditions acetylcholine is released from the presynaptic neuron, it travels to the heart and activates receptors causing the heart rate to slow, etc.

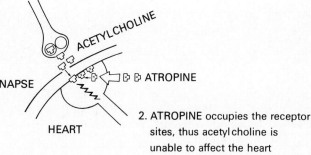

ACETYLCHOLINE

SYNAPSE

ATROPINE

HEART

2. ATROPINE occupies the receptor sites, thus acetylcholine is unable to affect the heart

Figure 4–31

28. TRUE: Atropine should not be administered in doses of less than 0.5 mg as it may actually slow the heart rate.

29. TRUE: Since heart rate is a major determinate of MVO$_2$ (myocardial oxygen consumption), an increase in the heart rate following atropine administration may result in a subsequent extension of myocardial ischemia.

30. FALSE: In bradycardia, atropine is administered in 0.5 to 1.0-mg doses every 5 minutes to a total of 2.0 mg. In asystole, atropine is administered in 1.0-mg doses every 5 minutes to a total of 2.0 mg.

31. Atropine's vagolytic action on the conduction system of the heart results in (1) accelerated rate of discharge of the SA node and (2) improved AV conduction.

32. Atropine may be used in asystole because, in some cases, severe vagal overtone may be the cause of cardiac arrest. Atropine can block this vagal tone and allow the sympathetic nervous system to resume spontaneous cardiac electrical activity.

33. Results of atropine administration: **a.** Sinus bradycardia, conversion to sinus rhythm due to blockage of vagal tone at SA node. **b.** Second-degree AV block, sinus without AV block due to diminished vagal tone at the SA node and AV junction causing an indirect increase in SA automaticity and AV conduction speed. (Figure 4–32). **c.** Asystole, initiation of spontaneous rhythm due to vagal blockade, which allows the SA node to resume normal pacemaking activity (Figure 4–33).

34. Figure 4–34 indicates the initial dosage range of atropine for a patient with hemodynamically compromising bradycardia (syringe contains 1.0 mg/10 ml): 5 to 10 ml; usual dose is 0.5 mg or 5.0 ml.

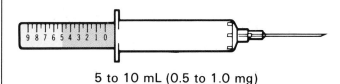

**5 to 10 mL (0.5 to 1.0 mg)
should be administered**

Figure 4–34

35. Figure 4–35 indicates the repeat dosage of atropine for a patient with hemodynamically compromising bradycardia: 5 to 10 ml; maximum of 2.0 mg.

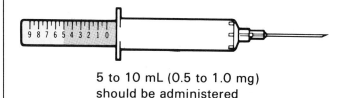

**5 to 10 mL (0.5 to 1.0 mg)
should be administered**

Figure 4–35

36. TRUE: The dosage for atropine in asystole is 1 mg. It can be repeated in 5 minutes to a total of 2.0 mg.

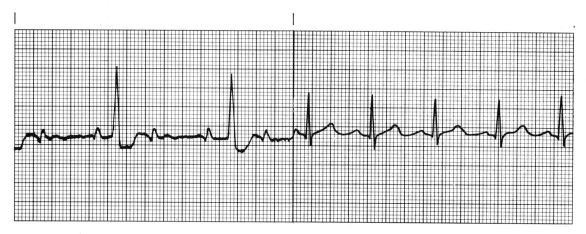

b. **Figure 4–32**

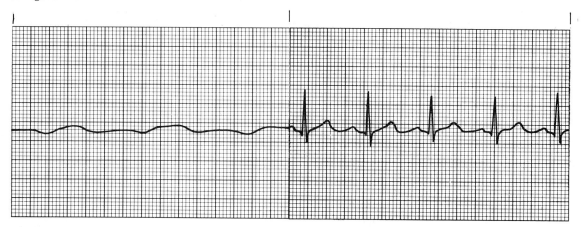

c. **Figure 4–33**

37. TRUE: Atropine can be administered via endotracheal tube.

38. FALSE: Isoproterenol is a nearly pure beta receptor stimulator.

39. FALSE: Isoproterenol increases the heart rate and the force of myocardial contraction and decreases preload by peripheral vasodilation. See Figure 4–36.

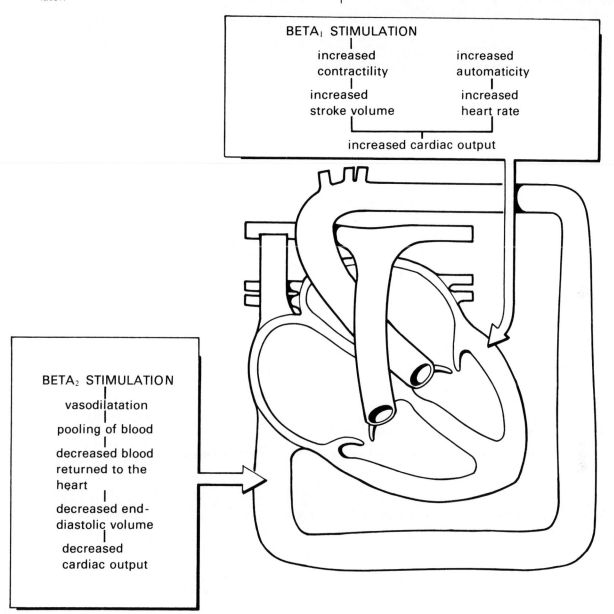

BETA₁ STIMULATION

increased contractility — increased stroke volume

increased automaticity — increased heart rate

increased cardiac output

BETA₂ STIMULATION

vasodilatation — pooling of blood — decreased blood returned to the heart — decreased end-diastolic volume — decreased cardiac output

Figure 4–36

40. Isoproterenol infusion: 1 mg diluted in 500 ml of 5% dextrose in water, producing a concentration of 2 μg/ml; recommended infusion rate is 2 to 10 μg/minute titrated to the desired heart rate and rhythm response.

41. TRUE: Because of its beta stimulating properties, isoproterenol may cause an increase in MVO_2, which may lead to exacerbation of ischemia (increase the extent of ischemia and infarction) and arrhythmias in patients with ischemic heart disease. Thus it has limited use in myocardial infarction (MI). See Figure 4–37.

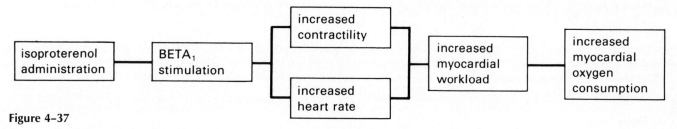

isoproterenol administration → BETA₁ stimulation → increased contractility / increased heart rate → increased myocardial workload → increased myocardial oxygen consumption

Figure 4–37

42. FALSE: Isoproterenol is a pure beta stimulator. Stimulation of beta 2 receptors on peripheral blood vessels has a vasodilatory effect, which reduces peripheral resistance and arterial blood pressure. Because beta 1 stimulation causes increased contractility and increased heart rate, cardiac output is not adversely affected. See Figure 4–38.

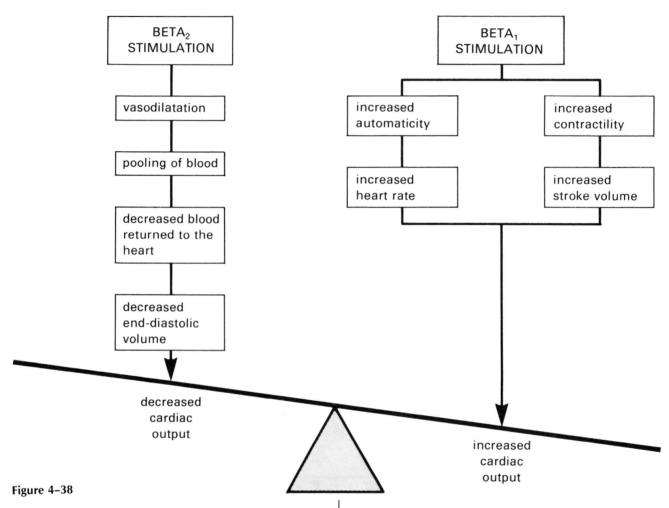

Figure 4–38

43. TRUE: Isoproterenol increases cardiac output by increasing the heart rate and strength of myocardial contraction.

44. TRUE: If atropine does not resolve bradycardia in a patient with a pulse, isoproterenol may be temporarily employed until a pacemaker is available.

45. FALSE: Isoproterenol is no longer recommended for asystole or EMD.

46. TRUE: The dosage for isoproterenol is 2 to 10 μg/minute continuous IV infusion.

47. TRUE: Electrical pacing is preferred over isoproterenol. Isoproterenol is considered to be a "temporary measure."

48. FALSE: When administering isoproterenol, the desired heart rate is approximately 60 per minute.

49. Results of isoproterenol administration: **a.** Third-degree AV block to second/first-degree AV block, possibly sinus rhythm due to beta 1 stimulation and enhanced automaticity and conductivity at SA node and AV junction.

50. One of the side effects of isoproterenol is increased ventricular ectopic automaticity, which may precipitate ventricular tachycardia or fibrillation. Any sign of ventricular ectopic activity, therefore, should prompt the reduction or termination of isoproterenol administration.

51. TRUE: In ventricular fibrillation, some medications (particularly epinephrine) may help improve cardiac output and subsequently increase the chance for successful resuscitation.

52. TRUE: In asystole there is total absence of ventricular electrical and mechanical activity. Medications such as epinephrine and atropine are given to improve cardiac output and initiate an effective spontaneous electromechanical rhythm.

53. FALSE: There is no cardiac output in EMD.

54. TRUE: In EMD there is coordinated electrical activity, but no mechanical response.

55. TRUE: Epinephrine is given to improve cardiac output, increase peripheral vascular resistance, and increase myocardial contractility. If bradycardia (relative or absolute) is seen with EMD, attempts to increase the heart rate are appropriate.

56. FALSE: Presently, epinephrine is considered an acceptable treatment modality in EMD, whereas calcium chloride and isoproterenol are not.

57. FALSE: Epinephrine increases both compression perfusion and spontaneous cardiac compressions.

58. TRUE: Epinephrine has both alpha 1 (increased systemic vascular resistance, increased arterial pressure) and beta 1 (increased heart rate, increased myocardial contractile force, increased myocardial oxygen requirements MVO$_2$, increased automaticity and speed of conduction) stimulating properties. See Figure 4–39.

59. TRUE: Its vasoconstrictor action increases the perfusion pressure generated during cardiac compression to better perfuse vital organs such as the heart, brain, and kidneys.

60. TRUE: Epinephrine can be effectively and efficiently administered endotracheally.

61. TRUE: When delivering epinephrine endotracheally, the full 1-mg dose (10 ml) must be administered to achieve an equivalent pressor response as lesser doses of epinephrine administered intravenously.

62. TRUE: Although it is true that epinephrine may not function effectively in an acidotic medium, the pH must be below 7.1 before epinephrine is rendered ineffective.

63. FALSE: In the doses used during cardiac arrest, epinephrine will cause coronary vasodilation.

64. TRUE: The repeat time for epinephrine administration during cardiac arrest is 5 minutes.

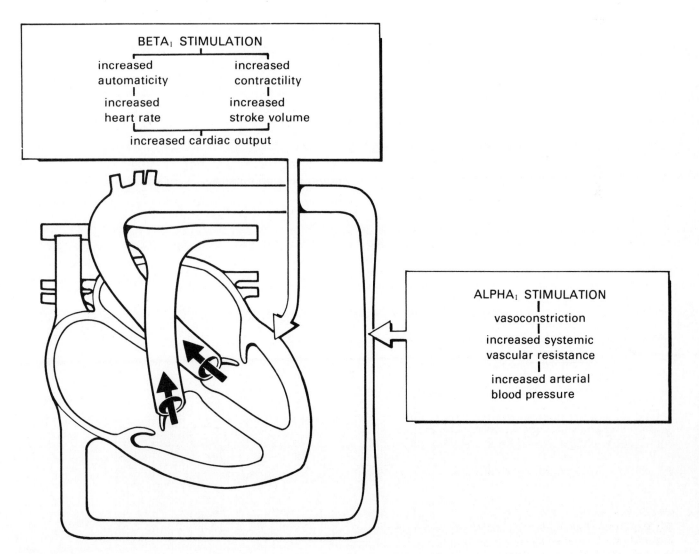

Figure 4–39

65. TRUE: Although it is not considered a first-line agent, epinephrine can be used as a pressor agent via continuous infusion.

66. Epinephrine may be used to treat (1) ventricular fibrillation, (2) ventricular standstill (asystole), (3) pulseless idioventricular rhythm and other forms of EMD, and (4) hypotension secondary to pump failure.

67. Epinephrine is given before $NaHCO_3$ in cardiac arrest because (1) restoration of spontaneous circulation (with epinephrine) is necessary for accurate correction of acidosis; (2) if bicarbonate were given first, a time delay would occur before epinephrine could be administered because the IV tubing would need to be flushed; (3) since epinephrine can be administered endotracheally, there is no need to wait for an IV line to be established before its administration; and (4) epinephrine is considered a first-line treatment modality for cardiac arrest, whereas sodium bicarbonate is not.

68. Figure 4–40 indicates the initial dosage range of epinephrine for a cardiac arrest victim (each syringe contains 10 ml of 1:10,000 solution or 0.1 mg/ml): 5 to 10 ml (0.5 to 1.0 mg).

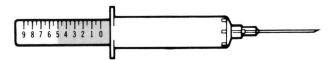

5 to 10 mL (0.5 to 1.0 mg)
should be administered   **Figure 4–40**

69. Figure 4–41 indicates the repeat dosage range of epinephrine: 5 to 10 ml (0.5 to 1.0 mg).

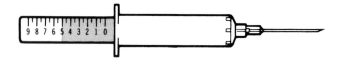

5 to 10 mL (0.5 to 1.0 mg)
should be administered   **Figure 4–41**

70. Results of epinephrine administration: **a.** Asystole, initiation of a spontaneous rhythm due to increased automaticity (Figure 4–42). **b.** Fine ventricular fibrillation, conversion to coarse ventricular fibrillation due to increased automaticity (Figure 4–43). **c.** Sinus rhythm with electromechanical dissociation (EMD), sinus rhythm with palpable pulses due to increased contractility and arterial blood pressure (Figure 4–44). **d.** Idioventricular rhythm with EMD, junctional or sinus rhythm with palpable pulses due to stimulation of automaticity of higher pacemakers (Figure 4–45). **e.** Sinus bradycardia, sinus rhythm due to enhanced automaticity at the SA node.

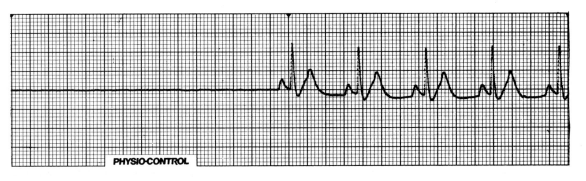

a. **Figure 4–42**

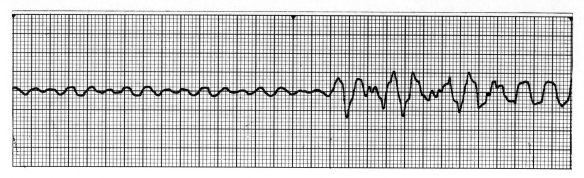

b. **Figure 4-43**

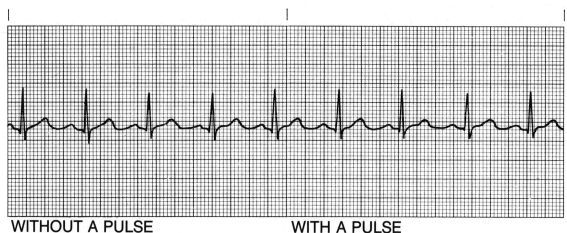

WITHOUT A PULSE   WITH A PULSE

c. **Figure 4-44**

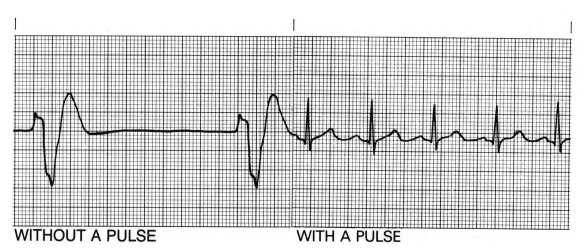

WITHOUT A PULSE   WITH A PULSE

d. **Figure 4-45**

71. Epinephrine can be administered via IV infusion by adding 1 mg to 250 ml of 5% dextrose in water. Start at 1 μg/minute and titrate to effect.

72. TRUE: Hemodynamically significant hypotension may be defined as a systolic blood pressure of less than 90 mm of Hg with accompanying signs of inadequate perfusion.

73. TRUE: The danger of hypotension is that perfusion to the vital organs may be significantly decreased.

74. TRUE: Hypotension can result from diminished stroke volume as seen with depressed ventricular function secondary to severe acute myocardial infarction.

75. FALSE: Inotropic agents (e.g., dobutamine) may be useful in the treatment of hypotension that is caused by depression of the left ventricular function.

76. TRUE: Inappropriate systemic vascular resistance can cause hypotension.

77. FALSE: Norepinephrine has both alpha and beta stimulating properties.

78. a, b, d, e (see Figure 4–46).

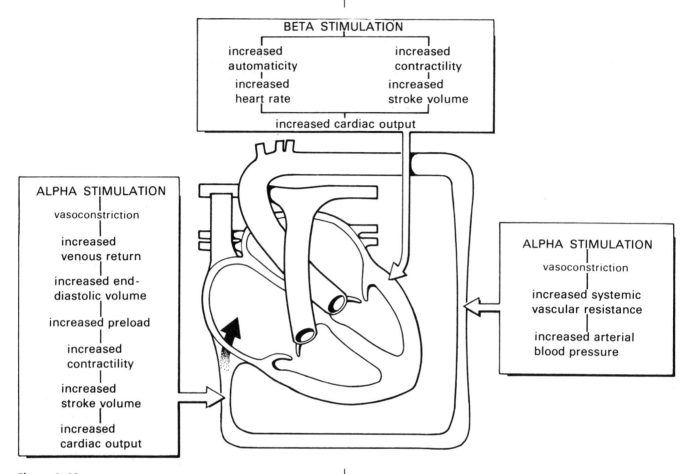

Figure 4–46

79. TRUE: Norepinephrine is indicated for the treatment of patients experiencing severe hypotension and low total peripheral resistance.

80. FALSE: One of the primary indications for norepinephrine is cardiogenic shock.

81. FALSE: Norepinephrine may increase MVO$_2$.

82. FALSE: Because of its alpha stimulating properties, norepinephrine may cause coronary vasoconstriction. This is usually a transient response; however, due to increased metabolic activity of the heart and increased perfusion pressures caused by peripheral vasoconstriction.

83. TRUE: Norepinephrine raises the blood pressure more rapidly than other catecholamines.

84. Norepinephrine may improve cardiac output when vasoconstriction is extreme because of its positive inotropic and chronotropic properties.

85. Cardiac output often increases once an optimal blood pressure has been restored with norepinephrine because coronary perfusion is improved and the heart has more oxygen available with which to work.

86. Norepinephrine can be particularly deleterious in the patient with myocardial ischemia and/or infarction because myocardial oxygen requirements may be increased as contractility, heart rate, and left ventricular wall tension are increased.

87. When administering norepinephrine, the following types of monitoring should be provided: (1) blood pressure check every 2 to 5 minutes, (2) ECG monitored continuously, and (3) arterial monitoring when available. It must be noted that standard blood pressure measurements may be inaccurately low when high doses of vasoconstrictive agents are used and thus intraarterial pressure monitoring is necessary for accurate interpretation of the patient's response.

88. b

89. c: The initial dosage of norepinephrine is 8 to 16 µg/ml, IV infusion, titrated to effect.

90. c: Norepinephrine administration should be adjusted to maintain a systolic blood pressure at or above 90 mm of Hg.

91. See Figure 4–47 for the correct preparation and administration of norepinephrine.

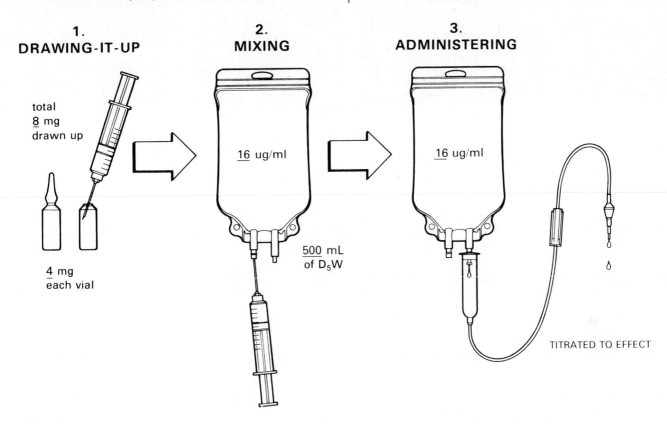

1.
DRAWING-IT-UP

total
8 mg
drawn up

4 mg
each vial

2.
MIXING

16 ug/ml

500 mL
of D₅W

3.
ADMINISTERING

16 ug/ml

TITRATED TO EFFECT

Figure 4–47

92. Extravasation of norepinephrine: phentolamine 5 to 10 mg in 10 to 15 ml of saline solution; infiltrate as soon as possible into area of extravasation.

93. b: Dopamine has the following properties: alpha stimulation (high doses), beta stimulation (medium doses), and dopaminergic stimulation (low doses).

94. a, b, d, e: Dopamine causes venous constriction and increased venous return, increases myocardial contractility, increases automaticity, and raises arterial blood pressure through arterial vasoconstriction. See Figure 4–48.

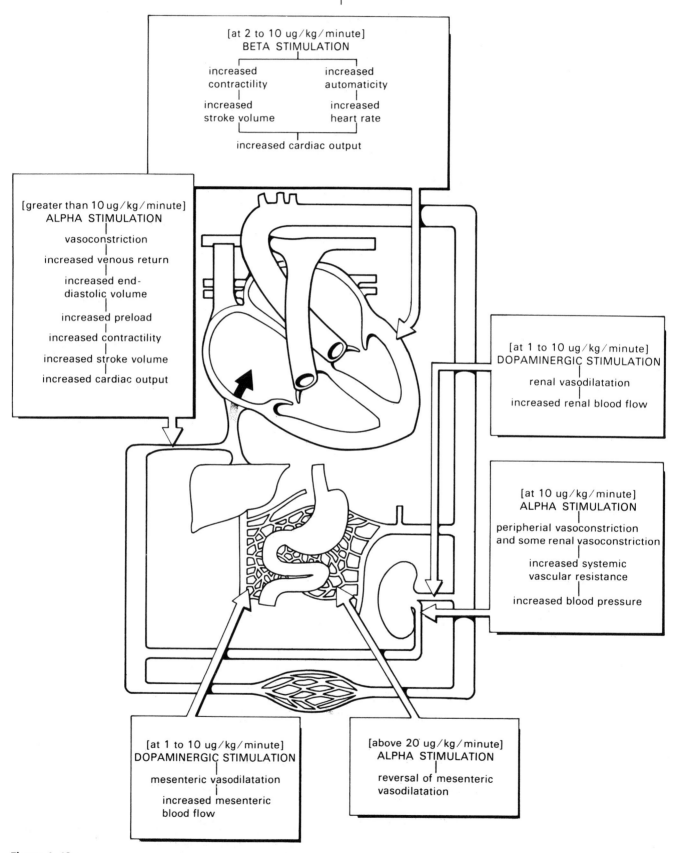

[at 2 to 10 ug/kg/minute]
BETA STIMULATION

increased   increased
contractility   automaticity

increased   increased
stroke volume   heart rate

increased cardiac output

[greater than 10 ug/kg/minute]
ALPHA STIMULATION

vasoconstriction

increased venous return

increased end-
diastolic volume

increased preload

increased contractility

increased stroke volume

increased cardiac output

[at 1 to 10 ug/kg/minute]
DOPAMINERGIC STIMULATION

renal vasodilatation

increased renal blood flow

[at 10 ug/kg/minute]
ALPHA STIMULATION

peripherial vasoconstriction
and some renal vasoconstriction

increased systemic
vascular resistance

increased blood pressure

[at 1 to 10 ug/kg/minute]
DOPAMINERGIC STIMULATION

mesenteric vasodilatation

increased mesenteric
blood flow

[above 20 ug/kg/minute]
ALPHA STIMULATION

reversal of mesenteric
vasodilatation

Figure 4–48

95. FALSE: The actions of dopamine are dose-dependent and may differ with the individual patient.

96. FALSE: The primary indications for dopamine in the emergency setting are cardiogenic shock and hemodynamically significant hypotension.

97. FALSE: The initial dosage for dopamine is 2 to 5 μg/kg/minute and, subsequently, titrated to effect. The infusion rate should be increased until blood pressure, urine output, and other parameters of organ perfusion show response.

98. Figure 4–49 shows the correct preparation and administration of dopamine.

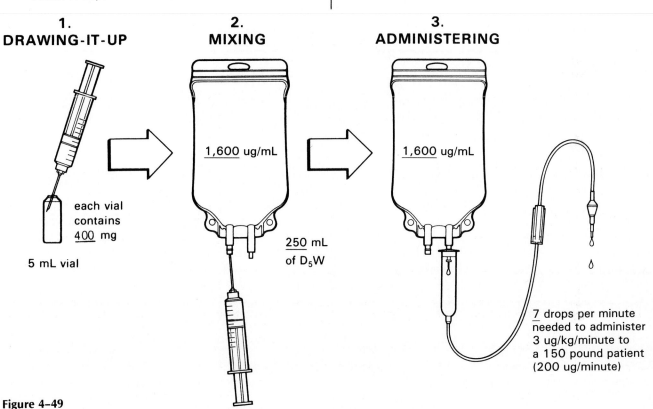

1.
DRAWING-IT-UP

5 mL vial
each vial contains <u>400</u> mg

2.
MIXING

1,600 ug/mL

<u>250</u> mL of D$_5$W

3.
ADMINISTERING

1,600 ug/mL

<u>7</u> drops per minute needed to administer 3 ug/kg/minute to a 150 pound patient (200 ug/minute)

Figure 4–49

99. The lowest possible dosage of dopamine should be used because its dopaminergic effects are achieved only at lower dosages. Higher dosages cause renal and mesenteric vasoconstriction and raise myocardial workload.

100. a. 1 to 2 μg/kg/minute: dilates renal and mesenteric vessels

b. 2 to 10 μg/kg/minute: beta stimulation increases cardiac output

c. >10 μg/kg/minute: alpha stimulation with peripheral constriction

d. >20 μg/kg/minute: alpha stimulation may reverse dilation of renal and mesenteric blood vessels

101. Side effects of dopamine include (1) tachydysrhythmias, (2) undesirable degrees of vasoconstriction at high doses, (3) vasodilation at low doses, (4) ectopic beats, (5) nausea and vomiting, (6) myocardial ischemia, (7) tissue necrosis and sloughing.

102. FALSE: Dobutamine is a beta 1 stimulator.

103. TRUE: Dobutamine increases cardiac output by increasing myocardial contractility.

104. c: Dobutamine differs from norepinephrine at usual doses, because dobutamine may induce peripheral vasodilation.

105. b: Dobutamine differs from isoproterenol in that dobutamine rarely causes tachycardia.

106. TRUE: The use of sodium nitroprusside results in decreased peripheral resistance (decreased afterload, reduced myocardial workload, decreased MVO$_2$), while coronary perfusion pressure can be maintained with dobutamine.

107. TRUE: The usual dosage range for dobutamine is from 2.5 to 10 μg/kg/minute.

108. TRUE: Higher doses of dobutamine may cause tachycardia. This may exacerbate myocardial ischemia.

109. Figure 4–50 shows the correct preparation and administration of dobutamine.

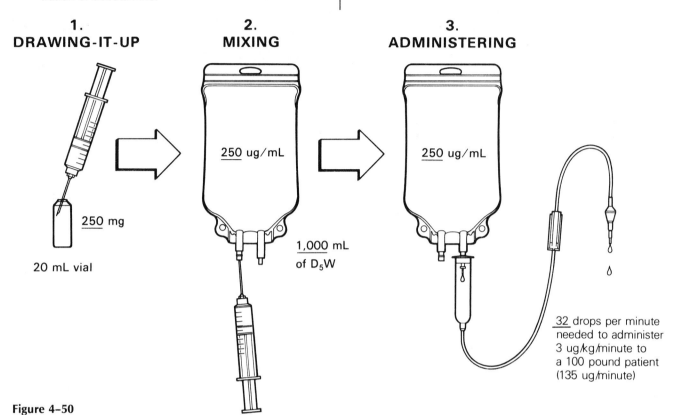

1.
DRAWING-IT-UP

250 mg

20 mL vial

2.
MIXING

250 ug/mL

1,000 mL of D_5W

3.
ADMINISTERING

250 ug/mL

32 drops per minute needed to administer 3 ug/kg/minute to a 100 pound patient (135 μg/minute)

Figure 4–50

110. c: Dobutamine is used to treat refractory congestive heart failure due to depressed ventricular function.

111. FALSE: Amrinone is a nonadrenergic cardiotonic agent.

112. TRUE: Amrinone acts similarly to dobutamine, increasing cardiac output by enhancing myocardial contractility.

113. FALSE: The usual dosage range of amrinone is a 0.75-mg/kg dose, which is given initially over 2 to 3 minutes, followed by an infusion of 5 to 10 μg/kg/minute.

114. TRUE: Amrinone may exacerbate myocardial ischemia.

115. FALSE: When afterload is increased, the myocardial workload and MVO$_2$ are increased; this has a deleterious effect on the heart when the patient has coronary artery disease, ischemia, and/or myocardial infarction.

116. TRUE: Increases in peripheral vascular resistance will increase afterload and can have a deleterious effect on the heart when the patient has coronary artery disease, ischemia, and/or myocardial infarction.

117. b: Actions of morphine sulfate include an analgesic effect and a vasodilatory effect.

118. a: Morphine sulfate reduces myocardial oxygen consumption by reducing left ventricular end-diastolic dimensions and wall stress, slowing heart rate, and decreasing myocardial contractility and perfusion pressures.

119. Indications for morphine sulfate administration are (1) acute MI and (2) pulmonary edema.

120. TRUE: The dosage for morphine sulfate is 2 to 5 mg slow IV push every 5 to 30 minutes until desired effects are achieved.

121. Hemodynamic effects of morphine sulfate include (1) increased venous capacitance, (2) decreased left ventricular end-diastolic dimensions and wall stress (re- duced MVO₂), and (3) reduced systemic vascular resis- tance (reduced afterload and myocardial workload). See Figure 4–51.

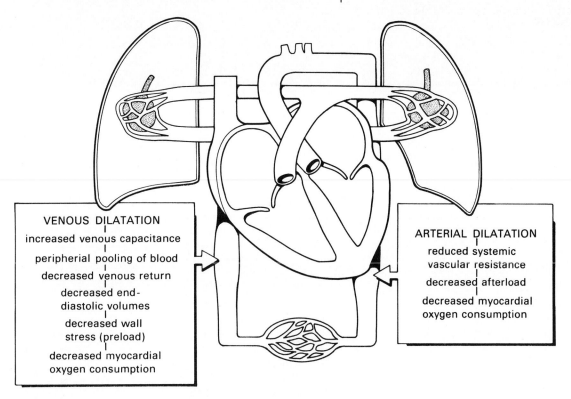

VENOUS DILATATION

increased venous capacitance

peripherial pooling of blood

decreased venous return

decreased end-
diastolic volumes

decreased wall
stress (preload)

decreased myocardial
oxygen consumption

ARTERIAL DILATATION

reduced systemic
vascular resistance

decreased afterload

decreased myocardial
oxygen consumption

Figure 4–51

122. Morphine sulfate may assist in relieving pulmonary con- gestion by increasing venous capacitance, thereby pooling blood peripherally and reducing venous return.

123. Side effects of morphine sulfate include (1) respiratory depression and (2) hypotension.

124. TRUE: Nitroglycerin dilates coronary arteries and sys- temic veins. See Figure 4–52.

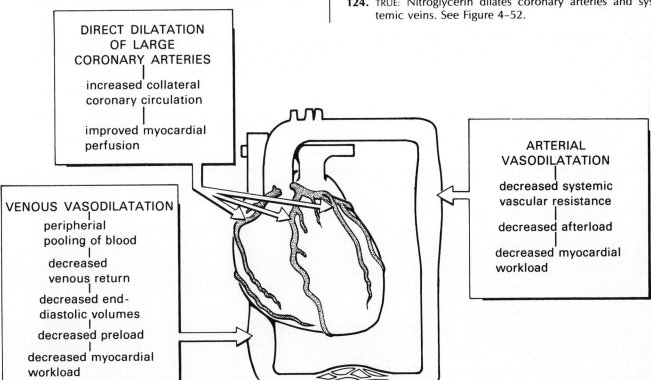

**DIRECT DILATATION
OF LARGE
CORONARY ARTERIES**

increased collateral
coronary circulation

improved myocardial
perfusion

**ARTERIAL
VASODILATATION**

decreased systemic
vascular resistance

decreased afterload

decreased myocardial
workload

VENOUS VASODILATATION

peripherial
pooling of blood

decreased
venous return

decreased end-
diastolic volumes

decreased preload

decreased myocardial
workload

Figure 4–52

125. The two competing theories for nitroglycerin's mechanism of action are the increased supply theory and the decreased demand theory. See Figure 4–53.

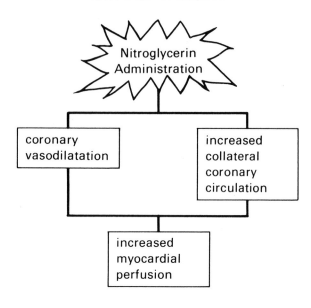

INCREASED SUPPLY THEORY

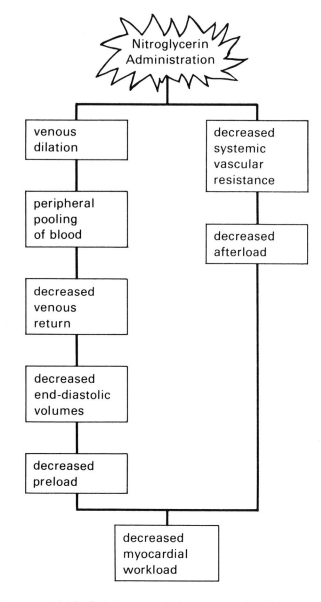

DECREASED DEMAND THEORY

Figure 4–53

126. TRUE: Nitroglycerin relieves coronary artery spasm.

127. FALSE: Nitroglycerin is the treatment of choice for anginal episodes.

128. TRUE: Nitroglycerin may be used for reducing pain and myocardial oxygen consumption in acute myocardial infarction.

129. TRUE: Nitroglycerin may produce maldistribution of coronary blood flow and reperfusion dysrhythmias in myocardial infarction patients.

130. TRUE: Following nitroglycerin administration, the patient should be monitored for an excessive drop in blood pressure. If the patient becomes hypotensive, place him or her in a recumbent position and elevate the legs.

131. TRUE: Initial administration of nitroglycerin should be at a dose of 0.3 to 0.4 mg.

132. TRUE: Nitroglycerin can be administered by IV.

133. The indications for IV administration of nitroglycerin include (1) congestive heart failure and (2) unstable angina.

134. The initial IV dosage for nitroglycerin is 10 μg/minute. This can be increased in 5- to 10-μg/minute increments as mandated by the response.

135. The two most common side effects of nitroglycerin are (1) headache and (2) hypotension.

136. FALSE: Sodium nitroprusside reduces preload by peripheral venous dilation and reduces afterload by peripheral arteriolar dilation.

137. FALSE: When an infusion of sodium nitroprusside is terminated, the effects of the medication cease immediately.

138. TRUE: Because cardiac output is typically sufficient to maintain the systemic arterial blood pressure.

139. The effects of sodium nitroprusside in pump failure associated with MI are illustrated in Figure 4–54.

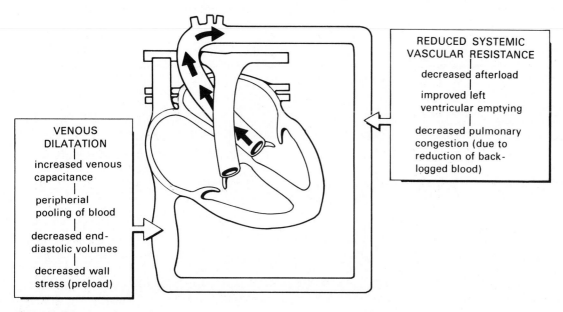

REDUCED SYSTEMIC
VASCULAR RESISTANCE

decreased afterload

improved left
ventricular emptying

decreased pulmonary
congestion (due to
reduction of back-
logged blood)

VENOUS
DILATATION

increased venous
capacitance

peripherial
pooling of blood

decreased end-
diastolic volumes

decreased wall
stress (preload)

Figure 4–54

140. a

141. TRUE: Nitroprusside is a rapid-acting direct peripheral vasodilator and thus is a preferred agent when immediate reduction in peripheral arterial resistance is necessary. Because of its potency and rapid action, sodium nitroprusside should be administered only by an infusion pump.

142. TRUE: Tachycardia following sodium nitroprusside administration is suggestive of hypotension or inadequate left ventricular filling pressure.

143. TRUE: Sodium nitroprusside may be more effective in combination with other agents than when it is used alone.

144. FALSE: Once sodium nitroprusside is prepared, it should be discarded after 4 hours.

145. TRUE: Only 5% dextrose should be used to dilute sodium nitroprusside.

146. Figure 4–55 shows the correct preparation and administration of sodium nitroprusside.

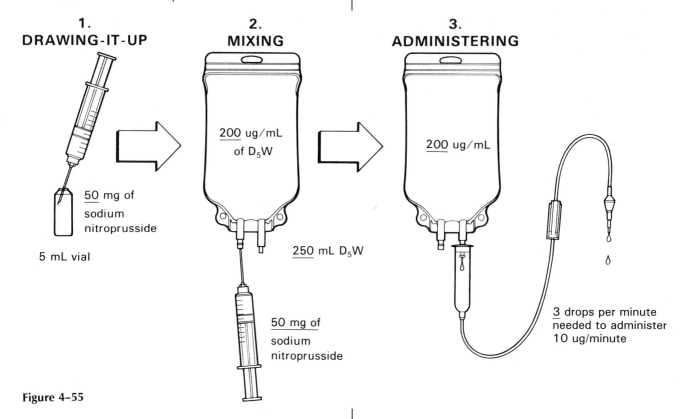

**1.
DRAWING-IT-UP**

50 mg of
sodium
nitroprusside

5 mL vial

**2.
MIXING**

200 ug/mL
of D₅W

250 mL D₅W

50 mg of
sodium
nitroprusside

**3.
ADMINISTERING**

200 ug/mL

3 drops per minute
needed to administer
10 ug/minute

Figure 4–55

147. FALSE: The current recommended initial dosage for sodium nitroprusside is 10 to 20 μg/minute.

148. FALSE: Sodium nitroprusside levels may become toxic
with dosages at or above 0.75 mg/kg/hour.

149. TRUE

150. TRUE: Circulatory overload may increase cardiac preload
as well as afterload. This increases myocardial workload
and subsequently MVO₂.

151. FALSE: Furosemide is potent diuretic agent. It also has
some direct venodilating effects, although it may cause
transient vasoconstriction in chronic heart failure.

152. FALSE: In emergency cardiac care, furosemide is the
treatment of choice for acute pulmonary edema and
cerebral edema after cardiac arrest.

153. TRUE: As sodium is excreted, water is also excreted.

154. FALSE: The onset of diuresis after furosemide administration usually begins within 5 minutes, peaks within 30
minutes, and lasts about 2 hours.

155. TRUE: Furosemide may reduce pulmonary edema by reducing preload through venous dilation.

156. FALSE: The current recommended initial dosage is 0.5 to
1.0 mg/kg injected slowly IV.

157. Side effects of furosemide include (1) dehydration and
blood volume depletion with circulatory collapse, (2)
potassium depletion, (3) sodium depletion, (4) hyperos-
molarity, (5) metabolic alkalosis, and (6) allergic reac-
tions.

158. Automaticity is the ability to spontaneously depolarize (initiate an electrical impulse) (Figure 4–56). The SA node normally has the fastest rate of automaticity, making it the normal pacemaker. Other potential pacemaker sites are normally suppressed by depolarization from the SA node. If the SA node fails to initiate an impulse, one of these lower pacemaker sites will usually do so (escape/default mechanism). If there is an acceleration of phase 4 in the action potential of these latent pacemaking sites (in lower pacemakers or ectopic pacemakers), their automaticity would be enhanced and premature beats or tachydysrhythmias may result. This condition could occur with myocardial injury or ischemia, increased catecholamines, or by the action of some drugs.

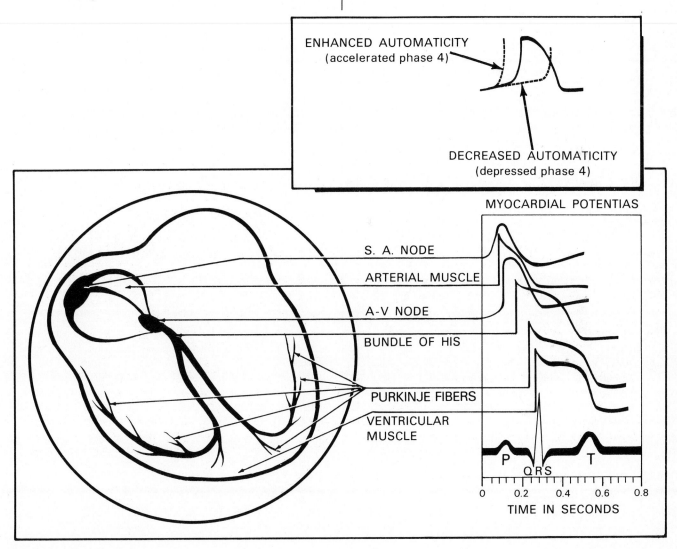

Figure 4–56

159. Reentry is a condition in which the cardiac impulse is delayed in a pathway of slowed conduction enough that it is still active when surrounding tissues have repolarized (Figure 4–57). Because the impulse is still active, it may reenter that surrounding tissue and propagate another impulse. Reentry may be caused by ischemia and hypoxia, and may occur in the ventricles, AV junctions, SA node, or atria. Focal reentry is a condition that may occur when neighboring fibers are activated simultaneously, but repolarize at different rates. This can result in a second beat being generated in the repolarized fibers by the area that is still depolarized. Focal reentry can be caused by ischemia, sympathetic stimulation, hypoxia, and other causes. Reentry may cause tachydysrhythmias, ectopic beats, and fibrillation.

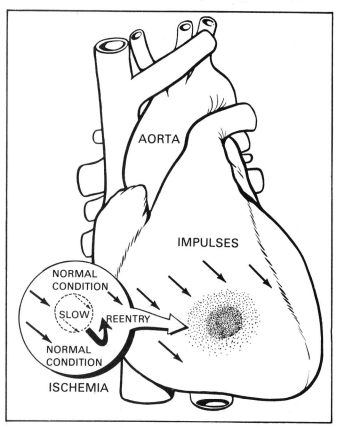

Figure 4–57

160. TRUE: A discrepancy in conduction times between normal and injured areas of the myocardium makes the heart prone to reentrant dysrhythmias.

161. FALSE: Ischemic heart muscle has a slower conduction time than normal tissue.

162. Medications that control dysrhythmias due to increased automaticity or reentry work by (1) controlling ion flow across the cell membrane, which reduces automaticity due to slowed spontaneous depolarization, (2) increasing the threshold level at which depolarization occurs, thereby making cells less sensitive to stimulation, and (3) prolonging the effective refractory period when the cell is unable to respond to another stimulus. These medications may also slow phase 4 depolarization, which increases the time required for depolarization. Reentry can be controlled by making repolarization times more uniform throughout normal and ischemic myocardium.

The four primary actions of antidysrhythmic drugs are (1) stabilization of the cell membrane by inhibiting ion movement through the fast sodium channel, (2) beta receptor blockade, (3) prolongation of the action potential duration, and (4) inhibition of ion movement through the slow calcium channel.

163. TRUE: Lidocaine is used to treat dysrhythmias originating from the ventricles.

164. FALSE: Lidocaine has no effect on conduction velocity. It increases the effective refractory period of infarcted tissue and decreases the degree of dispersion of recovery to raise the fibrillation threshold. See Figure 4–58.

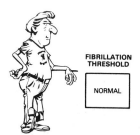

This person illustrates the normal myocardium, calm, non-irritable, relaxed, unlikely to go off the deep end (fibrillation). This may represent the non-ischemic myocardium or a patient who has received lidocaine to raise the fibrillation threshold.

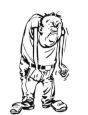
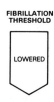

This person illustrates decreased fibrillation threshold, irritable, easily provoked into fibrillation. May be due to ischemia, increased catecholamines, etc.

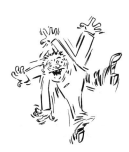

This person represents fibrillation, a chaotic action which is ineffective at best. Treatment will be directed toward converting this into effective action. Once effective function has been restored, lidocaine needs to be administered to raise the fibrillation threshold to prevent the patient from doing this again.

Figure 4–58

165. TRUE: Lidocaine is indicated for ventricular tachycardia, ventricular fibrillation, PVCs, and suspected myocardial ischemia.

166. FALSE: The initial IV push dosage for lidocaine is 1 mg/kg.

167. TRUE: In doses applied clinically, lidocaine has little effect on myocardial contractility or ventricular conduction velocity.

168. Results of lidocaine administration: **a.** Sinus rhythm with PVCs, conversion to sinus rhythm without PVCs due to the suppression of ventricular ectopy (Figure 4–59). **b.** Ventricular tachycardia, conversion to sinus rhythm due to the suppression of ventricular ectopy (Figure 4–60). **c.** Ventricular fibrillation, conversion to sinus rhythm due to an increase in the fibrillation threshold (Figure 4–61). (*Note:* Lidocaine administration alone will not likely restore effective sinus rhythm; however, it is believed to improve the heart's response to electrical therapy in ventricular fibrillation that is resistant to defibrillation.)

169. 7.5 ml

170. Lidocaine doses for each of the following weights: 90 lb = 41 mg; 168 lb = 76 mg; 300 lb = 136 mg

171. The preferred method for administering lidocaine: In cardiac arrest, a 1-mg/kg bolus is administered initially; this is followed by 0.5-mg/kg boluses every 8 to 10 minutes up to a total of 3 mg/kg. Only boluses should be used in the cardiac arrest setting. After successful resuscitation, a continuous infusion should be started at 2 to 4 mg per minute.

In cases where hemodynamics are more normal, boluses may be given every 2 or 3 minutes; an infusion should be started at 2 mg/minute and increased if necessary by 1 mg/minute after each additional bolus injection to a maximum of 4 mg/minute.

172. Drip rate: 2 mg/minute = 30 drops/minute

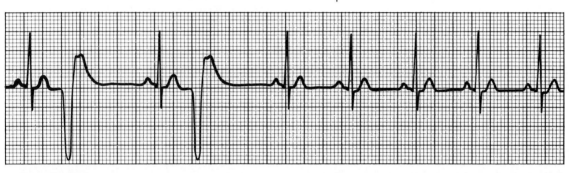

a. **Figure 4–59**

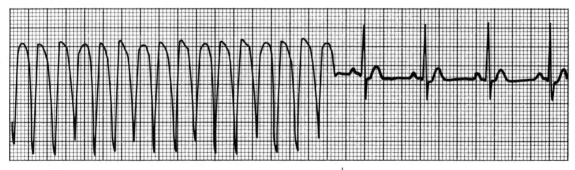

b. **Figure 4–60**

DEFIBRILLATION

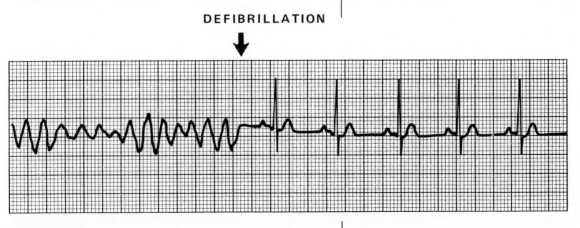

c. **Figure 4–61**

173. Prophylactic lidocaine should be administered for myocardial infarction and/or ischemia and following the termination of ventricular fibrillation or ventricular tachycardia. Lidocaine should be infused for up to 24 hours after termination of ventricular tachycardia or ventricular fibrillation.

174. Administer 0.5- to 1.0-mg boluses every 2 to 3 minutes and the infusion rate should be increased by 1 mg/minute after each additional bolus to a total of 4 mg/minute.

175. TRUE: Signs of lidocaine toxicity include disorientation, impaired hearing, paresthesia, and muscle twitching.

176. Seizures associated with lidocaine therapy are treated with CNS depressants such as barbiturates or diazepam.

177. FALSE: Unless it is followed by a continuous infusion, a single bolus of lidocaine will fall to subtherapeutic blood levels within 8 to 20 minutes.

178. TRUE: In the infarcted and ischemic tissue, lidocaine delays activation time (reduces conduction velocity) and prolongs the effective refractory period.

179. TRUE: Lidocaine suppresses reentry dysrhythmias by further depressing conduction in injured myocardium so impulses cannot conduct to adjacent normal tissue.

180. FALSE: Lidocaine toxicity is usually manifested in the central nervous system.

181. TRUE: After the initial 1-mg/kg bolus, additional 0.5-mg boluses can be given every 8 to 10 minutes to a total of 3 mg/kg.

182. TRUE: This will avoid development of lidocaine toxicity.

183. TRUE: In cases of heart failure or shock, lidocaine toxicity may develop after relatively short periods of time as circulation to the liver is diminished. Thus the dose of lidocaine should be reduced by approximately one-half in the presence of decreased cardiac output. The dosage for lidocaine should also be reduced in elderly patients and persons with hepatic dysfunction.

184. FALSE: Lidocaine may be used with conduction disturbances because it has little or no effect on AV or intraventricular conduction.

185. TRUE: Lidocaine may be administered endotracheally.

186. c: Procainamide or bretylium can be used to treat PVCs refractory to lidocaine.

187. TRUE: Procainamide reduces automaticity by suppressing phase 4 diastolic depolarization.

188. TRUE: Procainamide slows conduction velocity and produces a bidirectional block that terminates reentry mechanisms.

189. FALSE: Procainamide is used in the treatment of persistent PVCs and ventricular tachycardia that is refractory to lidocaine, but is no longer a recommended modality in ventricular fibrillation.

190. FALSE: Procainamide decreases ion flow through the myocardial membranes and thereby decreases automaticity in these cells.

191. Procainamide decreases the rate and amplitude of depolarization, thereby prolonging the action potential and reducing the speed of impulse conduction.

192. TRUE: Procainamide increases threshold potential.

193. TRUE

194. TRUE: Procainamide inhibits transportation of calcium ions across the cell membrane, thereby reducing myocardial contractility.

195. Indicators for termination of procainamide therapy are (1) the dysrhythmia is suppressed, (2) hypotension ensues, (3) the QRS complex widens by 50% or more of its original width, or (4) a total of 1 gm of the drug has been administered.

196. Amount of procainamide that should be administered every minute: 20 mg/minute or 100 mg/5 minutes. See Figure 4–62.

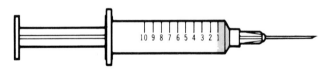

Figure 4–62

20 mg/minute
100 mg/5 minutes

197. Procainamide drops rate: 2 mg/minute = 30 gtts/minute

198. TRUE: Bretylium has postganglionic adrenergic blocking properties, antidysrhythmic effects, and a positive inotropic action.

199. TRUE: Initially, bretylium provokes a catecholamine release. See Figure 4–63.

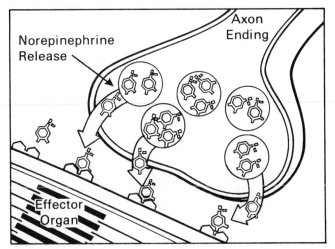

Bretylium provokes the release of norepinephrine from the axon ending

Figure 4–63

200. TRUE: A decline in arterial pressure following bretylium administration is due to the adrenergic blocking action of bretylium.

201. TRUE: Bretylium acts on the adrenergic nerve terminals. See Figure 4–64.

202. TRUE: Bretylium works by prolonging the action potential throughout the entire conduction system without affecting the infarcted areas; because all areas have slower conduction, reentry is less likely.

203. TRUE: Bretylium may be used to treat ventricular fibrillation, PVCs, and ventricular tachycardia that is refractory to other treatments.

204. FALSE: In ventricular fibrillation refractory to countershock, bretylium is administered as a 5-mg/kg initial IV bolus, repeated every 5 to 10 minutes at a dose of 10 mg/kg.

205. Side effects of bretylium administration are (1) postural hypotension and (2) nausea and vomiting.

206. FALSE: Bretylium raises the fibrillation threshold, making it less likely that the ventricles will fibrillate.

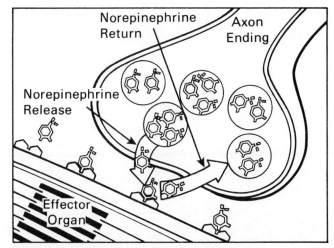

Normally norepinephrine is released and then taken back up at the axon ending

Figure 4–64

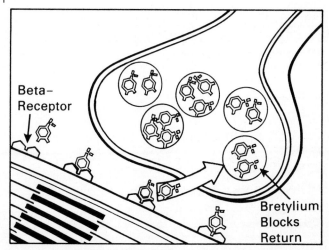

Bretylium blocks the return of norepinephrine to the axon ending

207. The amount of bretylium for a 350-mg dose is 7 ml. See Figure 4-65.

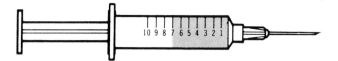

To deliver the correct dosage
<u>7</u> mL should be administered

Figure 4-65

208. Initial and repeat bretylium doses for the following weights:

Weight (lb)	Initial Dose (mg)	Repeat Dose (mg)
85	195	390
205	465	930
330	750	1500

209. d (see Figure 4-66)

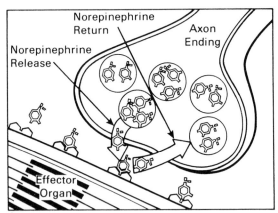

1. When the sympathetic nervous system is stimulated, norepinephrine is released

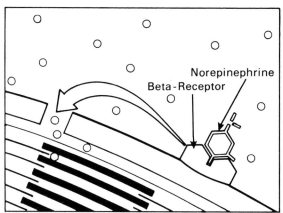

2. Norepinephrine interacts with a specific beta receptor

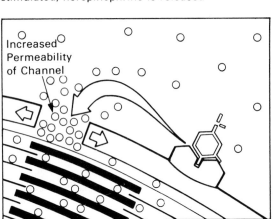

3. This interaction increases the permeability of ion channels allowing ions to enter the cells at a faster rate. This results in acceleration of the electrical processes of the heart. Additionally, more calcium ions can enter the cells and contractility can be increased.

Following propranolol administration. . . .

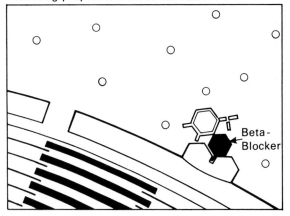

Propranolol occupies the beta receptor sites and subsequently prevents norepinephrine from affecting the cells.

Figure 4-66

210. Effects of propranolol: SA node, decrease in automaticity (phase 4) of pacemaker cells resulting from decreased amounts of calcium and sodium entering the cell. AV junction, reduced conduction velocity due to prolongation of the effective refractory period and action potential duration. Myocardial contractility, little effect unless contractility is being maintained by sympathetic stimulation; blocks the beta adrenergic receptors, producing a depressant effect on contractility. See Figure 4-67.

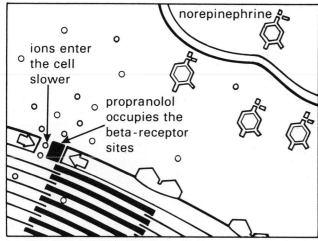

Following propranolol administration

Figure 4-67

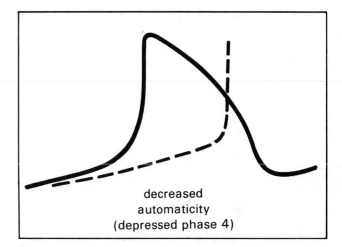

decreased
automaticity
(depressed phase 4)

211. TRUE: Effectiveness of propranolol depends on the degree of existing sympathetic stimulation because it only competes for sites that are actively being stimulated.

212. TRUE

213. FALSE: Propranolol must be used with extreme caution in patients with bronchospasm because blockade of beta 2 receptors located in the bronchioles precipitates further bronchoconstriction and bronchospasm.

214. TRUE

215. Use of propranolol with caution in patients (1) with dependence on beta stimulation (asthma, CHF), (2) when cardiac function is depressed, (3) with AV block or bradydysrhythmias, or (4) in acute myocardial infarction.

216. Atropine or isoproterenol should be used for bradycardia following propranolol administration.

217. TRUE

218. c

219. b

220. d

221. TRUE

222. FALSE: Verapamil eliminates abnormally slow responses by decreasing ion flow through the cell membrane. See Figure 4-68.

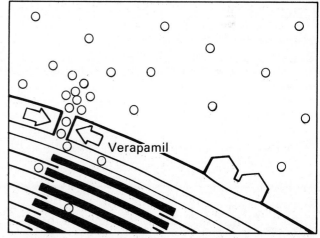

Verapamil depresses slow response fibers by inhibiting the movement of ions (calcium and possibly sodium) through the slow channels of the cell membrane

Figure 4-68

223. Matching actions of verapamil with effects:

   b: prolongs the relative refractory period of the AV junction: results in slowing of AV conduction

   e: causes vasodilation of the peripheral blood vessels; is counteracted by improved ventricular performance

   d: decreases peripheral resistance: improves ventricular performance and cardiac output

   a: relaxes coronary vascular smooth muscle; increases myocardial oxygen supply

   c: decreases myocardial contractility; results in decreases in myocardial workload and oxygen consumption

224. FALSE: Verapamil relaxes coronary and peripheral vascular smooth muscle by reducing the contractile tone. More specifically, it reduces inward movement of calcium ions across the cell membrane.

225. TRUE

226. TRUE

227. Initial and repeat doses of verapamil in the adult: initially, 5 mg should be administered IV; if the paroxysmal atrial tachycardia persists, 10 mg should be administered in 15 to 30 minutes if there has not been an adverse reaction to the initial dose.

228. Verapamil should be used in caution with patients with (1) hypotension, (2) severely compromised hemodynamics, or (3) sick sinus syndrome or AV block. It should not be used with patients receiving IV beta blockers.

229. c, d, e, f, g: ventricular fibrillation

   c, h, k: acute pulmonary edema

   a, c, l: symptomatic bradycardia

   a, c, d, e: asystole

   c, f, g, j: PVCs

   c, d, e: electromechanical dissociation

   d: metabolic acidosis

   c: hypoxia

   i: supraventricular tachycardia, atrial fibrillation or flutter, chronic angina

   b, c: cardiogenic shock

230. h: dopamine: in low doses, dilates renal and mesenteric blood vessels

   g: isoproterenol: a pure beta adrenergic receptor stimulator

   c: nitroglycerin: dilates coronary vessels directly and relaxes peripheral blood vessels

   d: propranolol: a beta receptor blocker

   i: norepinephrine: a potent peripheral vasoconstrictor as well as a powerful inotropic agent that initially causes coronary vasoconstriction; causes renal and mesenteric vasoconstriction

   f: dobutamine: a beta adrenergic receptor stimulating agent that seldom causes systemic arterial constriction or tachycardia

   a: furosemide: a potent diuretic that inhibits renal reabsorption of sodium

   e: amrinone: a nonadrenergic cardiotonic agent

231. f: dobutamine: refractory congestive heart failure due to depressed ventricular function and contractility

   g: isoproterenol: hemodynamically significant bradycardia that is refractory to atropine

   i: norepinephrine: symptomatic hypotension due to cardiogenic shock or low peripheral resistance

   h: dopamine: hemodynamically significant hypotension

   a: furosemide: cerebral edema after cardiac arrest and acute pulmonary edema

   b: sodium nitroprusside: hypertensive crisis or for immediate reduction of peripheral vascular resistance

   c: nitroglycerin: angina and some cases of myocardial infarction

   e: morphine sulfate: acute myocardial infarction and acute pulmonary edema

232. furosemide: 0.5 to 1.0 mg/kg injected slowly IV

   sodium nitroprusside: 10 to 20 microgram μg minute

   nitroglycerin (sublingual): 0.3 to 0.4 mg

   propranolol: 1 to 3 mg, slow IV push

   dobutamine: 2.5 to 10.0 μg/kg/minute, IV infusion

   isoproterenol: 2 to 10 μg/minute, IV infusion, titrated to heart rate and BP

   dopamine: 2 to 5 μg/kg, IV infusion, titrated to effect

   norepinephrine: 8 to 16 μg/ml, IV infusion, titrated to effect

233.

TABLE 4–3

	Afterload	Preload	MVO₂	Contractility	Heart Rate
Morphine sulfate	↓	↓	↓	← ↓	↑ ↓ ←
Nitroglycerin	↓	↓	↓	←	← ↑
Furosemide	←	↓	↓	←	←
Sodium nitroprusside	↓	↓	↓	←	← ↑
Isoproterenol	↓	↓	↑	↑	↑
Norepinephrine	↑	↑	↑	↑	↑
Dopamine	← ↑	← ↑	← ↑	← ↑	← ↑
Dobutamine	←	←	↑	↑	←
Propranolol	← ↓	← ↓	← ↓	← ↓	← ↓

234.

TABLE 4–4

	Angina	Myocardial infarction	Acute pulmonary edema	Congestive heart failure	Refractory CHF	Hypertensive crisis	Cardiogenic shock	Bradycardia	Premature ventricular complexes (PVCs)	Ventricular tachycardia	Ventricular fibrillation	Rapid supraventricular tachycardia	Asystole	Electromechanical dissociation (EMD)
Atropine								×					×	
Isoproterenol								×						
Oxygen	×	×	×	×	×	×	×	×	×	×	×	×	×	×
Morphine sulfate		×	×											
Nitroglycerin	×	×												
Furosemide			×	×										
Sodium nitroprusside					×	×								
Norepinephrine							×							
Dopamine							×							
Dobutamine				×			×							
Lidocaine		×							×	×	×			
Bretylium									×	×	×			
Procainamide									×	×				
Propranolol												×		
Verapamil												×		
Epinephrine							×				×		×	×

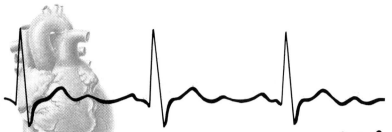

Chapter 5

Acid–Base Balance

OBJECTIVES

Upon completion of this chapter, you will be able to:

- Distinguish aerobic from anaerobic metabolism.

- Recognize the components and normal values in an arterial blood gas report.

- Differentiate between respiratory and metabolic derangements of acid–base balance.

- Describe the carbonic acid–bicarbonate buffer system.

- Explain the treatment(s) appropriate for managing oxygenation problems and acid–base abnormalities.

- Describe the relationships among arterial carbon dioxide levels, arterial pH, and the adequacy of alveolar ventilation.

1. Briefly describe the roles of glucose and oxygen in normal cellular metabolism.

2. Metabolism that occurs in the presence of oxygen is called _____ metabolism; metabolism that occurs without oxygen is called

   _____ metabolism

3. The two types of acids normally produced by aerobic metabolism are _____

   and _____ acids.
   a. lactic and pyruvic
   b. lactic and hydrochloric
   c. carbonic and metabolic
   d. carbonic and bicarbonate

4. Write a formula that illustrates how the combination of sodium bicarbonate ($NaHCO_3$) and hydrogen ion (H^+) produces carbonic acid.

   _____

   _____

   _____

True or False

5. T F Acid–base status is usually quite static; adjustments are rarely necessary and values are precisely balanced.

6. T F Some acids are produced as normal waste products of cellular energy production.

7. T F Cellular metabolism is enhanced when the intracellular environment becomes highly acidic.

8. Match the following terms with their appropriate definition.

   Term

   _____ H_2CO_3

   _____ $NaHCO_3$

   _____ pH

   _____ acidosis

   _____ alkalosis

   Definition
   a. mathematical expression of the hydrogen ion concentration
   b. pH less than 7.35
   c. carbonic acid (volatile acid)
   d. sodium bicarbonate; buffers metabolic acid
   e. pH greater than 7.45

9. Match the following body systems with their respective function in acid–base physiology.

   Body System

   _____ kidneys

   _____ buffers

   _____ lungs

   Function in Acid–Base Physiology
   a. eliminate carbonic acid by exhalation of carbon dioxide
   b. convert metabolic acids into weak acids and their neutral salts
   c. excrete metabolic acids

10. In the body, carbon dioxide (CO_2) combines with water (H_2O) to form
    a. sodium bicarbonate
    b. carbonic acid
    c. lactic acid
    d. pyruvate

True or False

11. T F Carbonic acid levels have little or no effect on the pH.

12. T F Carbonic acid levels decrease as ventilation increases.

13. T F Hyperventilation may be used as a protective compensatory mechanism to raise the pH in metabolic acidosis.

14. Explain the role of the kidneys in maintaining a normal pH.

    _____

    _____

    _____

    _____

15. Name the weak acid and salt (base) components of the most important buffering system of the body.

_____

_____

16. Figure 5–1 is an illustration of the buffering process of metabolic acids. Fill in the missing components of this process.

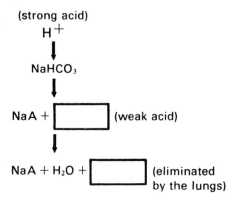

(strong acid)

H $^+$

↓

NaHCO$_3$

↓

NaA + ⬚ (weak acid)

↓

NaA + H$_2$O + ⬚ (eliminated by the lungs)

Figure 5–1

17. Which of the following is depleted in the metabolic acid buffering process?

    a. H_2CO_3
    b. H_2O
    c. $NaHCO_3$
    d. CO_2

18. The normal sodium bicarbonate to carbonic acid ratio is _____ to _____

    a. 5:1
    b. 4:2
    c. 20:1
    d. 25:30
    e. 1:1

19. Which of the following may result in acidosis?

    a. depletion of base (bicarbonate)
    b. accumulation of metabolic acids
    c. increase in $PaCO_2$
    d. shortage in H_2CO_3

20. Which of the following illustrations in Figure 5–2 depicts ANAEROBIC metabolism?

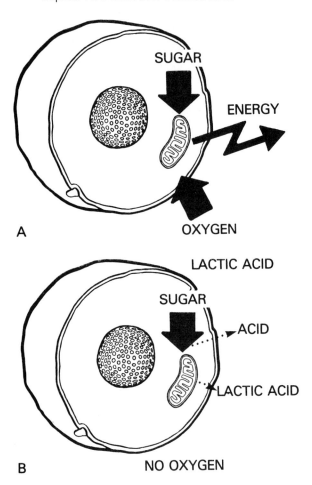

Figure 5–2

21. Which of the following is the most effective diagnostic aid for evaluating and treating disturbances of acid–base balance?

    a. blood pressure
    b. capillary wedge pressure
    c. arterial blood gas analysis
    d. respiratory rate and depth

22. Which of the following are considered part of an arterial blood gas (ABG) report?

    a. PaO_2 and hemoglobin
    b. pH, PaO_2, $PaCO_2$
    c. $PaCO_2$ and H^+
    d. hematocrit and FiO_2

23. The tension of oxygen and/or carbon dioxide is measured in units of _____

    a. degrees
    b. milliliters
    c. mm Hg (torr)
    d. cm H_2O

24. Match the following terms with their respective definition and normal values. (Each term will have two answers.)

Term	Definition	Normal Values
PaO_2	_____	_____
$PaCO_2$	_____	_____
pH	_____	_____
base	_____	_____
deficit	_____	_____

a. H^+ concentration
b. 80 to 100 mm Hg
c. 7.35 to 7.45
d. arterial oxygen tension
e. arterial carbon dioxide tension
f. 35 to 45 mm of Hg
g. depletion or excess of bicarbonate
h. zero (none)

True or False

25. T   F   If hypoxia is present, it must be corrected.

26. T   F   Hypoxia can cause metabolic acidosis.

27. T   F   The arterial oxygen content depends on the arterial oxygen tension and the hemoglobin level.

28. T   F   During resuscitation, a PaO_2 of at least 80 mm of Hg is optimal

29. T   F   100% oxygen is seldom necessary in cardiac arrest situations.

30. What should be done if the PaO_2 is below acceptable levels during resuscitation?

_____

_____

_____

_____

31. Which of the following are true regarding the $PaCO_2$ level?

a. normally has a mean value of 40 mm of Hg
b. normally ranges between 35 and 45 mm of Hg
c. decreases with an increase in ventilation
d. below normal level, is considered hyperventilation and alkalosis

32. An increase in $PaCO_2$ causes a (an)

a. decrease in H_2CO_3
b. decrease in pH
c. increase in $NaHCO_3$
d. increase in bicarbonate combined with carbonic acid

True or False

33. T   F   When assessing ventilations, medical personnel need only be concerned about the patient's ventilatory rate.

34. T   F   Increases in $PaCO_2$ may decrease myocardial contractility.

35. T   F   As alveolar ventilation increases, the $PaCO_2$ also increases.

36. Match the following changes in $PaCO_2$ with their results. (More than one response will be correct.)

PaCO₂ Change

_____ an increase in $PaCO_2$ to 50 mm of Hg

_____ a decrease in $PaCO_2$ to 30 mm of Hg

Result

a. respiratory acidosis
b. hyperventilation
c. respiratory alkalosis
d. hypoventilation
e. results in pH of 7.48
f. results in pH of 7.32

37. Explain what should be done if the $PaCO_2$ is above 40 torr (mm of Hg).

_____

_____

_____

_____

_____

38. Why is it important to evaluate the degree to which the PaCO$_2$ level has influenced the pH before administering sodium bicarbonate?

_____

_____

_____

_____

_____

_____

_____

_____

True or False

39. T   F   The pH reflects only the metabolic acid concentration of the arterial blood.

40. T   F   The amount of sodium bicarbonate administered should be determined by the patient's pH.

41. Place a check mark beside the pH levels listed that indicate acidosis.

_____ 7.56

_____ 7.12

_____ 7.38

_____ 7.22

_____ 6.80

_____ 7.42

True or False

42. T   F   A base deficit is due to loss of bicarbonate; bicarbonate is located primarily in the extracellular fluid (ECF).

43. T   F   The ECF consists of only intravascular fluid.

44. On Figure 5–3, place an × beside the name of the body fluid compartment(s) where sodium bicarbonate is primarily located.

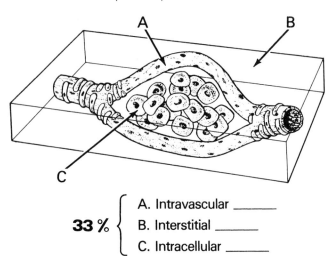

33 % { A. Intravascular _____
          B. Interstitial _____
          C. Intracellular _____

Figure 5–3

45. On Figure 5–4, darken in the percentage of body weight that corresponds to the amount that extracellular fluid represents.

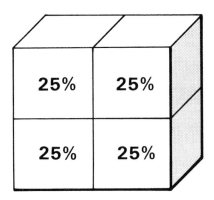

Figure 5–4

46. List three results of overzealous administration of bicarbonate.

1) _____

2) _____

3) _____

47. What is the recommended *initial* and *subsequent* dosage of sodium bicarbonate in the adult patient when arterial blood gases are NOT available?

_____

_____

_____

48. Which of the following is true for the patient with chronic obstructive pulmonary disease and CO_2 retention?

    a. There is compensatory accumulation of bicarbonate to maintain a near normal pH.

    b. Hypoventilation is often present.

    c. Metabolic alkalosis is often present.

    d. ABGs would likely show a low $PaCO_2$ and a high HCO_3 level.

    e. The pH is often extremely low.

49. Your patient's $PaCO_2$ is 55 and his pH is 7.36. With which of the following conditions might a report such as this be seen?

    a. a COPD patient with chronic CO_2 retention

    b. a previously healthy patient who was overloaded with bicarbonate and who is being hyperventilated

    c. a patient with nasogastric suction

    d. a patient in diabetic ketoacidosis who is hyperventilating

    e. a patient who is hyperventilating and who has not received sufficient bicarbonate.

50. Match the following conditions with their appropriate treatment.

Condition

_____ respiratory acidosis

_____ metabolic acidosis

_____ cardiac arrest

Treatment

a. improve ventilation

b. $NaHCO_3$, oxygen, improve ventilation

ANSWER KEY

1. Glucose is the primary energy source of the body. When glucose enters the cell, it is split into two pyruvic acid molecules. This process occurs *without* the presence of oxygen and is called ANAEROBIC metabolism. When the pyruvic acid molecules reach the mitochondria of the cell, oxygen must be available for further breakdown of pyruvic acid in the Krebs cycle. Cellular metabolism that requires the presence of oxygen is called AEROBIC metabolism. The metabolism of glucose through the Krebs cycle produces three byproducts: carbon dioxide, water, and—most importantly—energy (see Figure 5–5).

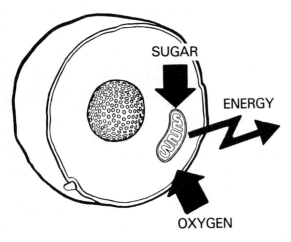

Figure 5–5

2. Aerobic metabolism requires oxygen; anaerobic metabolism occurs in absence of oxygen.

3. c

4. Production of carbonic acid:

$$\left(\begin{array}{c}\text{hydrogen}\\\text{ion}\end{array}\right) \left(\begin{array}{c}\text{sodium}\\\text{bicarbonate}\end{array}\right) \qquad \left(\begin{array}{c}\text{sodium}\\\text{ion}\end{array}\right) \left(\begin{array}{c}\text{carbonic}\\\text{acid}\end{array}\right)$$
$$H^+ + NaHCO_3 \longleftrightarrow Na^+ + H_2CO_3$$

5. FALSE: The acid–base balance of the body is highly dynamic, varying with intake and removal of acids and bases. Because of this variance, key body systems must continually readjust acid and base concentrations to maintain acid–base balance.

6. TRUE

7. FALSE: Acidosis depresses cellular metabolism.

8. H_2CO_3: c   acidosis: b
   $NaHCO_3$: d   alkalosis: e
   pH: a

9. kidneys: c
   buffers: b
   lungs: a

10. b($CO_2 + H_2O = H_2CO_3$)

11. FALSE: Increases in carbonic acid lower the pH (acidosis) (Figure 5–6), whereas decreases in carbonic acid raise the pH (alkalosis). Acidosis depresses cellular function and eventually causes cellular death.

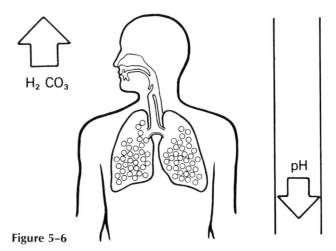

$H_2 CO_3$ pH

Figure 5–6

12. TRUE: Since carbonic acid levels are directly related to the concentration of carbon dioxide and CO_2 is directly related to the adequacy of alveolar ventilation; increased ventilation results in decreased carbonic acid (Figure 5–7).

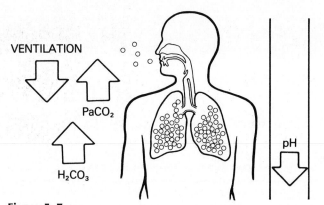
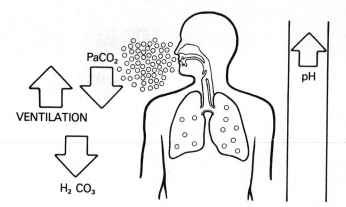

Figure 5–7

13. TRUE: An increase in ventilation decreases the $PaCO_2$ and helps restore the pH toward normal. Hyperventilation results in a respiratory alkalosis that compensates the metabolic acidosis (Figure 5–8).

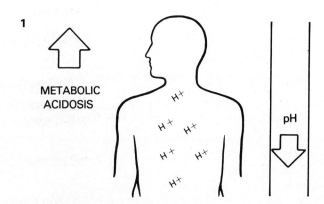

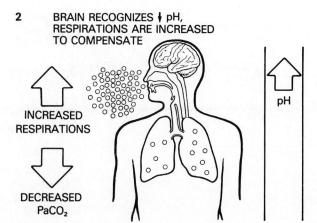

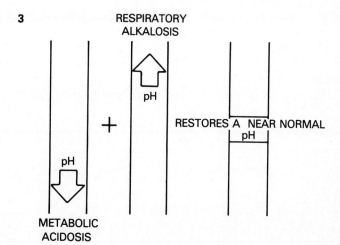

Figure 5–8

14. The kidneys assist in maintaining a normal pH by excreting large metabolic acids and by regulating the excretion and absorption of hydrogen ions, sodium, potassium, bicarbonate, and water.

15. The weak acid is carbonic acid and the salt of this weak acid (base) is sodium bicarbonate.

16. Components in buffering of metabolic acid (Figure 5–9):

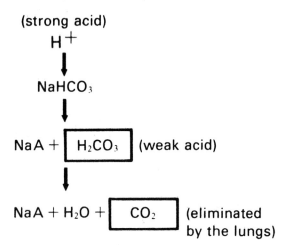

(strong acid)

H^+

$\downarrow$

$NaHCO_3$

$\downarrow$

$NaA + \boxed{H_2CO_3}$ (weak acid)

$\downarrow$

$NaA + H_2O + \boxed{CO_2}$ (eliminated by the lungs)

Figure 5–9

17. c

18. c

19. a, b, c: Normally there is a 20:1 ratio of bicarbonate to carbonic acid (see Figure 5–10). Acidosis occurs whenever this ratio is lowered. Apnea or inadequate ventilation allows carbon dioxide to accumulate in the arterial blood, resulting in a respiratory acidosis. The treatment for respiratory acidosis is to improve ventilation. Effective ventilation causes exhalation of CO_2 and lowered carbonic acid; this restores the 20:1 ratio needed to maintain a normal pH. If bicarbonate levels are lowered (e.g., by buffering metabolic acids), sodium bicarbonate may need to be administered to restore the 20:1 ratio.

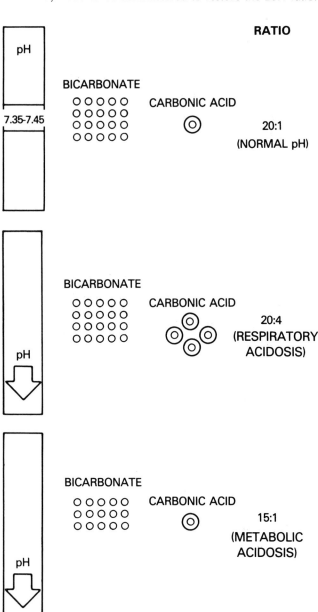

Figure 5–10

20. Figure 5–11 shows anaerobic metabolism.

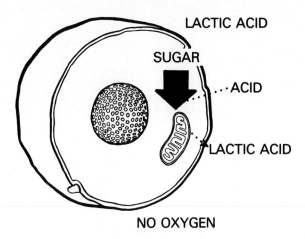

NO OXYGEN

ANAEROBIC METABOLISM
(without oxygen)

Figure 5–11

21. c

22. b (see Figure 5–12)

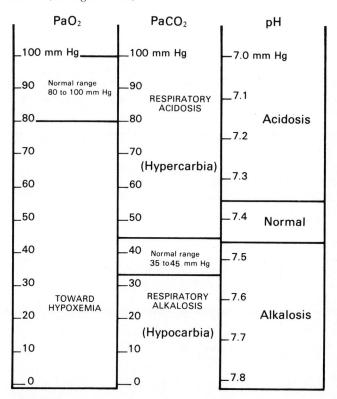

Figure 5–12

23. c

24. PaO₂: b and d;   PaCO₂: e and f
pH: a and c   base deficit: g and h

25. TRUE: Without adequate oxygen, cells produce metabolic acids via anaerobic metabolism. Hypoxia and (metabolic) acidosis reduce the likelihood of successful resuscitation.

26. TRUE: When oxygen is unavailable at the cellular level, anaerobic metabolism cannot proceed and pyruvic acids are converted to lactic acid. Lactic acid lowers the pH in three ways: (1) lactic acid is a metabolic acid in itself, (2) lactic acid will be buffered by bicarbonate, thereby depleting bicarbonate stores, causing a base deficit, and reducing the bicarbonate : carbonic acid ratio, and (3) buffering of metabolic acids increases carbonic acid ($NaHCO_3 + H^+ = Na^+ + H_2CO_3$), which lowers the pH.

This is why it is crucial that hypoxia be eliminated in metabolic acidosis. The patient does not have to be in cardiac arrest to have this situation exist. Any condition that interferes with oxygen reaching the cells (shock, myocardial infarction, respiratory failure) can result in hypoxia-induced metabolic acidosis. See Figure 5–13.

HYPOXIA

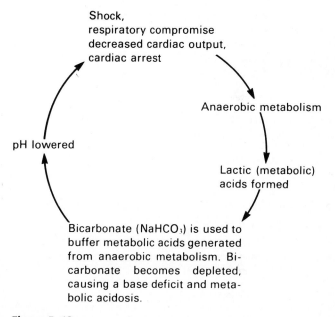

Figure 5–13

27. TRUE

28. TRUE: A PaO₂ of less than 80 mm of Hg indicates a need for supplemental oxygen.

29. FALSE: 100% oxygen should always be used in the treatment of cardiac arrest.

30. When the PaO₂ is less than 80 mm of Hg during resuscitation, the cause for the hypoxia must be discovered and corrected. The airway, ventilatory status, and inspired oxygen concentration should be checked as well as the adequacy of chest compressions and the pulmonary and cardiac causes of hypoxia.

31. All these statements are true of PaCO₂.

32. b

33. FALSE: Both ventilatory rate and depth (volume) affect the adequacy of ventilation. Excessively fast or slow rates and shallow breathing all reduce ventilation.

34. TRUE

35. FALSE: As ventilation increases, the PaCO₂ decreases (see Figure 5–14).

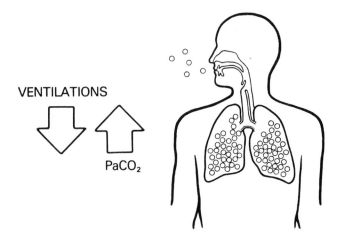
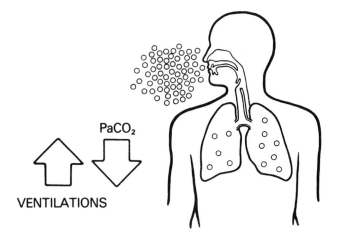

Figure 5–14

36. PaCO₂ 50 mm of Hg: a, d, f
PaCO₂ 30 mm of Hg: b, c, e

37. If the PaCO₂ is above 40 torr, the effectiveness of ventilation needs to be improved. When the patient is being ventilated, either the rate or volume may need to be increased to improve the minute volume. If the patient is breathing spontaneously, airway patency and exchange should be verified and, if necessary, improved.

38. It is important to evaluate the degree to which PaCO₂ has influenced the pH because CO_2 combines with water to form carbonic acid (H_2CO_3). Increases in carbonic acid lower the pH and produce respiratory acidosis; decreases in carbonic acid raise the pH and produce respiratory alkalosis. If the pH indicates acidosis, the cause may be respiratory, metabolic, or both. Since sodium bicarbonate will only be useful for treating *metabolic* acidosis, the respiratory component of an acidosis should be determined before treating the acidosis so that inappropriate administration of bicarbonate for a respiratory acidosis can be avoided.

39. FALSE: The pH reflects both respiratory (H_2CO_3) and metabolic acid (H^+) concentrations in the blood.

40. FALSE: Bicarbonate administration should be based on the patient's base deficit.

41. Acidotic pH levels: 7.12, 7.22, 6.80

42. TRUE

43. FALSE: Extracellular fluid consists of both intravascular as well as interstitial fluids.

44. Fluid compartments where sodium bicarbonate is primarily located are shown in Figure 5–15.

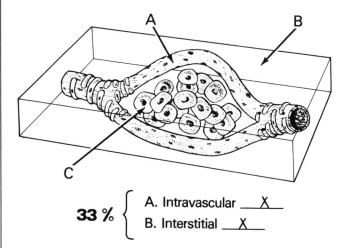

33 % { A. Intravascular ___X___
           B. Interstitial ___X___

Figure 5–15

45. Percentage of body weight composed of extracellular fluid (Figure 5–16):

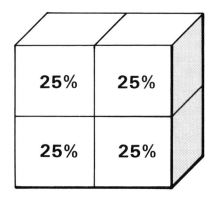

Figure 5–16

46. Overzealous use of bicarbonate may result in (1) metabolic alkalosis with impaired oxygen release from hemoglobin, (2) hypokalemia and dysrhythmias, and (3) marked hyperosmolality.

47. Dosage of $NaHCO_3$ when ABGs are not available: an initial dose of 1 mEq/l and subsequent doses every 10 minutes at half the initial dose.

48. a: There is compensatory accumulation of bicarbonate to maintain a near normal pH, and b: hypoventilation is often present (see Figure 5–17).

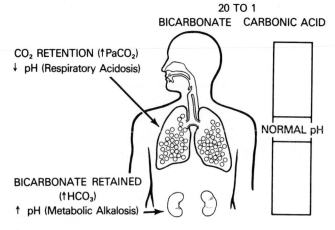

20 TO 1
BICARBONATE CARBONIC ACID

CO_2 RETENTION (↑$PaCO_2$)
↓ pH (Respiratory Acidosis)

NORMAL pH

BICARBONATE RETAINED
(↑HCO_3)
↑ pH (Metabolic Alkalosis)

Figure 5–17

49. a

50. respiratory acidosis: a;
cardiac arrest: c

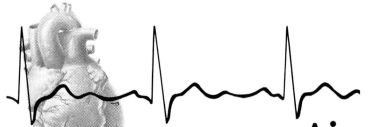

Chapter 6

Airway Management and Ventilation

OBJECTIVES

Upon completion of this chapter, you will be able to:

- Describe the definitive treatment of hypoxia in emergency cardiac care.
- Distinguish differences in management of hypoxia for patients with COPD.
- Explain how to perform various techniques for securing and maintaining a patent airway.
- Differentiate among the components, functions, and insertion techniques for various airway devices used in advanced life support.
- Specify how to manage hazards of endotracheal intubation.
- Describe how to use selected pieces of oxygen therapy equipment.
- Identify recommended procedures for airway suctioning.
- Describe the procedures for ventilating a patient with various adjuncts for ventilation.

True or False

1. T   F   The Venturi mask is the preferred device for administering oxygen to patients with chronic obstructive pulmonary disease (COPD).

2. T   F   Patients with chest pain do not need supplemental oxygen unless they show signs of respiratory distress.

3. T   F   Hypoxia may be present even when the patient isn't cyanotic or short of breath.

4. T   F   100% oxygen should be used in all cases of cardiac arrest.

5. Match the following oxygen devices and liter flows with the oxygen concentration each delivers:

O2 Device, Liter Flow	Delivered % O2
_____ nasal cannula, 2 to 6 lpm	a. 35 to 60
_____ simple face mask, 6 to 10 lpm	b. 80 to 100
_____ nonrebreather mask, 10 to 15 lpm	c. 40 to 50
_____ bag-valve-mask, 10 lpm (without a reservoir)	d. 17 to 22
	e. 24 to 44

6. COPD patients in respiratory arrest should be ventilated with

a. room air, manual resuscitator, 21% oxygen
b. manual resuscitator, 2 to 3 liters, 24 to 30% oxygen
c. manual resuscitator, 10 liters, 60% oxygen
d. manual resuscitator, 100% oxygen

7. Match the following airway problems with the appropriate technique for managing each:

Airway Problem

_____ upper airway obstruction due to foreign material

_____ posterior displacement of the tongue

_____ absence of spontaneous breathing

Management Technique

a. artificial ventilation via mouth-to-mouth, pocket mask, bag-valve-mask, etc.
b. suctioning or other methods of clearing the airway
c. positioning of the head: head tilt, chin lift, jaw thrust, oropharyngeal airway, etc.

8. For Figures 6–1 and 6–2, circle the letter of the one which shows an "open" airway.

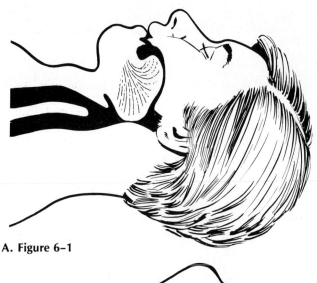

A. Figure 6–1

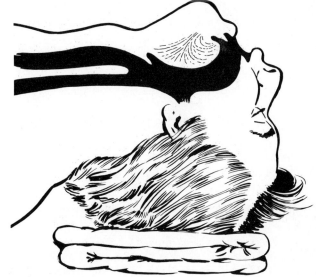

B. Figure 6–2

9. Briefly describe the technique for performing each of the following airway procedures:

HEAD TILT/CHIN LIFT

_____

_____

_____

_____

_____

_____

_____

JAW-THRUST

_____

_____

_____

_____

_____

_____

_____

_____

10. Match the airway devices in Figures 6–3 through 6–7 with their description.

Airway Device

Description

a. A long plastic tube open at the top and closed at the distal end; distal end is inserted into the esophagus; distal cuff occludes esophagus; ventilated air exits tube through air holes located at level of trachea; prevents aspiration while allowing adequate lung ventilation.

b. A soft rubber or plastic 15 mm-tube that is open at both ends; inserted along floor of nostril into the posterior pharynx behind tongue, allowing passage of air into lower pharynx.

c. A semicircular apparatus that fits over the tongue and rests in the lower posterior pharynx; holds the tongue away from the posterior oral pharynx.

d. A long plastic tube open at both ends that is placed directly into the trachea; when the distal cuff is inflated, the trachea is sealed and protected from aspiration.

e. A long plastic tube open at both ends; on the mask there is a port connecting to the tube

through which a gastric tube can be passed to decompress the stomach; the lungs can be ventilated via a separate mask port; allows esophageal occlusion while providing a mechanism for gastric suction.

Airway Device

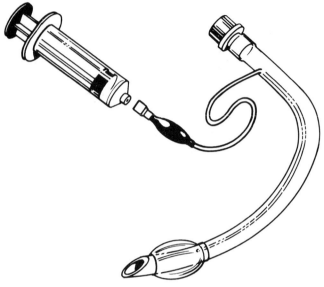

_____ **Figure 6–3**   ENDOTRACHEAL TUBE

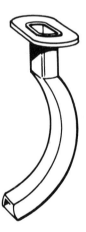

_____ **Figure 6–4**   OROPHARYNGEAL AIRWAY

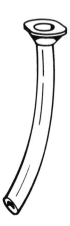

_____ **Figure 6–5**   NASOPHARYNGEAL AIRWAY

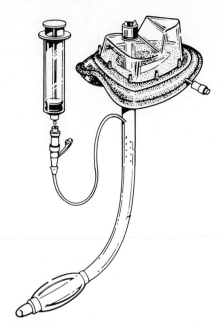

ESOPHAGEAL OBTURATOR AIRWAY

_____   **Figure 6–6**

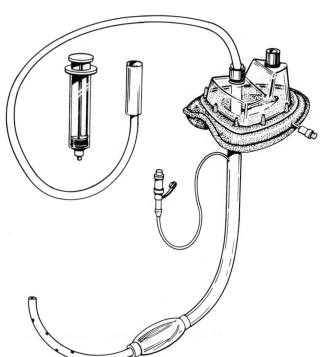

ESOPHAGEAL GASTRIC TUBE AIRWAY

_____   **Figure 6–7**

11. Describe the technique used for inserting an oropharyngeal airway.

_____

_____

_____

_____

_____

True or False

12. T   F   The oropharyngeal airway can be used in both conscious and unconscious patients.

13. T   F   A complication of an improperly inserted oropharyngeal airway is that it may push the patient's tongue back against the posterior oropharynx.

14. T   F   The head must be maintained in hyperextension even after insertion of an oropharyngeal airway.

15. Describe the technique for inserting a nasopharyngeal airway.

_____

_____

_____

_____

16. Briefly explain the primary reason for using the nasopharyngeal airway.

_____

_____

_____

17. In Figure 6–8, label each component of the esophageal obturator airway with the letter of the function it performs.

a. allows air to exit the tube and pass into the trachea

b. when inflated, it blocks the distal esophagus to prevent regurgitation

c. provides a seal between the patient's face and the plastic portion of the mask housing

d. bag-valve-mask attaches here

e. is the housing for the tube and face cushion; prevents the forced ventilation from regurgitating back out of the patient's mouth

f. connects to the distal cuff; serves as the passageway for air from the syringe to fill the distal cuff

g. used to fill the distal cuff and face cushion

h. snaps in place to hold the EOA tube in place

i. inflates when the distal cuff is inflated so that the health professional can be sure the distal cuff remains inflated

j. is inserted into the esophagus; serves as the air passageway

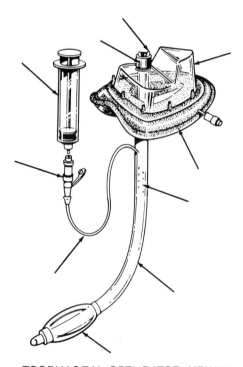

ESOPHAGEAL OBTURATOR AIRWAY

Figure 6–8

18. When inserting the esophageal airway, the patient's head should be placed in a _____ position.

a. sniffing
b. hyperextended
c. neutral
d. flexed

True or False

19. T   F   The airway must be visualized to insert an esophageal airway.

20. T   F   Prior to inserting an esophageal airway, the mask should be attached to the tube.

21. T   F   The esophageal airway helps minimize gastric distension during artificial ventilation.

22. Number the correct sequence for securing the airway with an esophageal airway:

_____ Inflate the distal cuff with 30 to 35 ml of air.

_____ Attach the mask to the tube.

_____ Insert the tube in the midline, following the natural curvature of the pharynx.

_____ Pass the tube directly into the esophagus and advance it until the mask rests on the patient's face.

_____ Use the tongue-jaw lift to prepare for insertion.

_____ Check to see if the EOA is in the proper location; verify ventilation.

_____ Insert the tube blindly into the mouth.

_____ Hyperventilate the patient with a bag-valve-mask and 100% O_2.

_____ Recheck for proper location of the EOA.

True or False

23. T   F   The EOA eliminates the need to maintain hyperextension of the neck during assisted ventilation.

24. T   F   It is necessary to check the EOA for proper placement before and after inflation of the distal cuff.

25. List possible hazards associated with use of the EOA.

_____

_____

_____

26. Briefly explain why the EOA should only be used in unconscious patients.

_____

_____

_____

27. List three contraindications for use of an EOA.

1) _____

_____

2) _____

_____

3) _____

_____

28. T   F   The EOA can be removed as soon as the patient is admitted to the hospital.

29. In Figure 6–9, label each esophageal gastric tube airway component with the letter of the function that it performs:

   a. when inflated, it blocks the distal esophagus to prevent regurgitation
   b. provides a seal between the patient's face and the plastic portion of the mask housing
   c. bag-valve-mask attaches here
   d. the housing for the tube, air port, and face cushion
   e. is inserted into the stomach to relieve excess pressure and unwanted substances
   f. connects to the distal cuff; serves as passageway for air from the syringe to fill the distal cuff
   g. used to fill the distal cuff and face cushion with air
   h. snaps in place to hold the tube in place
   i. the housing for the esophageal tube
   j. is inserted into the esophagus
   k. inflates when the distal cuff is inflated so that the health professional can be sure the distal cuff remains inflated

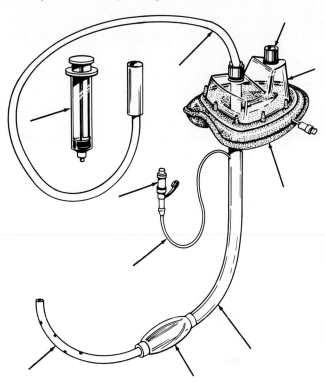

ESOPHAGEAL GASTRIC TUBE AIRWAY

Figure 6–9

30. Match the following characteristics with each of the devices listed. Some characteristics may apply to both devices.

Device

   a. EOA (esophageal obturator airway)
   b. EGTA (esophageal gastric tube airway)

Characteristics

_____ ventilate through the esophageal tube

_____ ventilate through the face mask

_____ inflate distal cuff with 30 to 35 ml air

_____ gastric distention can be relieved when distal cuff is inflated

_____ a tight mask to face seal must be maintained to provide adequate forced ventilation

_____ the face mask must be removed before endotracheal intubation can be performed

31. Describe the technique for removing the EOA/EGTA mask prior to endotracheal intubation.

_____

_____

_____

32. Which of the following are true about endotracheal intubation?

   a. should always be performed as a first step in CPR

   b. should always be preceded by oxygenation of the lung by other methods of ventilation

   c. allows adequate lung inflation without causing gastric distention

   d. should not be attempted by persons inexperienced in the technique

   e. may be improperly performed so that only one lung is ventilated

   f. is preferred over EOA/EGTA intubation

33. Endotracheal intubation should not be attempted (more than one may be correct):

   a. unless it can be completed in less than 30 seconds

   b. in a conscious patient

   c. while an EOA/EGTA is in place

   d. if there are not adequate means to suction the patient for regurgitation

   e. until all necessary equipment is prepared

34. Label Figure 6–10.

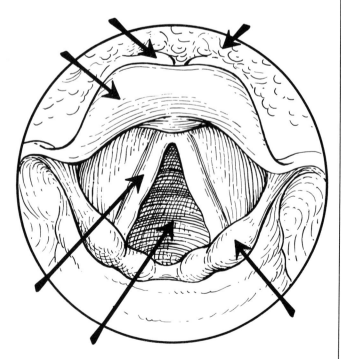

Figure 6–10

35. Label each component of the laryngoscope (Figure 6–11).

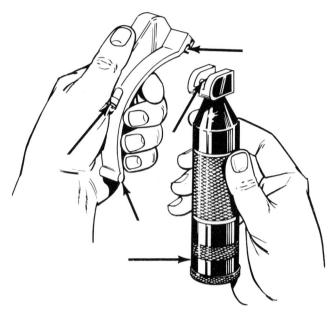

Figure 6–11

36. In Figure 6–12, label each endotracheal tube component with the letter of the function it performs:

   a. when inflated, it seals and protects the trachea from aspiration of foreign materials

   b. bag-valve-mask attaches here

   c. inflates when the distal cuff is inflated so that the health professional can be sure that the distal cuff remains properly filled

   d. connects to the distal cuff; serves as passageway for air from the syringe to fill the distal cuff

   e. is inserted into the trachea

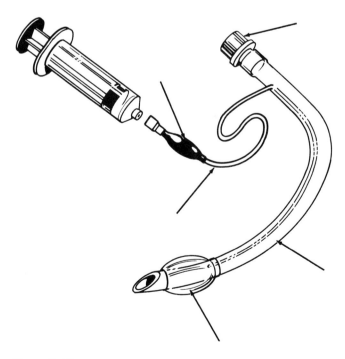

Figure 6–12

37. Describe what is meant by the "sniffing position."

_____

_____

_____

38. List the advantages of endotracheal intubation.

1) _____

2) _____

3) _____

4) _____

39. Number the correct sequence for securing the airway with an endotracheal tube:

_____ Position the patient's head.

_____ Insert the tube into the trachea until the cuff is past the vocal cords.

_____ Insert the blade of the laryngoscope along the right side of the tongue at the base and displace the tongue to the left.

_____ Visualize the vocal cords.

_____ Hyperventilate the patient with 100% oxygen.

_____ Check placement of the endotracheal tube and then inflate the distal cuff with 10 ml of air.

_____ Lift the laryngoscope handle slightly upward and forward to displace the jaw.

_____ Ventilate the patient and tape the endotracheal tube in place.

_____ Recheck the placement of the endotracheal tube.

_____ Hyperventilate the patient again with 100% oxygen.

40. Which of the following statements about the laryngoscope are true?

a. It is used to lift the tongue out of the way so the glottis may be visualized.

b. Its blades come in only one size and/or style.

c. Attachment of the blade to the handle is done by inserting the U-shaped indentation of the blade onto the small bar at the top of the handle.

d. "Locking" the blade onto the handle can be done by pressing the blade backward against and onto the handle's bar.

e. It is held with the left hand.

41. Before insertion of an endotracheal tube, the distal cuff should be checked for:

a. firmness

b. compliance

c. leakage

d. easy deflation

True or False

42. T F The reason for recessing the end of a malleable stylette at least one-half inch from the endotracheal tube opening is to prevent damaging the distal cuff during tube insertion.

43. Number the correct sequence for endotracheal intubation when an esophageal airway is in place:

_____ Connect the blade and handle.

_____ Visualize the epiglottis and vocal cords.

_____ Inflate the distal cuff with 5 to 10 ml of air.

_____ Check for proper placement of the endotracheal tube.

_____ Hyperventilate the patient and remove the EOA.

_____ Hold the laryngoscope in the left hand.

_____ Insert the laryngoscope into the right side of the mouth.

_____ Move the tongue and EOA to the left.

_____ Hyperventilate the patient with 100% oxygen.

_____ Lift the laryngoscope handle slightly upward and forward to displace the jaw.

_____ Recheck placement of the endotracheal tube and hyperventilate with 100% oxygen; then tape the tube in place.

_____ Remove the EOA mask.

_____ Insert the endotracheal tube between the vocal cords.

44. Match the list of standards below with their most fitting description:

Description

_____ standard 15-mm adaptor

_____ average adult-size endotracheal tube

_____ endotracheal tube size for children

_____ amount of air to inflate distal endotracheal tube cuff in adults

_____ amount of air to inflate distal endotracheal tube cuff in children over 8 years old

_____ amount of air to inflate distal endotracheal tube cuff for children less than 8 years old

Standard

a. 12.0-mm ID
b. no cuff used
c. 8.0-mm ID
d. attaches to bag-valve-mask device
e. 5 to 10 ml
f. 30 to 35 ml
g. same as outside diameter of patient's little finger
h. 5 ml

45. Match the means of recognizing and treating each hazard of endotracheal intubation:

Hazard	Recognition	Treatment
esophageal intubation	_____	_____
right bronchial intubation	_____	_____
time delay induced hypoxia	_____	_____

Recognition

a. failure of the chest to rise during ventilation, absence of breath sounds, gurgling of epigastrum upon auscultation
b. poor patient color, failure to respond to appropriate treatment
c. adequate lung sounds on right side of chest, but diminished or absent sounds on left side during ventilation
d. gurgling sounds heard upon auscultation, frothy sputum regurgitating back through the endotracheal tube

Treatment

e. allow only 15 to 20 seconds for each intubation attempt; hyperventilate with 100% oxygen before and after each attempt
f. withdraw the endotracheal tube until adequate lung sounds are heard
g. remove endotracheal tube and reattempt intubation after adequately ventilating and oxygenating the patient
h. suction endotracheal tube and hyperventilate again with 100% oxygen

True or False

46. T   F   Once an endotracheal tube is in place, ventilations should be synchronized with chest compressions.

47. In Figure 6–13, label the components of the bag-valve-mask unit with the letter of their description of each:

  a. face mask

  b. oxygen reservoir

  c. nonrebreathing valve

  d. oxygen supply

  e. intake valve/oxygen reservoir valve

  f. compressible, self-filling bag

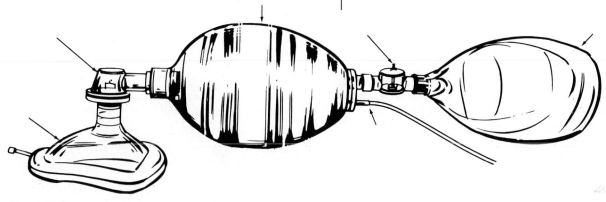

Figure 6–13

48. Which of the following are true statements about bag-valve-mask devices?

  a. should only be used by trained personnel

  b. should be designed to deliver 100% oxygen

  c. can be applied effectively by one person

  d. usually provide better ventilation than mouth-to-mouth

  e. should have a self-expanding bag and transparent mask

49. A bag-valve-mask device will deliver 100% oxygen when it is supplied with:

  a. 2 to 3 liters of supplemental oxygen

  b. 6 to 10 liters of supplemental oxygen

  c. 10 to 15 liters of supplemental oxygen

  d. 10 to 15 liters of supplemental oxygen and a reservoir bag with tubing

50. Number the correct sequence for ventilating a patient with a bag-valve-mask device.

_____ Hyperextend the patient's head to maintain an open airway.

_____ Attach a 100% oxygen supply line to the device.

_____ With one hand, hold the mask to the patient's face and make a tight seal.

_____ Position yourself behind the patient's head.

_____ Squeeze the bag as completely as possible to force air into the lungs.

_____ Select the proper-size mask.

_____ Position the mask over the patient's face with the apex of the mask over the bridge of the nose and the base resting between the lower lip and the chin projection.

_____ Clear the airway if necessary.

51. In Figure 6–14, label the components of the pocket mask with the letter of that part.

    a. face mask
    b. oxygen inlet nipple
    c. ventilation port
    d. head strap

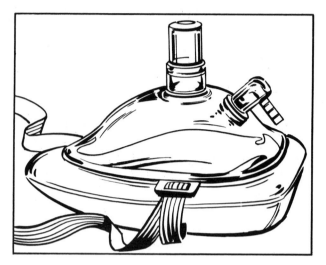

Figure 6–14

52. Number the correct sequence for ventilating a patient with a pocket mask.

    _____ Insert an oropharyngeal airway.

    _____ Establish a seal with the mask.

    _____ Connect the oxygen tubing to the mask; set at 10 to 15 liters.

    _____ Establish an airway with a head tilt.

    _____ Ventilate the patient with at least 800 ml of air in each breath.

53. In Figure 6–15, label the components of the oxygen-powered breathing device with the letter of that part:

    a. face mask
    b. nonrebreathing patient valve
    c. oxygen source
    d. control button

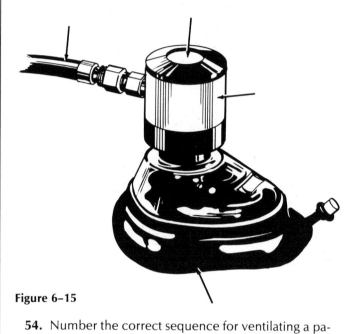

Figure 6–15

54. Number the correct sequence for ventilating a patient with an oxygen-powered breathing device.

    _____ Open the reducing valve.

    _____ Connect regulator to oxygen source.

    _____ Establish a seal with the mask.

    _____ Establish an airway with a head tilt.

    _____ Select the appropriate-size mask.

    _____ Insert an oropharyngeal airway.

    _____ Ventilate the patient with at least 800 ml of air in each ventilation.

55. The upper limit for airway suctioning duration is _____ seconds.

    a. 5
    b. 10
    c. 30
    d. 60

56. Number the correct sequence for suctioning the airway.

_____ Allow airflow to return.

_____ Withdraw catheter, rotating it between fingertips.

_____ Hyperventilate the patient.

_____ Measure the catheter from the patient's earlobe to his lips to determine the depth of insertion.

_____ Insert catheter to predetermined length.

_____ Apply suction for no more than recommended duration.

ANSWER KEY

1. TRUE

2. FALSE: Chest pain alone or in combination with respiratory distress should be treated with oxygen.

3. TRUE

4. TRUE

5. nasal cannula: e (Figure 6–16)
   simple face mask: a (Figure 6–17)
   nonrebreather mask: b (Figure 6–18)
   bag-valve-mask: c (Figure 6–19)

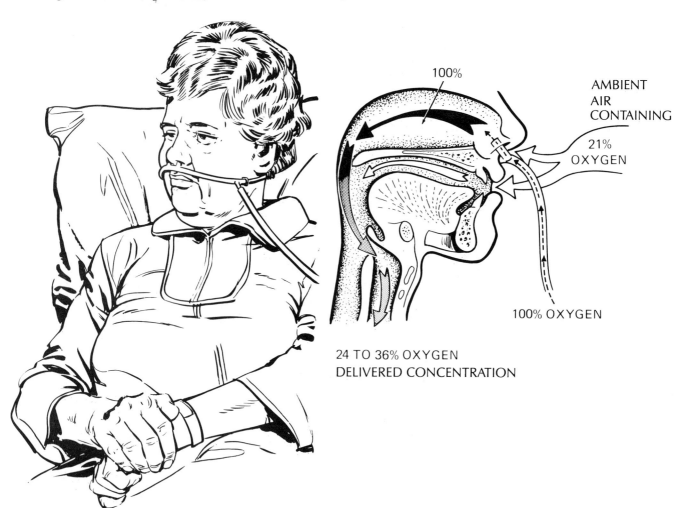

Figure 6–16

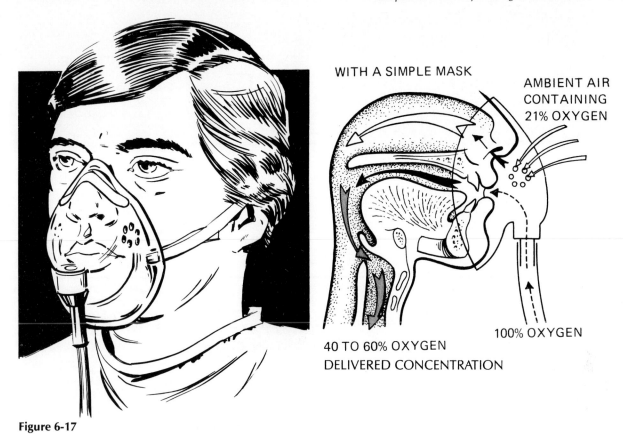

WITH A SIMPLE MASK

AMBIENT AIR CONTAINING 21% OXYGEN

40 TO 60% OXYGEN DELIVERED CONCENTRATION

100% OXYGEN

Figure 6-17

nonrebreather mask: b;

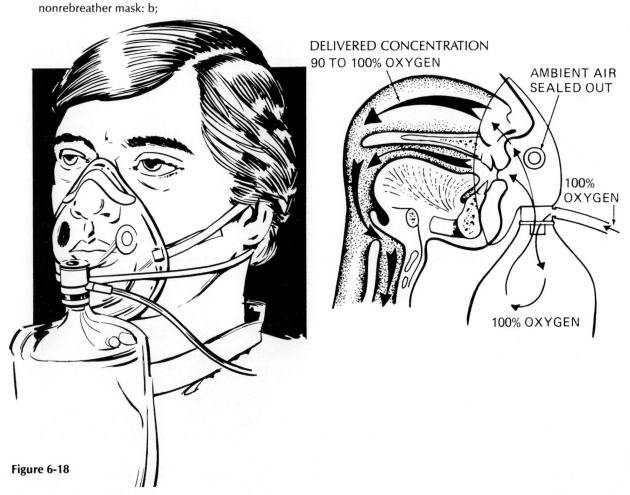

DELIVERED CONCENTRATION 90 TO 100% OXYGEN

AMBIENT AIR SEALED OUT

100% OXYGEN

100% OXYGEN

Figure 6-18

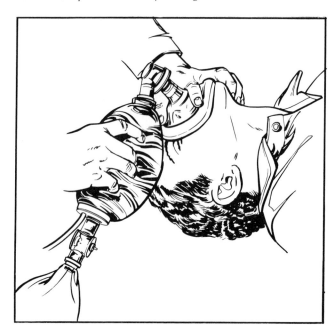

Figure 6-19

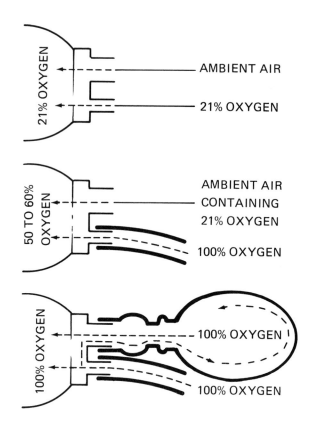

- 21% OXYGEN — AMBIENT AIR
- 21% OXYGEN

- 50 TO 60% OXYGEN — AMBIENT AIR CONTAINING
- 21% OXYGEN
- 100% OXYGEN

- 100% OXYGEN — 100% OXYGEN
- 100% OXYGEN — 100% OXYGEN

6. d

7. upper airway obstruction due to foreign material: b
posterior displacement of the tongue: c
absence of spontaneous breathing: a

8. Figure B has an open airway (Figure 6-20)

9. HEAD TILT/CHIN LIFT: Place one hand on the forehead and apply firm, backward pressure with the palm to tilt the head back. Place the fingers of the other hand under the bony part of the lower jaw near the chin and lift the chin forward. This will pull the tongue away from the posterior oropharynx and open the airway. See Figure 6-21.

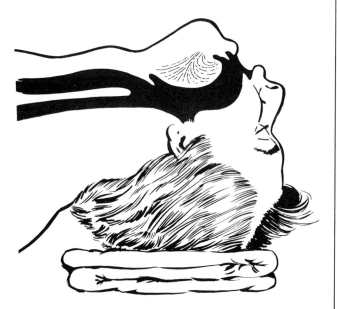

Figure 6-20

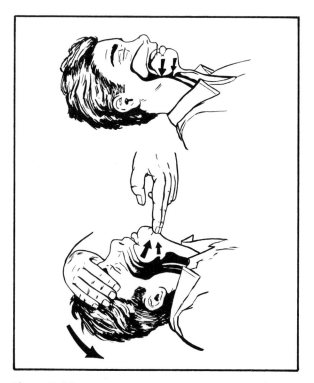

Figure 6-21

JAW THRUST: The index fingers should be bent to conform to the angles of the jaw. The jaw can then be lifted upward by pulling up on the angles of the jaw. This motion will lift the chin forward and displace the tongue away from the posterior oropharynx. See Figure 6–22.

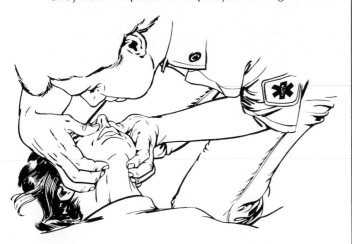

Figure 6–22

10. endotracheal tube: d   oropharyngeal airway: c
    nasopharyngeal airway: b   esophageal obturator: a
    esophageal gastric tube airway: e

11. Insert the oropharyngeal airway into the pharynx in a backward (rotated) position (Figure 6–23). As the airway traverses the oral cavity and approaches the posterior wall of the pharynx near the base of the tongue, rotate the airway 180 degrees into its proper anatomical position (Figure 6–24).

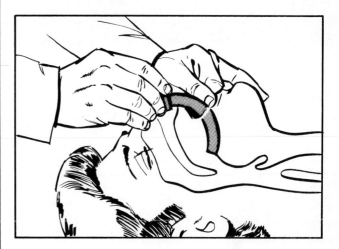

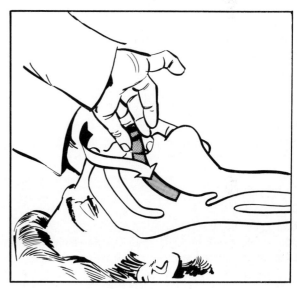

Figure 6–23 and Figure 6–24

12. FALSE: The oropharyngeal airway should be used only in unconscious patients.

13. TRUE

14. TRUE

15. To insert a nasopharyngeal airway, lubricate the tube for ease of insertion. Place the airway into a nostril and, with gentle pressure, insert the airway toward the medial aspect until the flange comes to rest against the nares. If resistance is met, remove the airway and reinsert it into the other nostril; never force the airway against resistance.

16. The primary reason for using the nasopharyngeal airway is that it is better tolerated in responsive patients.

17. Components and functions of an esophageal obturator airway are given in Figure 6–25.

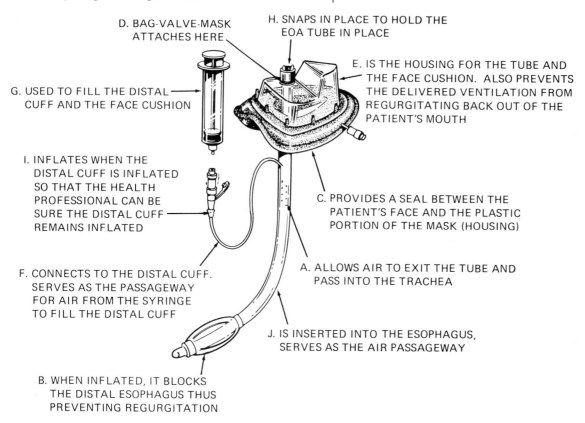

D. BAG-VALVE-MASK ATTACHES HERE

H. SNAPS IN PLACE TO HOLD THE EOA TUBE IN PLACE

E. IS THE HOUSING FOR THE TUBE AND THE FACE CUSHION. ALSO PREVENTS THE DELIVERED VENTILATION FROM REGURGITATING BACK OUT OF THE PATIENT'S MOUTH

G. USED TO FILL THE DISTAL CUFF AND THE FACE CUSHION

I. INFLATES WHEN THE DISTAL CUFF IS INFLATED SO THAT THE HEALTH PROFESSIONAL CAN BE SURE THE DISTAL CUFF REMAINS INFLATED

C. PROVIDES A SEAL BETWEEN THE PATIENT'S FACE AND THE PLASTIC PORTION OF THE MASK (HOUSING)

F. CONNECTS TO THE DISTAL CUFF. SERVES AS THE PASSAGEWAY FOR AIR FROM THE SYRINGE TO FILL THE DISTAL CUFF

A. ALLOWS AIR TO EXIT THE TUBE AND PASS INTO THE TRACHEA

J. IS INSERTED INTO THE ESOPHAGUS, SERVES AS THE AIR PASSAGEWAY

B. WHEN INFLATED, IT BLOCKS THE DISTAL ESOPHAGUS THUS PREVENTING REGURGITATION

Figure 6–25

18. c

19. FALSE: The esophageal airway can be inserted into the esophagus "blindly" (i.e., without visualization).

20. TRUE: Attachment is difficult following insertion and uses time that could be better spent in ventilating the patient.

21. TRUE

22. Esophageal airway insertion is shown in Figure 6–26.

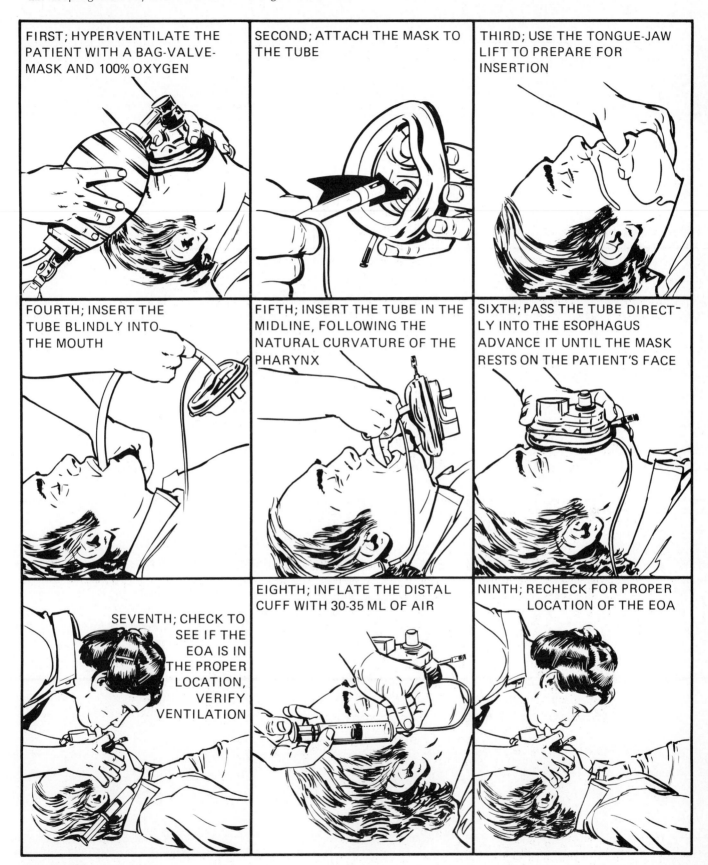

Figure 6–26

23. TRUE: Though the rescuer will find that ventilation is more effective when hyperextension is maintained.

24. TRUE

25. Possible hazards with EOA: (1) esophageal lacerations, rupture and (2) inadvertent endotracheal intubation. Endotracheal intubation is the most common and dangerous complication of an EOA.

26. The EOA should only be used in unconscious patients because the airway may stimulate the patient's gag reflex and cause regurgitation and aspiration.

27. Contraindications for use of EOA: (1) patients under 16 years of age or less than 5 feet tall, (2) known cases of esophageal disease, (3) when caustic poisons have been ingested, or (4) when victim is conscious or spontaneously breathing.

28. FALSE: The EOA should only be removed if the patient regains spontaneous breathing or consciousness, or after endotracheal intubation with an endotracheal tube.

29. Components and functions of the esophageal gastric tube airway are shown in Figure 6–27.

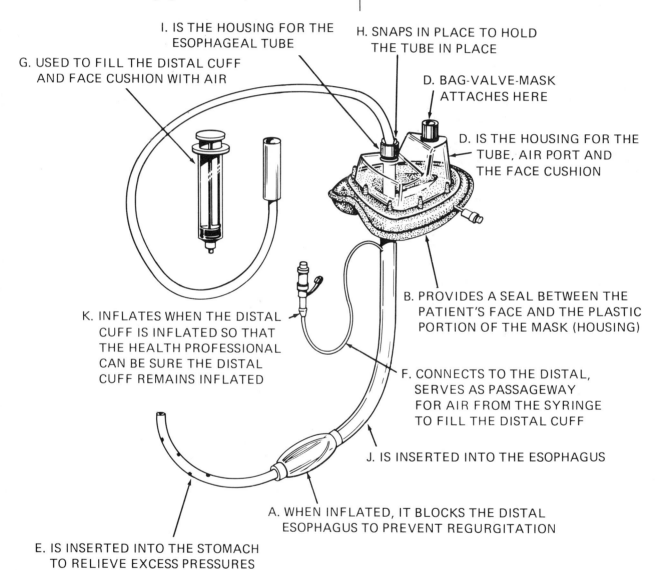

I. IS THE HOUSING FOR THE ESOPHAGEAL TUBE

G. USED TO FILL THE DISTAL CUFF AND FACE CUSHION WITH AIR

H. SNAPS IN PLACE TO HOLD THE TUBE IN PLACE

D. BAG-VALVE-MASK ATTACHES HERE

D. IS THE HOUSING FOR THE TUBE, AIR PORT AND THE FACE CUSHION

K. INFLATES WHEN THE DISTAL CUFF IS INFLATED SO THAT THE HEALTH PROFESSIONAL CAN BE SURE THE DISTAL CUFF REMAINS INFLATED

B. PROVIDES A SEAL BETWEEN THE PATIENT'S FACE AND THE PLASTIC PORTION OF THE MASK (HOUSING)

F. CONNECTS TO THE DISTAL, SERVES AS PASSAGEWAY FOR AIR FROM THE SYRINGE TO FILL THE DISTAL CUFF

J. IS INSERTED INTO THE ESOPHAGUS

A. WHEN INFLATED, IT BLOCKS THE DISTAL ESOPHAGUS TO PREVENT REGURGITATION

E. IS INSERTED INTO THE STOMACH TO RELIEVE EXCESS PRESSURES AND UNWANTED SUBSTANCES

Figure 6–27

30. Both EOA and EGTA: Inflate the distal cuff with 30 to 35 ml of air. A tight mask-to-face seal must be maintained to provide adequate forced ventilation. The face mask must be removed before endotracheal intubation can be performed.

EGTA: Ventilate through the face mask. Gastric distention can be relieved when the distal cuff is inflated.

EOA: Ventilate through the esophageal tube.

31. To remove the EOA/EGTA mask, squeeze the plastic prongs of the tube together where they project through the mask and slide the mask up and off the tube.

32. b, c, d, e, f

33. a, d, e

34. Figure 6–28 shows the glottic opening.

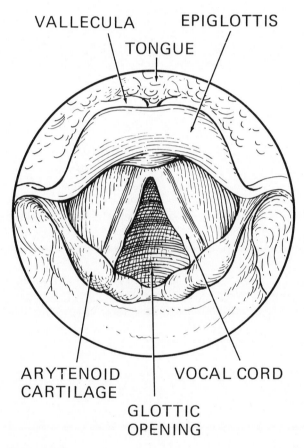

Figure 6–28

35. Components of the laryngoscope are shown in Figure 6–29.

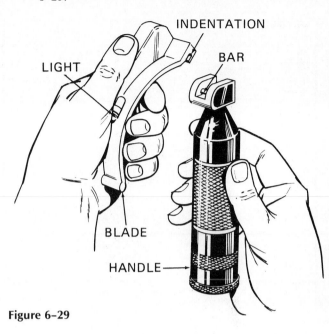

Figure 6–29

36. Components and functions of the endotracheal tube are shown in Figure 6–30.

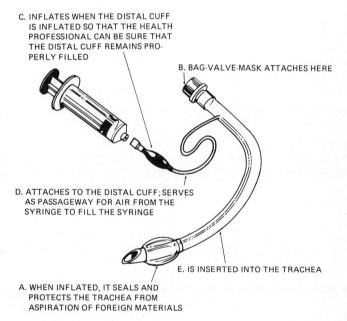

C. INFLATES WHEN THE DISTAL CUFF IS INFLATED SO THAT THE HEALTH PROFESSIONAL CAN BE SURE THAT THE DISTAL CUFF REMAINS PROPERLY FILLED

B. BAG-VALVE-MASK ATTACHES HERE

D. ATTACHES TO THE DISTAL CUFF; SERVES AS PASSAGEWAY FOR AIR FROM THE SYRINGE TO FILL THE SYRINGE

E. IS INSERTED INTO THE TRACHEA

A. WHEN INFLATED, IT SEALS AND PROTECTS THE TRACHEA FROM ASPIRATION OF FOREIGN MATERIALS

Figure 6–30

37. The "sniffing position" is with the neck flexed forward and the head extended backward (see Figure 6–31).

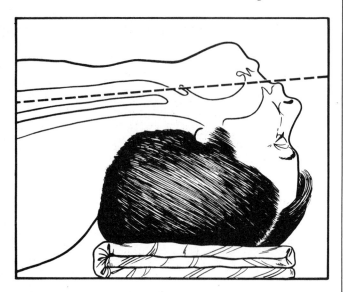

Figure 6–31

38. Advantages of endotracheal intubation are that it (1) protects the airway from aspiration, (2) allows for intermittent ventilation with 100% oxygen, (3) makes the trachea available for suctioning, and (4) eliminates the potential for gastric distention.

39. The sequence for endotracheal intubation is shown in Figure 6–32.

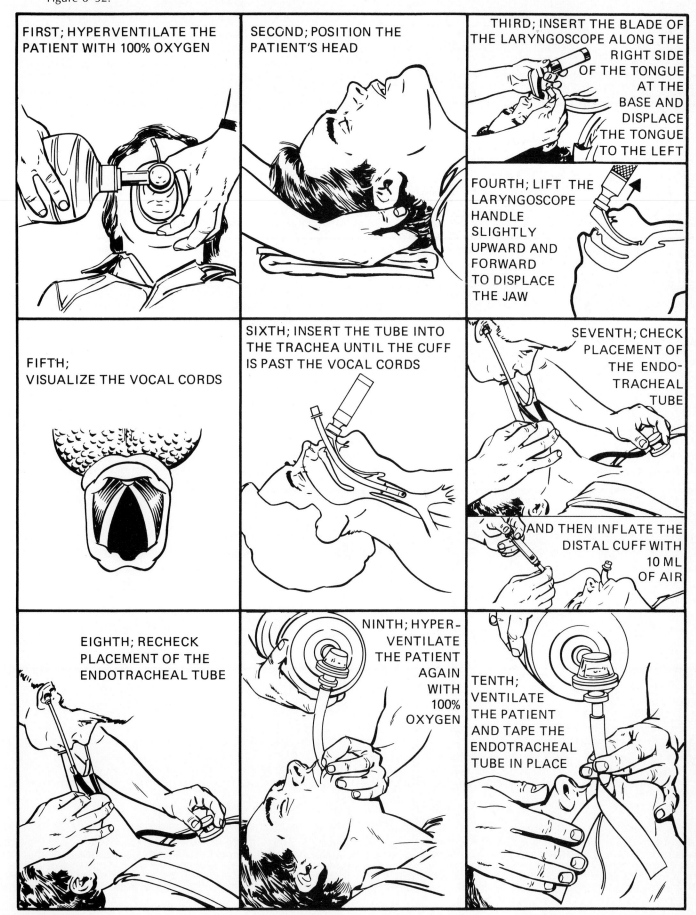

FIRST; HYPERVENTILATE THE PATIENT WITH 100% OXYGEN

SECOND; POSITION THE PATIENT'S HEAD

THIRD; INSERT THE BLADE OF THE LARYNGOSCOPE ALONG THE RIGHT SIDE OF THE TONGUE AT THE BASE AND DISPLACE THE TONGUE TO THE LEFT

FOURTH; LIFT THE LARYNGOSCOPE HANDLE SLIGHTLY UPWARD AND FORWARD TO DISPLACE THE JAW

FIFTH; VISUALIZE THE VOCAL CORDS

SIXTH; INSERT THE TUBE INTO THE TRACHEA UNTIL THE CUFF IS PAST THE VOCAL CORDS

SEVENTH; CHECK PLACEMENT OF THE ENDOTRACHEAL TUBE

AND THEN INFLATE THE DISTAL CUFF WITH 10 ML OF AIR

EIGHTH; RECHECK PLACEMENT OF THE ENDOTRACHEAL TUBE

NINTH; HYPERVENTILATE THE PATIENT AGAIN WITH 100% OXYGEN

TENTH; VENTILATE THE PATIENT AND TAPE THE ENDOTRACHEAL TUBE IN PLACE

Figure 6–32

40. a, c, e

41. c

42. FALSE: The malleable stylette is recessed at least one-half inch from the endotracheal tube opening to prevent pharyngeal, laryngeal, or tracheal trauma from the stylette during intubation.

43. Sequence for endotracheal intubation with an esophageal airway in place.

1st: Hyperventilate the patient with 100% oxygen.
2nd: Connect the blade and handle.
3rd: Remove the EOA mask.
4th: Hold the laryngoscope in the left hand.
5th: Insert the laryngoscope into the right side of the mouth.
6th: Move the tongue and EOA to the left.
7th: Lift the laryngoscope handle slightly upward and forward to displace the jaw.
8th: Visualize the epiglottis and vocal cords.
9th: Insert the endotracheal tube between the vocal cords.
10th: Check for proper placement of the endotracheal tube.
11th: Inflate the distal cuff with 5 to 10 ml of air.
12th: Recheck placement of the endotracheal tube and hyperventilate with 100% oxygen; then tape the tube in place.
13th: Hyperventilate the patient and remove the EOA.

44. d: standard 15-mm adapter
c: average-size adult endotracheal tube
g: average-size endotracheal tube for children
e: amount of air to inflate distal endotracheal tube cuff for adults
h: amount of air to inflate distal endotracheal tube cuff for children over 8 years old
b: amount of air to inflate distal endotracheal tube cuff for children less than 8 years old

45.

Hazard	Recognized by	Treatment
esophageal intubation	a	g
right bronchial intubation	c	f
time delay induced hypoxia	b	e

46. FALSE: Once endotracheal intubation is completed, ventilations do *not* need to be synchronized with chest compressions, but should be provided asynchronously at 12 to 15 per minute.

47. Components of bag-valve-mask device are shown in Figure 6–33.

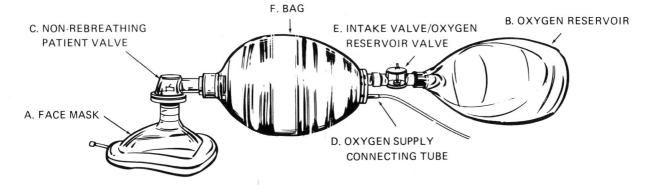

C. NON-REBREATHING PATIENT VALVE
F. BAG
E. INTAKE VALVE/OXYGEN RESERVOIR VALVE
B. OXYGEN RESERVOIR
A. FACE MASK
D. OXYGEN SUPPLY CONNECTING TUBE

Figure 6–33

48. a, b, c, e

49. d

50. The sequence for ventilating with a bag-valve-mask device is shown in Figure 6–34.

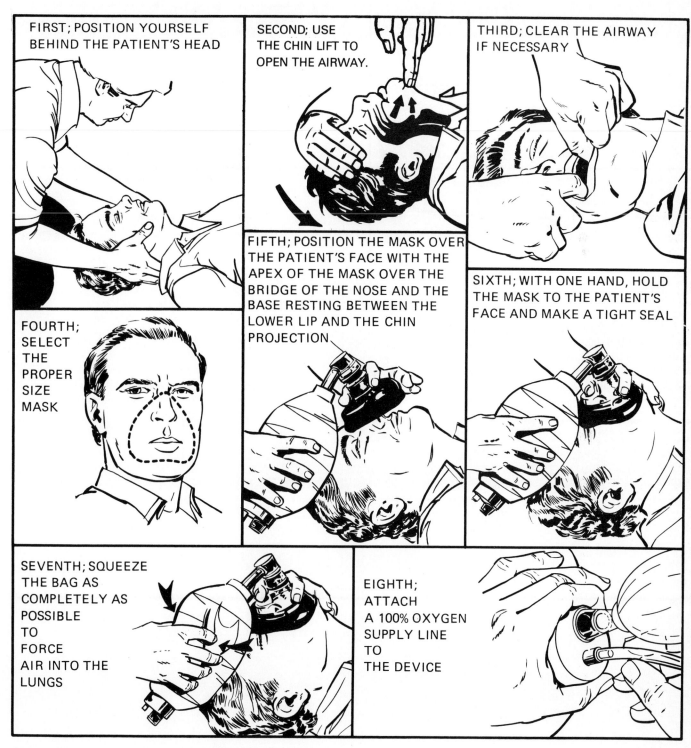

Figure 6–34

51. Components of the pocket mask are shown in Figure 6–35.

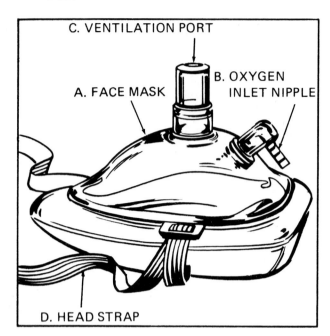

Figure 6–35

52. Sequence for ventilating with a pocket mask:
    1st: Insert an oropharyngeal airway.
    2nd: Establish a seal with the mask.
    3rd: Establish an airway with a head tilt.
    4th: Ventilate the patient with at least 800 ml of air in each breath.
    5th: Connect the oxygen tubing to the mask; set at 10 to 15 liters.

53. Components of an oxygen-powered breathing device are shown in Figure 6–36.

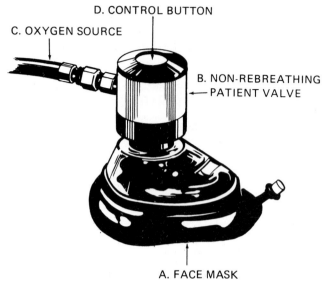

Figure 6–36

54. Sequence for ventilating with an oxygen-powered breathing device:
    1st: Connect regulator to oxygen source.
    2nd: Open the reducing valve.
    3rd: Select the appropriate-size mask.
    4th: Insert an oropharyngeal airway.
    5th: Establish a seal with the mask.
    6th: Establish an airway with a head tilt.
    7th: Ventilate the patient with at least 800 ml of air in each ventilation.

55. a

56. The sequence for upper airway suctioning is shown in
   Figure 6–37.

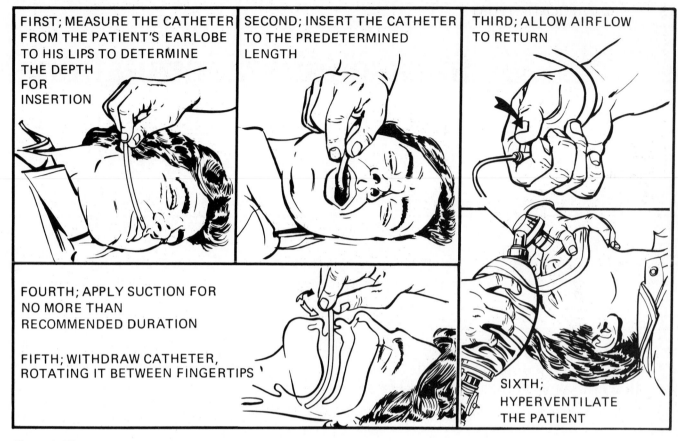

FIRST; MEASURE THE CATHETER FROM THE PATIENT'S EARLOBE TO HIS LIPS TO DETERMINE THE DEPTH FOR INSERTION

SECOND; INSERT THE CATHETER TO THE PREDETERMINED LENGTH

THIRD; ALLOW AIRFLOW TO RETURN

FOURTH; APPLY SUCTION FOR NO MORE THAN RECOMMENDED DURATION

FIFTH; WITHDRAW CATHETER, ROTATING IT BETWEEN FINGERTIPS

SIXTH; HYPERVENTILATE THE PATIENT

Figure 6–37

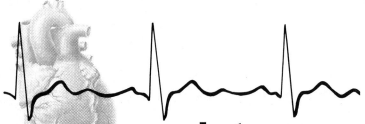

Chapter 7

Intravenous Cannulation–
Supporting Circulation–
Defibrillation

OBJECTIVES

Upon completion of this chapter, you will be able to:

- Describe the preferred sites, means, and practices for parenteral administration of medications in emergency cardiac care.

- Identify the anatomical landmarks used for peripheral and central intravenous cannulation in advanced life support.

- Delineate the recommended procedures for cannulation of peripheral and central veins.

- List the advantages, disadvantages, and complications of peripheral and central venous cannulations.

- Specify how mechanical adjuncts can assist circulation in victims of cardiac arrest.

- Explain the indications and procedures for using MAST trousers in emergency cardiac care.

- Recognize factors that enhance the likelihood of successful cardiac defibrillation.

- Distinguish between the uses of defibrillation and cardioversion in emergency cardiac care.

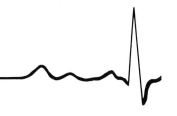

1. List three indications for intravenous cannulation in a cardiac arrest situation.

   1) _____

   2) _____

   3) _____

2. Give two reasons why intravenous administration is preferred over intramuscular injection for a cardiac arrest victim.

   1) _____

   _____

   _____

   2) _____

   _____

   _____

True or False

3. T   F   Plastic catheters are generally preferred over hollow needles in advanced life support.

4. T   F   In emergency cardiac care, intracardiac injections are considered hazardous and may cause cardiac tamponade.

5. T   F   The preferred sites for IV cannulation during cardiac arrest are the external jugular and subclavian veins.

6. A plastic IV bag can be kept running during patient transport by

   a. lowering it below the level of the IV site
   b. closing off the IV flow adjustment
   c. placing the bag under the patient's shoulder
   d. detaching the IV line from the IV cannula

7. Label the veins in Figure 7–1.

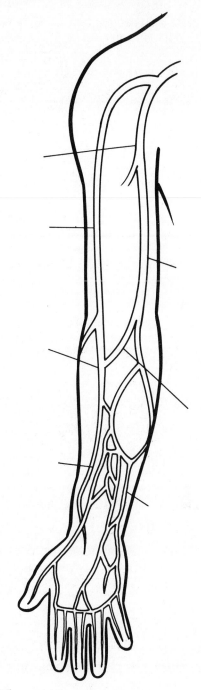

Figure 7–1

True or False

8. T   F   Antecubital veins should always be used first because they are the largest veins in the arm.

9. T   F   If the long saphenous vein is utilized, it should be entered at its most distal point.

10. T   F   A vein should be entered at its junction with another vein.

11. Number the correct sequence for initiating IV therapy in an arm or a leg vein.

_____ Anesthetize the skin if a large-bore cannula is to be inserted in an awake patient; select as large a catheter as possible.

_____ Note blood return and advance catheter either over or through the needle depending on the device employed.

_____ Remove the tourniquet.

_____ Withdraw and remove the needle and attach the infusion tubing.

_____ Apply a tourniquet proximally.

_____ Puncture the skin with the bevel of the needle upward about 0.5 to 1.0 cm from the vein; enter the vein from the top or side.

_____ Hold the vein in place by applying pressure on it distal to the point of entry.

_____ Locate the vein and cleanse the overlying skin with alcohol or povidone iodine.

_____ Cover the site with povidone iodine ointment and a sterile dressing; tape dressing and catheter in place.

12. List three advantages of antecubital venipuncture.

1) _____

2) _____

3) _____

13. Describe two disadvantages of distal extremity venipuncture.

_____

_____

_____

14. Label the anatomical structures in Figure 7–2.

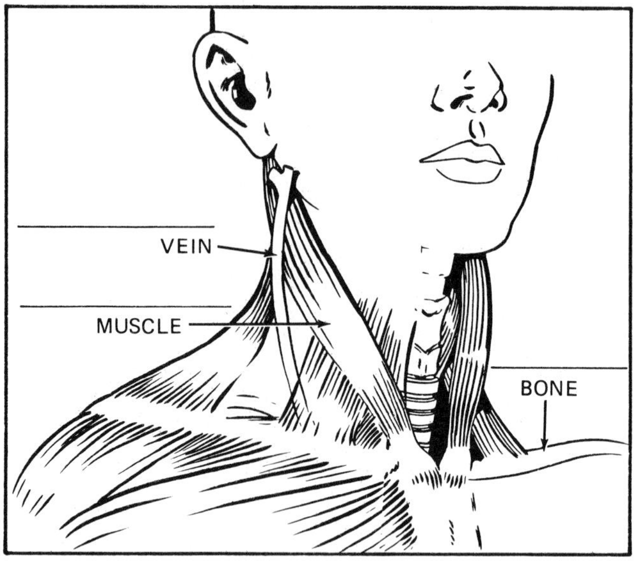

VEIN

MUSCLE

BONE

Figure 7–2

15. Number the correct sequence for initiating IV therapy in the external jugular vein.

_____ Make the venipuncture midway between the angle of the jaw and the midclavicular line.

_____ Tourniquet the vein lightly with one finger above the clavicle.

_____ Locate the vein and cleanse the overlying skin with alcohol or povidone iodine.

_____ Place the patient in a supine, head-down position to fill the vein; turn the patient's head toward the opposite side.

_____ Anesthetize the skin if a large-bore cannula is to be inserted in an awake patient.

_____ Note blood return and advance the catheter.

_____ Align the cannula in the direction of the vein with the point aimed toward the ipsilateral shoulder.

_____ Withdraw and remove the needle and attach the infusion tubing.

_____ Hold the vein in place by applying pressure on the vein distal to the point of entry at the angle of the mandible.

_____ Puncture the skin with the bevel of the needle upward about 0.5 to 1.0 cm from the vein; enter the vein from the top or side.

_____ Cover the site with povidone-iodine and a sterile dressing; tape the dressing and catheter in place.

The next four questions refer to Figure 7–3.

16. The rescuer's left index finger is used to:

a. hold the vein stable
b. tourniquet the vein
c. provide a reference point
d. hold the clavicle steady

17. The rescuer's left thumb is used to:

a. hold the vein stable
b. tourniquet the vein
c. provide a reference point
d. stabilize the muscle

18. The needle tip is aimed toward the:

a. angle of the mandible
b. ipsilateral shoulder
c. tracheal notch
d. sternal notch

19. The cannula is aligned parallel to the:

a. jugular vein
b. sternomastoid muscle
c. clavicle
d. chin

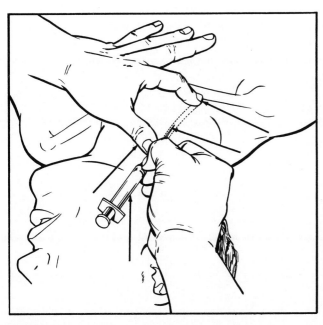

Figure 7–3

20. Label the anatomical structures on Figure 7–4.

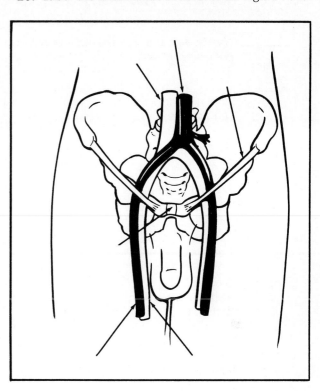

Figure 7–4

True or False

21. T   F   Below the inguinal ligament, the femoral vein runs medial to the femoral artery.

22. T   F   The femoral artery runs directly across the midpoint between the anterior iliac spine and the symphysis pubis.

23. List two ways the femoral artery can be located.

1) _____

2) _____

24. Number the correct sequence for cannulation of the femoral vein.

_____ Locate the femoral artery by either its pulsation or by landmarks.

_____ Lower the needle more parallel to the frontal plane; remove the syringe and insert the catheter.

_____ Infiltrate the skin with lidocaine if the patient is awake.

_____ Maintain suction on the syringe and pull the needle back slowly until blood appears in the syringe.

_____ Cleanse the overlying skin with povidone iodine.

_____ Puncture the skin with the needle attached to a 5- or 10-ml syringe two fingers-breadth below the inguinal ligament, medial to the artery, directing the needle cephalad at a 45- or 90-degree angle, until the needle will go no farther.

_____ Attach the infusion tubing; cover the site with povidone iodine ointment and a sterile dressing; secure the catheter in place.

_____ Withdraw the needle, leaving the catheter in place; remove the stylette.

The next four questions relate to Figure 7–5.

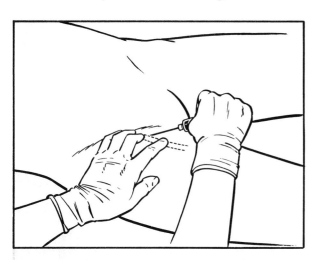

Figure 7–5

True or False

25. T   F   The needle tip is aimed toward the patient's heart.

26. T   F   The skin is punctured medial to the femoral artery.

27. T   F   The needle should be inserted until it will go no farther.

28. T   F   Negative pressure should be maintained on the syringe as the needle is slowly pulled backward until blood appears in the syringe upon entry into the vein.

29. List three advantages of using the femoral vein cannulation in cardiac arrest situations.

1) _____

_____

2) _____

_____

3) _____

_____

30. What are two disadvantages of using femoral vein cannulation in cardiac arrest situations?

1) _____

_____

2) _____

_____

31. Name three specific complications of using femoral veins for IV therapy.

1) _____

2) _____

3) _____

32. Label the anatomical structures in Figure 7–6.

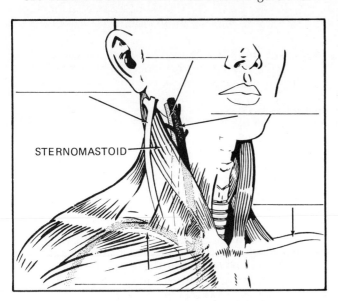

STERNOMASTOID

Figure 7–6

33. Label the anatomical structures in the sagittal view of the medial clavicle as illustrated in Figure 7–7.

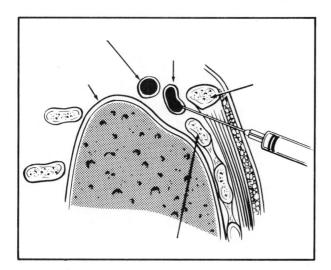

Figure 7–7

34. Which of the following are TRUE statements regarding the subclavian vein?

a. It may remain patent when peripheral veins have collapsed.

b. It can be used to provide access for measuring central venous pressure.

c. It cannot be used to administer hypotonic or irritating solutions.

d. It can be used to pass catheters into the heart or pulmonary circulation.

e. It is generally cannulated by a catheter-over-needle device.

35. Label the anatomical landmarks in Figure 7–8 used to determine catheter placement.

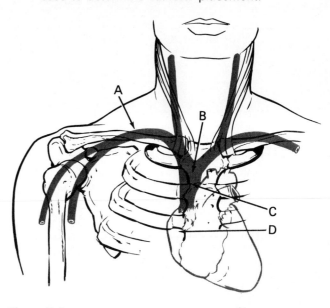

Figure 7–8

36. T   F   The proper catheter and needle size for cannulating the subclavian vein is a 14-gauge needle at least 6 cm long with a 16-gauge, 15- to 20-cm-long catheter.

37. What should be done if bright red blood suddenly appears in the syringe and pushes the plunger up during an attempt to cannulate the subclavian vein?

_____

_____

_____

38. What should be done if the subclavian vein is not entered despite insertion of the needle to the proper depth?

_____

_____

_____

39. After entering the subclavian vein, why is it necessary to occlude the needle opening following removal of the syringe?

_____

_____

40. Why is it dangerous to pull an IV catheter backward when using a catheter-through-needle system?

_____

_____

_____

41. Number the correct sequence for initiating IV therapy using the subclavian vein.

_____ Hold the syringe and needle parallel to the frontal plane.

_____ Establish a point of reference by firmly pressing the fingertip of the opposite hand into the suprasternal notch to locate the deep side of the superior aspect of the clavicle.

_____ Direct the course of the needle slightly behind the fingertip.

_____ Direct the needle medially and slightly cephalad toward the superior aspect of the sternal end of the clavicle.

_____ Once the vein is entered, rotate the bevel of the needle caudally and clockwise 90 degrees.

_____ Place the patient in a supine, head-down position of at least 15 degrees.

_____ Introduce the needle 1 cm below the junction of the middle and medial thirds of the clavicle.

_____ Remove the syringe and insert the catheter.

_____ Infiltrate the skin with lidocaine if the patient is awake.

_____ Maintain suction of the syringe and advance the needle until blood appears in the syringe, indicating that the lumen of the vein has been entered.

_____ Withdraw the needle, leaving the catheter in place; remove the stylette.

_____ Cleanse the overlying skin with povidone iodine.

_____ Attach the infusion tubing, cover the site with povidone iodine ointment and a sterile dressing; secure the catheter and infusion tubing in place.

42. T   F   The left subclavian vein is preferred over the right subclavian vein for emergency cannulation.

43. Place an ✕ on Figure 7–9 to denote where the needle should be introduced when cannulating the subclavian vein.

A - LATERAL THIRD OF CLAVICLE
B - MIDDLE THIRD OF CLAVICLE
C - MEDIAL THIRD OF CLAVICLE

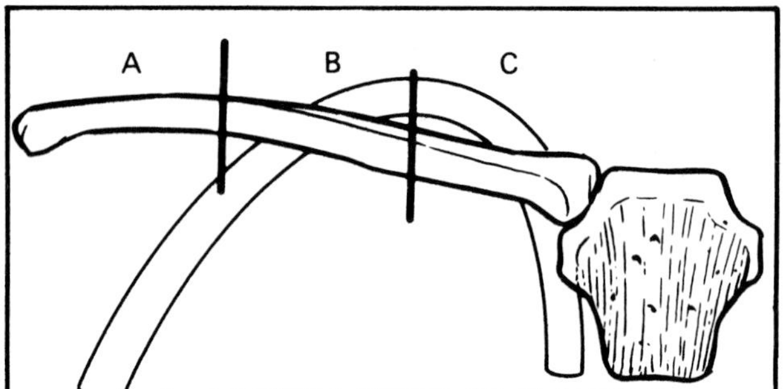

Figure 7–9

44. List three disadvantages of subclavian venipuncture.

1) _____

_____

2) _____

_____

3) _____

_____

45. List three systemic complications of subclavian venipuncture.

1) _____

2) _____

3) _____

46. Which of the following can help to minimize infectious complications of intravenous therapy?

a. careful aseptic technique during insertion
b. using IV bottles rather than IV bags
c. removal of the cannula after three days
d. changing administration set every 48 hours
e. infiltrating the skin with lidocaine

47. The major hazard associated with a catheter-through-needle system is:

   a. infection
   b. hematoma
   c. catheter fragment embolism
   d. extravasation of infused fluid

48. List three reasons why the mechanical chest compressor can be an effective adjunct for CPR.

1) _____

   _____

2) _____

   _____

3) _____

   _____

True or False

49. T   F   The automatic chest compressor and ventilator should not interrupt CPR for more than 5 to 10 seconds to be applied and can produce severe injuries if incorrectly applied.

50. T   F   The medical antishock trousers (MAST) can be used to provide a reversible fluid challenge for patients during the postresuscitation period.

51. T   F   MAST trousers are useful for treating acute pulmonary edema.

52. T   F   MAST trousers must be removed for a patient to be x-rayed.

53. T   F   As soon as a patient's blood pressure is raised and stabilized, the MAST trousers should be removed.

54. T   F   When deflating MAST trousers, the abdominal section should be deflated before the leg sections.

55. MAST trousers are indicated for patients with clinical signs of shock who have systolic blood pressures less than _____ mm of Hg.

   a. 150
   b. 120
   c. 100
   d. 90

56. Label the components of the MAST trousers illustrated in Figure 7–10 with the letter of that component.

   a. foot pump
   b. leg sections
   c. abdominal section
   d. tubing
   e. shut-off valve for left leg
   f. shut-off valve for right leg
   g. control box
   h. shut-off valve for abdominal section

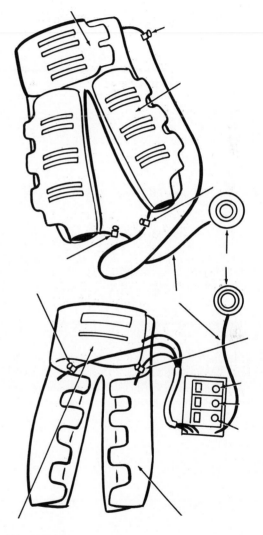

Figure 7–10

57. Number the correct sequence for applying the MAST trousers.

_____ Unfold the garment; lay it flat and smooth out the wrinkles.

_____ Close off the stopcocks (valves).

_____ Logroll the patient onto garment, or slip it under him; upper edge of the garment should be just below the rib cage.

_____ Open the stopcocks (valves).

_____ Enclose the left leg, securing Velcro straps.

_____ Use the foot pump to inflate compartments simultaneously.

_____ Check the patient's blood pressure.

_____ Enclose the abdomen and pelvis, securing the Velcro straps.

_____ Enclose the right leg, securing the Velcro straps.

_____ Check both extremities for distal pulse.

_____ Check the tubes leading to the compartments and the foot pumps.

_____ Monitor and record the vital signs every 5 minutes.

58. Which of the following terms best describes the process of passing electrical current through the heart to depolarize the heart cells and allowing them to repolarize uniformly?

a. precordial thump
b. defibrillation
c. intubation
d. ECG monitoring
e. external cardiac pacing

59. Which of the following statements are TRUE?

a. A "critical mass" is required to maintain ventricular fibrillation.
b. Successful defibrillation depends on depolarization of a sufficient portion of the fibrillating ventricles.
c. The entire myocardium must be depolarized for defibrillation to be successful.
d. Energy requirements for defibrillation are the same regardless of patient size or age.
e. The major determinant of survival in cardiac arrest secondary to ventricular fibrillation is the rapidity with which defibrillation is provided.
f. Defibrillation should always be preceded by CPR.

True or False

60. T   F   The longer ventricular fibrillation persists, the less likely electrical defibrillation will succeed.

61. T   F   To maximize the likelihood that defibrillation will be successful, the electrical resistance of the skin must be reduced.

62. T   F   Repeated countershocks are more likely to be successful than single countershocks in the early management of ventricular fibrillation.

63. T   F   Firm paddle contact pressure can reduce the electrical resistance of the skin by up to 75%.

64. T   F   If ventricular fibrillation is not terminated by one precordial thump, a second precordial thump should be administered.

65. The energy level that should be used to initially defibrillate an adult patient is _____ joules.

a. 50
b. 75
c. 100
d. 200
e. 400

66. The energy level that should be used for the second defibrillation attempt (when the first is unsuccessful) is _____ to _____ joules.

a. 40 to 60
b. 70 to 100
c. 100 to 200
d. 200 to 300
e. 300 to 400

67. What should be done immediately if the second defibrillation attempt is unsuccessful?

_____

_____

_____

68. Number the correct sequence for defibrillating a patient in ventricular fibrillation.

_____ Discharge the paddles.

_____ Order to stop CPR and tell others to "stand clear."

_____ Charge the defibrillator to 200 joules.

_____ Check the pulse and ECG; perform a second defibrillation at 200 to 300 joules if the rhythm is still ventricular fibrillation.

_____ Remove the paddles and continue CPR if a palpable pulse is not present.

_____ Apply the paddles with 20 to 25 lb of pressure.

_____ Apply conductive medium.

_____ Turn defibrillator power on.

_____ Check that the synchronizer switch is off.

_____ Recheck rhythm on monitor before defibrillating.

_____ Defibrillate a third time at up to 360 joules.

True or False

69. T   F   Defibrillating on the patient's bare skin reduces the electrical resistance by up to 50%.

70. T   F   For most defibrillators to deliver a countershock, the buttons on BOTH defibrillator paddles must be depressed.

71. For which of the following conditions is synchronized countershock (cardioversion) indicated?

a. ventricular asystole
b. ventricular tachycardia
c. sinus bradycardia
d. hemodynamically compromising supraventricular tachycardia
e. ventricular fibrillation

72. If the patient suddenly develops ventricular fibrillation during cardioversion, what should be done immediately?

a. begin cardiac compressions
b. administer 75-mg lidocaine IV push
c. administer a synchronized countershock
d. deliver 100% oxygen via nonrebreather mask
e. turn off the synchronizer and defibrillate the patient

ANSWER KEY

1. Indications for intravenous cannulation in cardiac arrest are (1) to administer drugs or fluids, (2) to obtain blood specimens, and (3) for physiological monitoring and cardiac pacing.

2. The IV route is preferred over the IM route in cardiac arrest because (1) in low cardiac output states, blood is shunted away from the skin and muscle, thus diminishing the uptake and distribution of IM medications and (2) IM injections cause local muscle release of creatine phosphokinase (CPK) into the circulation, thereby altering the reliability of this enzyme as an indicator of myocardial necrosis.

3. TRUE: Because they can be better anchored and permit freer patient movement.

4. TRUE

5. FALSE: The preferred sites for IV cannulation during cardiac arrest are the peripheral veins. These veins can be cannulated without interrupting cardiac compressions. If no vein has been cannulated prior to the arrest, the antecubital vein in the arm is the preferred site. If a central line is necessary in an intubated patient, the internal jugular vein should interrupt CPR less than the subclavian vein site.

6. c

7. Veins of the upper extremity are shown in Figure 7–11.

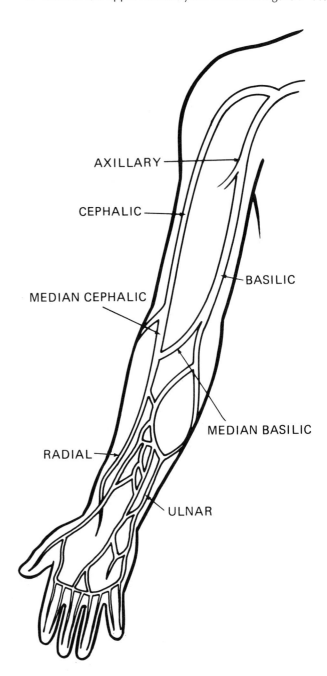

Figure 7–11

8. TRUE: The antecubital veins are among the largest in the arm. More distal veins are the least preferred IV sites because blood flow from distal extremities is markedly diminished during cardiac arrest.

9. TRUE

10. TRUE: Veins are more stabilized for cannulation at their junction with another vein (see Figure 7–12).

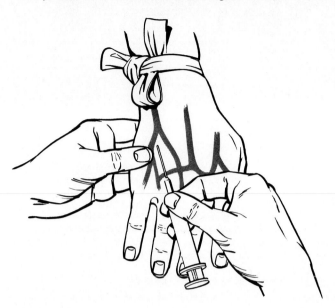

Figure 7–12

11. The sequence for initiating IV therapy in an arm or leg is shown in Figure 7–13.

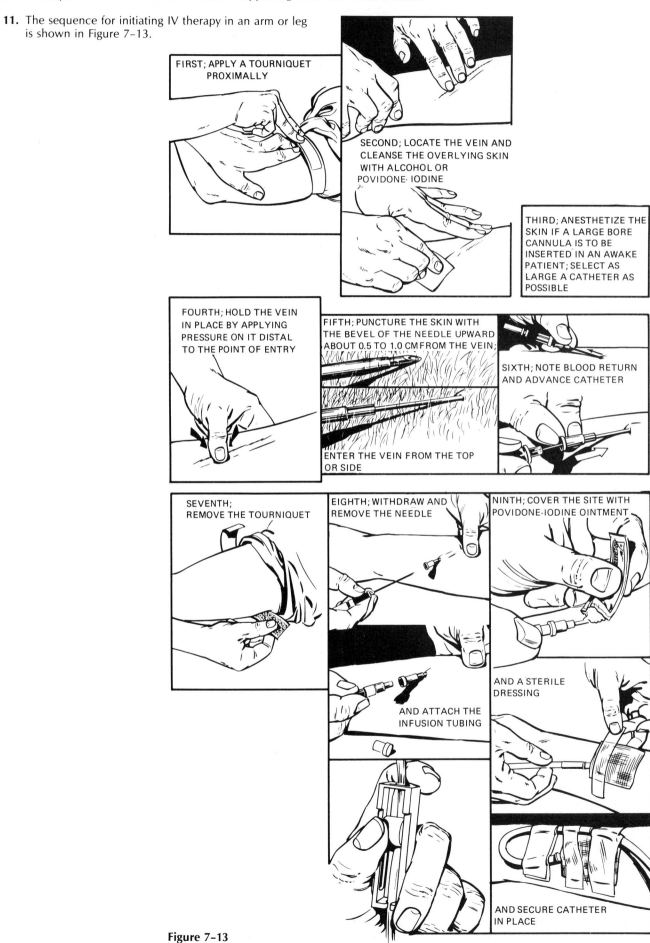

Figure 7–13

12. Advantages of antecubital venipuncture are that (1) it is easy to master, (2) it is an effective route for drug administration, and (3) it does not interfere with CPR procedures.

13. Disadvantages of peripheral venipuncture are (1) veins may be difficult or impossible to cannulate in circulatory collapse, (2) hypertonic or irritating solutions should not be administered through a peripheral vein since pain and phlebitis may result, and (3) delay in circulation of injected drugs.

14. Anatomical landmarks for the external jugular vein are shown in Figure 7–14.

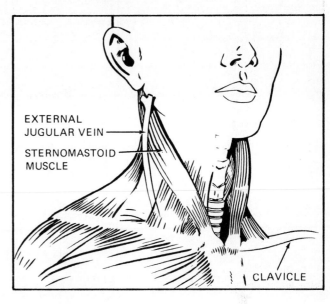

Figure 7–14

15. The sequence for cannulating the external jugular vein is shown in Figure 7–15.

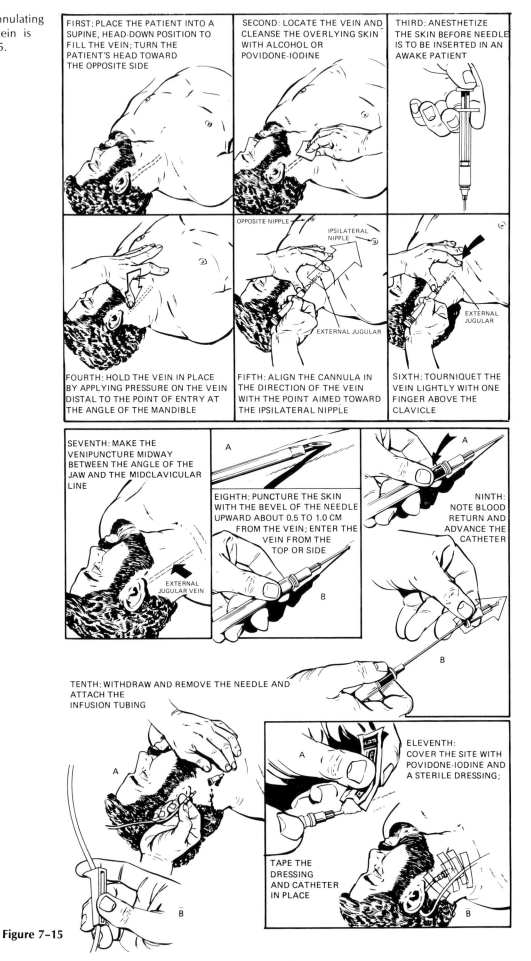

Figure 7–15

16. b (see Figure 7–16)

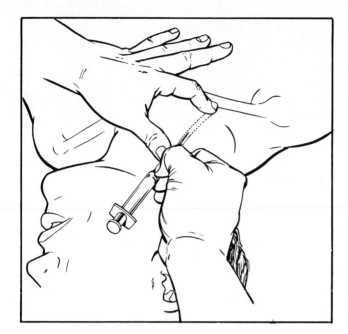

Figure 7–16

17. a

18. b

19. b

20. Anatomical landmarks for the femoral vein are shown in Figure 7–17.

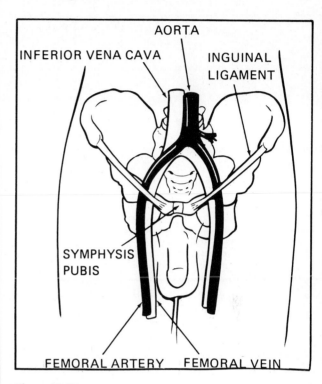

Figure 7–17

21. TRUE

22. TRUE

23. The femoral artery can be located by (1) directly palpating the vessel or by (2) using the appropriate anatomical landmarks (Figure 7–18). Remember that the reason for identifying the femoral artery is to locate the femoral vein, which lies medial to the artery.

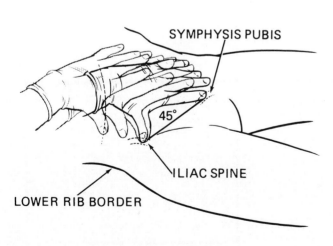

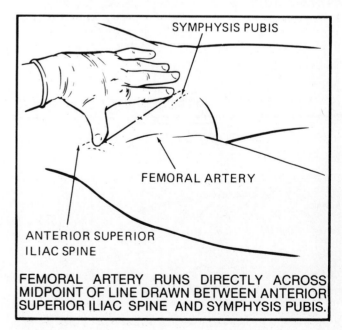

Figure 7–18

24. The sequence for cannulating the femoral vein is shown
in Figure 7–19.

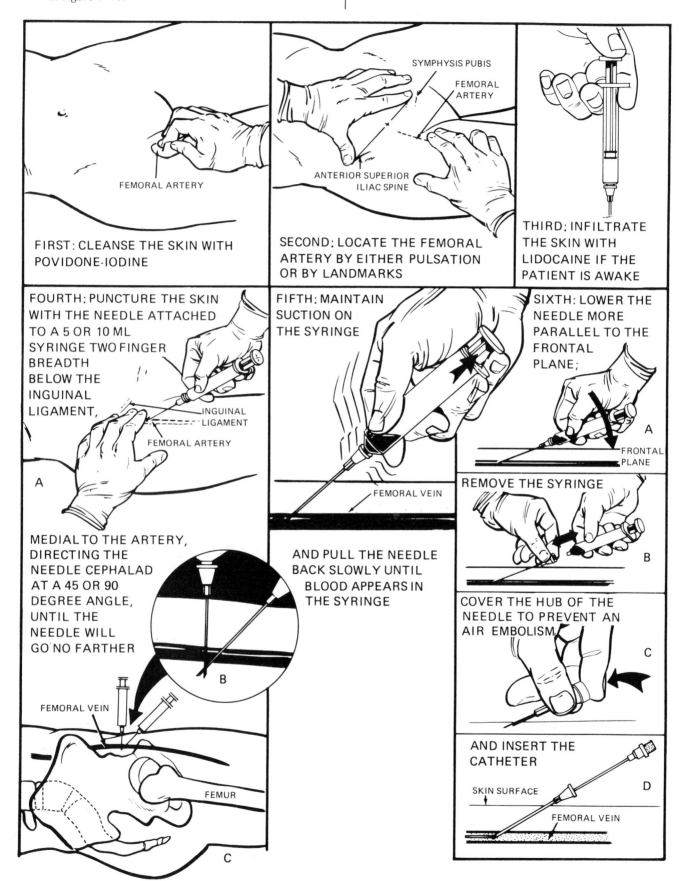

FIRST: CLEANSE THE SKIN WITH POVIDONE-IODINE

SECOND: LOCATE THE FEMORAL ARTERY BY EITHER PULSATION OR BY LANDMARKS

SYMPHYSIS PUBIS
FEMORAL ARTERY
ANTERIOR SUPERIOR ILIAC SPINE

THIRD: INFILTRATE THE SKIN WITH LIDOCAINE IF THE PATIENT IS AWAKE

FOURTH: PUNCTURE THE SKIN WITH THE NEEDLE ATTACHED TO A 5 OR 10 ML SYRINGE TWO FINGER BREADTH BELOW THE INGUINAL LIGAMENT,

INGUINAL LIGAMENT
FEMORAL ARTERY
A

MEDIAL TO THE ARTERY, DIRECTING THE NEEDLE CEPHALAD AT A 45 OR 90 DEGREE ANGLE, UNTIL THE NEEDLE WILL GO NO FARTHER

FEMORAL VEIN
FEMUR
B
C

FIFTH: MAINTAIN SUCTION ON THE SYRINGE

FEMORAL VEIN

AND PULL THE NEEDLE BACK SLOWLY UNTIL BLOOD APPEARS IN THE SYRINGE

SIXTH: LOWER THE NEEDLE MORE PARALLEL TO THE FRONTAL PLANE;

FRONTAL PLANE
A

REMOVE THE SYRINGE
B

COVER THE HUB OF THE NEEDLE TO PREVENT AN AIR EMBOLISM,
C

AND INSERT THE CATHETER

SKIN SURFACE
FEMORAL VEIN
D

Figure 7–19

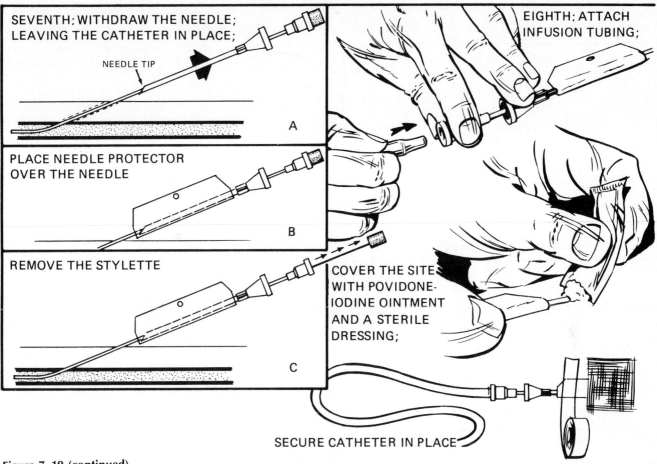

SEVENTH; WITHDRAW THE NEEDLE; LEAVING THE CATHETER IN PLACE;

NEEDLE TIP

A

PLACE NEEDLE PROTECTOR OVER THE NEEDLE

B

REMOVE THE STYLETTE

C

EIGHTH; ATTACH INFUSION TUBING;

COVER THE SITE WITH POVIDONE-IODINE OINTMENT AND A STERILE DRESSING;

SECURE CATHETER IN PLACE

Figure 7–19 (continued)

25. TRUE

26. TRUE

27. TRUE: Although the vein may be entered during needle advancement, many practitioners prefer to insert the needle until it will go no farther.

28. TRUE

29. Three advantages of femoral IV use are that the femoral vein (1) can be cannulated without interrupting CPR, (2) can be cannulated when more peripheral veins have collapsed, and (3) provides access to the central circulation.

30. Disadvantages of using the femoral vein are that (1) it may be difficult to locate without a palpable femoral artery pulse and (2) it has a higher complication rate than peripheral veins. Femoral veins should be avoided unless a long catheter can be passed above the diaphragm.

31. Complications of femoral venipuncture include (1) hematoma, (2) thrombosis and phlebitis, and (3) inadvertent cannulation of the femoral artery.

32. Anatomical landmarks for the subclavian vein are shown in Figure 7–20.

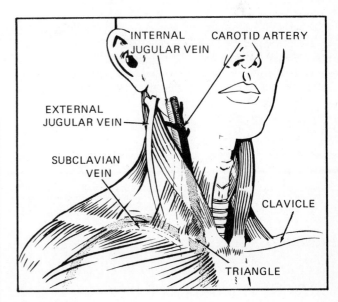

INTERNAL JUGULAR VEIN
CAROTID ARTERY
EXTERNAL JUGULAR VEIN
SUBCLAVIAN VEIN
CLAVICLE
TRIANGLE

Figure 7–20

33. The sagittal view of subclavian vein landmarks is shown in Figure 7–21.

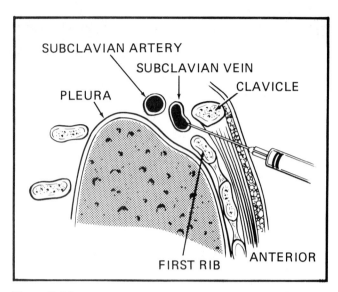

Figure 7–21

34. a, b, d

35. Anatomical landmarks for measuring catheter placement are given in Figure 7–22.

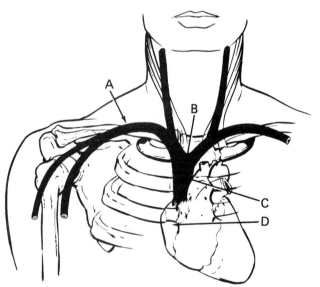

SURFACE MARKERS ON CHEST WALL TO DETERMINE DEPTH OF CATHETER PLACEMENT: STERNOCLAVICULAR JOINT—SUBCLAVIAN VEIN (A), MID-MANUBRIAL AREA—BRACHIOCEPHALIC VEIN (B), MANUBRIAL-STERNAL JUNCTION—SUPERIOR VENA CAVA (C), AND 5cm BELOW MANUBRIAL-STERNAL JUNCTION—RIGHT ATRIUM (D).

Figure 7–22

36. TRUE

37. Completely remove the needle and apply pressure to the puncture site for at least 10 minutes because these findings indicate that the subclavian artery has been entered.

38. Maintain negative pressure on the syringe plunger and slowly withdraw the needle. If blood does not appear, completely remove and reinsert the needle, taking a slightly different angle.

39. To prevent air embolism

40. Pulling the catheter backward may cause the needle tip to shear off the catheter, creating a catheter fragment embolism.

41. The sequence for cannulating the subclavian vein is shown in Figure 7–23.

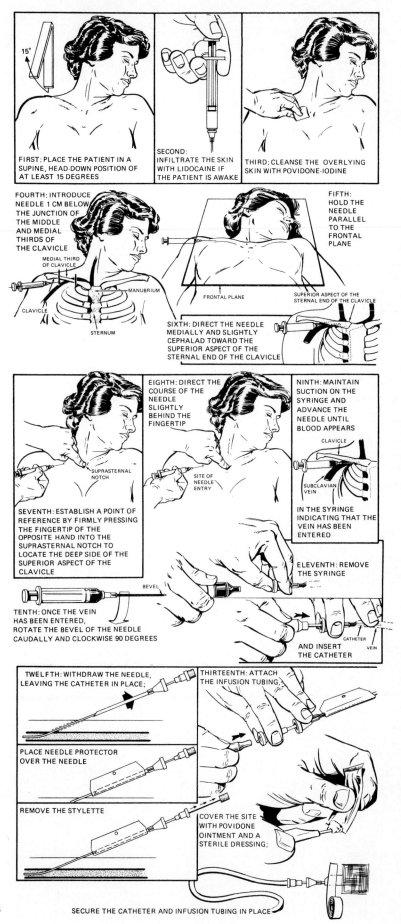

Figure 7–23

42. FALSE: The right subclavian vein is preferred over the left subclavian vein for two reasons: (1) the dome of the right lung and pleura are lower, reducing the chance of pneumothorax, and (2) the large thoracic duct in the left chest is avoided when the right subclavian is used.

43. Point of insertion for subclavian venipuncture: junction of medial and middle thirds of clavicle (see Figure 7–24).

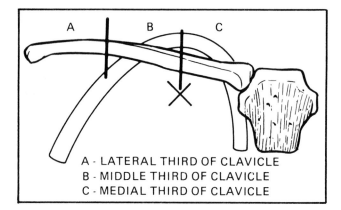

A - LATERAL THIRD OF CLAVICLE
B - MIDDLE THIRD OF CLAVICLE
C - MEDIAL THIRD OF CLAVICLE

Figure 7–24

44. Disadvantages of subclavian venipuncture are (1) the proximity of the subclavian artery, apical pleura, lymphatic ducts, and various nerves make these structures vulnerable to damage, (2) it requires more training and expertise than peripheral venipuncture and has a higher complication rate, and (3) it may require interruption of CPR.

45. Three systemic complications of subclavian venipuncture are (1) pneumothorax, hemothorax, infiltration of fluid into the mediastinum, (2) air embolism, and (3) dysrhythmias, perforation of the right atrium or right ventricle, cardiac tamponade.

46. a, c, d

47. c

48. The mechanical chest compressor can be effective for CPR because it (1) maintains optimal ventilation and compression by eliminating rescuer variability and fatigue, (2) frees rescuers to perform advanced life support procedures, and (3) assures the adequacy of chest compressions during transportation.

49. TRUE

50. TRUE

51. FALSE: MAST trousers are contraindicated in patients with pulmonary edema.

52. FALSE: MAST trousers can be left in place for x-rays.

53. FALSE: Deflating MAST trousers may result in an abrupt fall in the patient's blood pressure.

54. TRUE: This will allow gradual redistribution of blood volume and avoid trapping large volumes of blood in the legs.

55. d

56. Components of the MAST trousers system are shown in Figure 7–25.

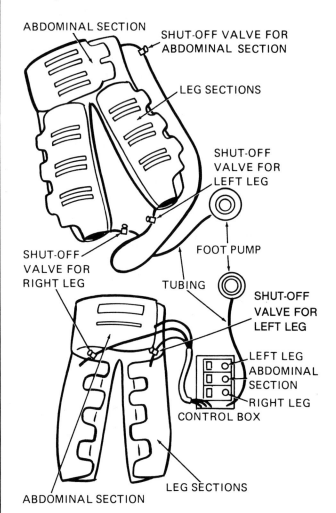

ABDOMINAL SECTION
SHUT-OFF VALVE FOR ABDOMINAL SECTION
LEG SECTIONS
SHUT-OFF VALVE FOR LEFT LEG
FOOT PUMP
SHUT-OFF VALVE FOR RIGHT LEG
TUBING
SHUT-OFF VALVE FOR LEFT LEG
LEFT LEG
ABDOMINAL SECTION
RIGHT LEG
CONTROL BOX
LEG SECTIONS
ABDOMINAL SECTION

Figure 7–25

57. The sequence for applying the pneumatic antishock trousers (MAST) is given in Figure 7–26.

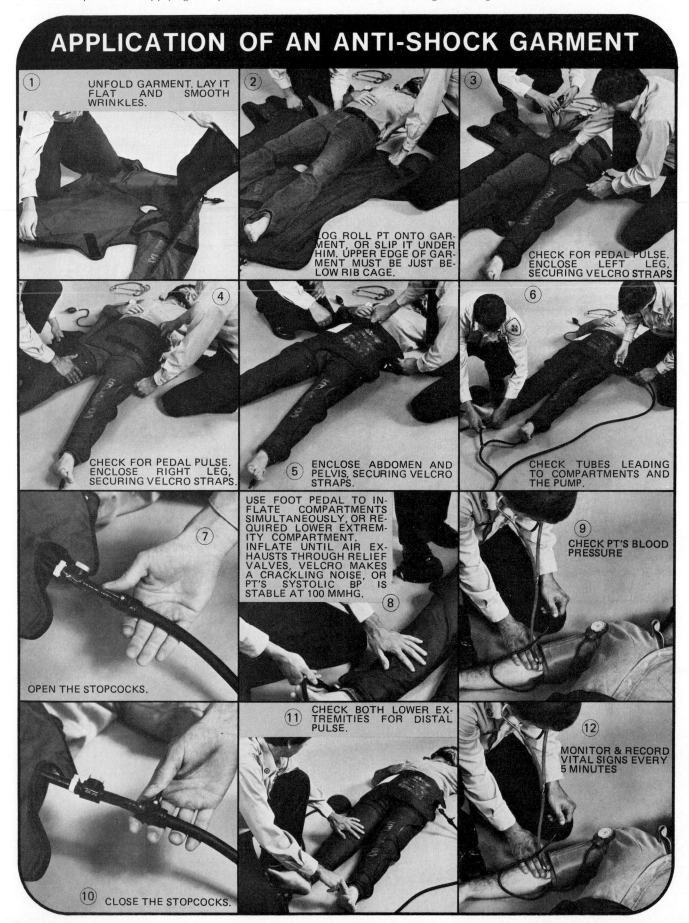

APPLICATION OF AN ANTI-SHOCK GARMENT

① UNFOLD GARMENT. LAY IT FLAT AND SMOOTH WRINKLES.

② LOG ROLL PT ONTO GARMENT, OR SLIP IT UNDER HIM. UPPER EDGE OF GARMENT MUST BE JUST BELOW RIB CAGE.

③ CHECK FOR PEDAL PULSE. ENCLOSE LEFT LEG, SECURING VELCRO STRAPS

④ CHECK FOR PEDAL PULSE. ENCLOSE RIGHT LEG, SECURING VELCRO STRAPS.

⑤ ENCLOSE ABDOMEN AND PELVIS, SECURING VELCRO STRAPS.

⑥ CHECK TUBES LEADING TO COMPARTMENTS AND THE PUMP.

⑦ OPEN THE STOPCOCKS.

⑧ USE FOOT PEDAL TO INFLATE COMPARTMENTS SIMULTANEOUSLY, OR REQUIRED LOWER EXTREMITY COMPARTMENT. INFLATE UNTIL AIR EXHAUSTS THROUGH RELIEF VALVES, VELCRO MAKES A CRACKLING NOISE, OR PT'S SYSTOLIC BP IS STABLE AT 100 MMHG.

⑨ CHECK PT'S BLOOD PRESSURE

⑩ CLOSE THE STOPCOCKS.

⑪ CHECK BOTH LOWER EXTREMITIES FOR DISTAL PULSE.

⑫ MONITOR & RECORD VITAL SIGNS EVERY 5 MINUTES

Figure 7–26

58. b

59. a, b, e

60. TRUE

61. TRUE: The more resistance there is, the less energy will be delivered.

62. TRUE

63. FALSE: Firm paddle pressure only reduces the resistance between the skin and defibrillator paddles by about 25%.

64. FALSE: If ventricular fibrillation is not terminated by one precordial thump, the patient should be immediately defibrillated.

65. d

66. d

67. If the second defibrillation is unsuccessful, a third shock of up to 360 joules should be administered.

68. The sequence for defibrillation is shown in Figure 7–27.

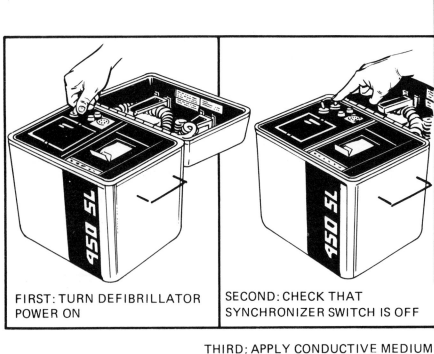

FIRST: TURN DEFIBRILLATOR POWER ON

SECOND: CHECK THAT SYNCHRONIZER SWITCH IS OFF

THIRD: APPLY CONDUCTIVE MEDIUM

Figure 7–27

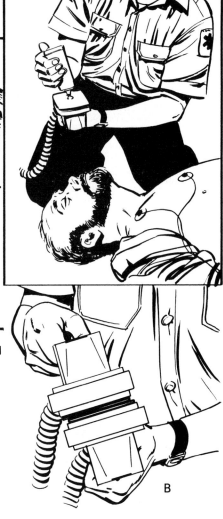

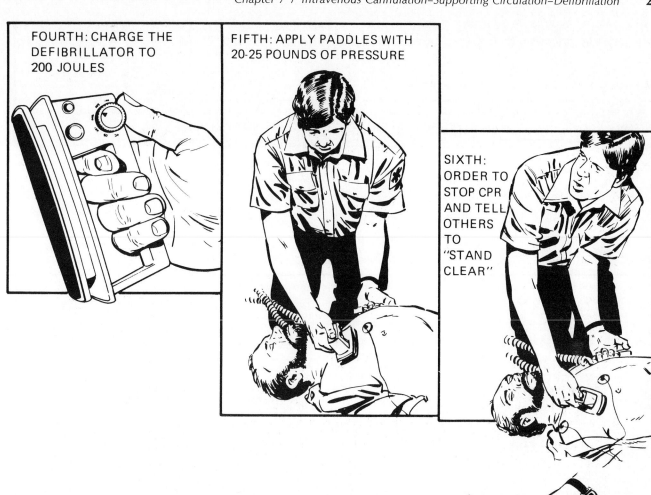

FOURTH: CHARGE THE DEFIBRILLATOR TO 200 JOULES

FIFTH: APPLY PADDLES WITH 20-25 POUNDS OF PRESSURE

SIXTH: ORDER TO STOP CPR AND TELL OTHERS TO "STAND CLEAR"

Figure 7–27 (continued)

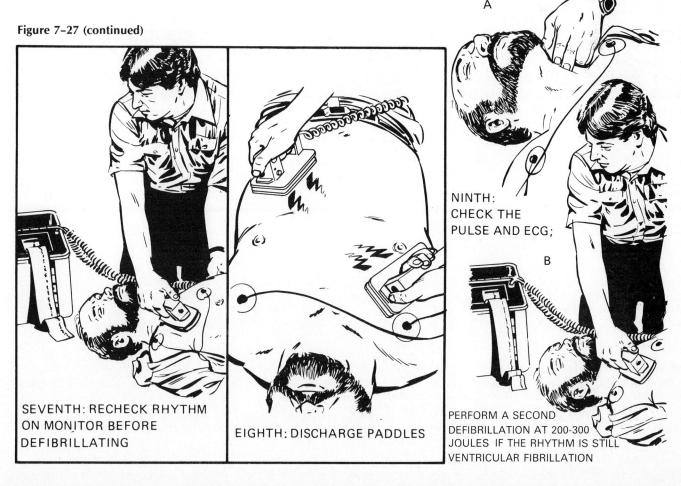

SEVENTH: RECHECK RHYTHM ON MONITOR BEFORE DEFIBRILLATING

EIGHTH: DISCHARGE PADDLES

A

NINTH: CHECK THE PULSE AND ECG;

B

PERFORM A SECOND DEFIBRILLATION AT 200-300 JOULES IF THE RHYTHM IS STILL VENTRICULAR FIBRILLATION

TENTH: IF THE PATIENT IS STILL PULSELESS AND IN VENTRICULAR
FIBRILLATION; DEFIBRILLATE A THIRD TIME AT UP TO 360 JOULES

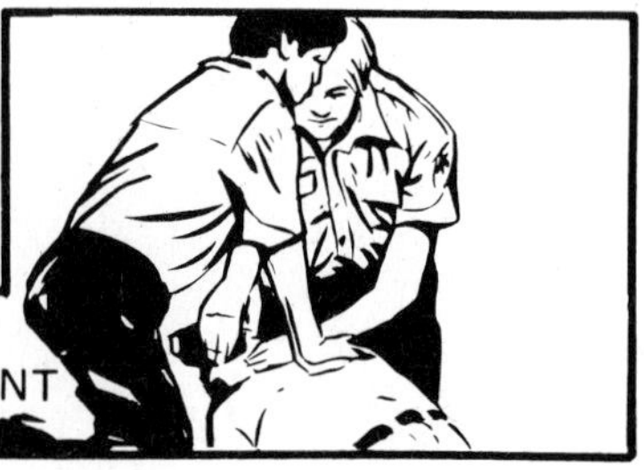

ELEVENTH:
REMOVE PADDLES AND CONTINUE CPR IF A PALPABLE PULSE IS NOT PRESENT

Figure 7–27 (continued)

69. FALSE: Defibrillating on bare skin will increase the resistance between the skin and paddles.

70. TRUE: This is a safety measure to prevent accidental defibrillation of the rescuer or others nearby.

71. b, d

72. e

Chapter 8

Myocardial Infarction

OBJECTIVES

Upon completion of this chapter, you will be able to:

- Describe the etiology, clinical course, and initial treatment of acute myocardial infarction (MI).

- Distinguish the indications and actions of drugs used in the management of acute MI.

- Specify drug therapy for broad categories of dysrhythmias and conduction defects commonly associated with acute MI.

- Differentiate among the clinical features and treatments used in cardiogenic shock and hyperdynamic states associated with acute MI.

- Identify the characteristics and management regimens for various shock syndromes seen following acute MI.

True or False

1. T   F   Myocardial infarction (MI) occurs when there is necrosis of heart muscle due to an inadequate blood supply to the heart.

2. T   F   Acute MI is always the result of severe atherosclerosis of the coronary arteries.

3. T   F   MI most often occurs during periods of moderate to heavy physical exertion.

4. On Figure 8–1, shade in the areas where the pain associated with acute MI is usually located. Include areas of pain radiation.

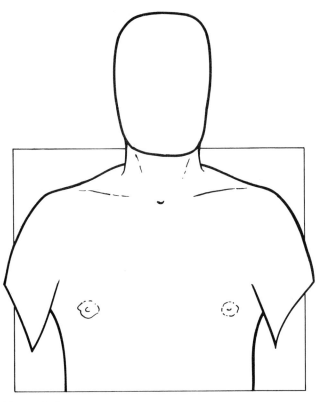

Figure 8–1

5. On Figure 8–2, shade in the time period when ventricular fibrillation is most likely to occur following the onset of symptoms from acute MI.

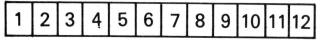

hours

Figure 8–2

6. Suspicion of acute MI should be based primarily on the patient's:

a. blood pressure
b. chest pain
c. electrocardiogram
d. history

7. Which of the following are appropriate treatments for patients with chest pain accompanied by diaphoresis?

a. monitor for dysrhythmias
b. reassure continually
c. give prophylactic isoproterenol IV push
d. provide supplemental oxygen
e. insert an IV lifeline

8. Which of the following are true regarding stabilization of cardiac patients outside a medical facility?

a. precedes transportation to the nearest medical facility
b. includes pain relief
c. includes control of life-threatening dysrhythmias
d. requires a physician in attendance
e. includes lights and siren transport to the hospital

9. Which of the following are actions of sublingual nitroglycerin?

a. reduces myocardial oxygen demand
b. increases coronary collateral blood flow
c. decreases susceptibility of ischemic myocardium to ventricular fibrillation
d. causes a reflex bradycardia
e. reduces mean arterial blood pressure

10. Which of the following are actions of morphine sulfate?

a. increases venous capacitance
b. reduces systemic vascular resistance
c. increases myocardial oxygen demand
d. inhibits catecholamine activity
e. causes reflex hypertension

11. T   F   Bradydysrhythmias that follow acute MI tend to protect against ventricular ectopic activity and decrease coronary perfusion.

12. T   F   Supraventricular bradydysrhythmias are particularly prevalent during the third hour following acute MI.

13. T   F   The most common bradydysrhythmias encountered after acute MI are sinus bradycardia, junctional (escape) rhythm, and AV block (AV Nodal level).

14. T   F   In the absence of ventricular ectopy and hypotension, bradycardias over 50 beats per minute usually do not require drug therapy.

15. T   F   There is no parasympathetic innervation of the ventricles.

16. T   F   In atropine refractory bradycardia, IV infusion of isoproterenol should maintain the heart rate at 100 beats per minute.

17. T   F   Management of sinus tachycardia is directed at identifying and correcting the underlying cause.

18. T   F   Analgesia and sedation may be sufficient to relieve sinus tachycardia due to pain and anxiety.

19. T   F   Young patients having their first acute MI are likely to have sinus tachycardia associated with a hyperdynamic state.

20. T   F   Excessive catecholamines may increase myocardial ischemia and cardiac workload, increase automaticity, and lower the fibrillation threshold.

21. Match the following dysrhythmias with one or more characteristics:

Dysrhythmia

a. atrial fibrillation or atrial flutter
b. hemodynamically compromising supraventricular tachycardia
c. premature atrial contractions (PACs)
d. junctional rhythm

Characteristic

_____ sequential AV pacing is treatment

_____ commonly occur with large anterior wall MI

_____ cardioversion, verapamil, or rapid atrial pacing is treatment

_____ associated with increased mortality

_____ does not require therapy, but may manifest occult heart failure or excess. adrenergic tone

_____ may be secondary to left atrial dilatation

_____ needs immediate conversion to sinus rhythm

_____ carotid stimulation or 10-mg edrophonium IV is treatment

_____ may compromise cardiac output by loss of atrial contribution to ventricular function

22. Which of the following are true statements regarding accelerated idioventricular rhythms?

a. They compromise cardiac function.
b. They may deteriorate into ventricular tachycardia.
c. They may represent an escape rhythm.
d. They may be successfully converted by a precordial thump.

23. Treatment for ventricular tachycardia may:

a. be delayed if the patient is hemodynamically stable
b. include bolus lidocaine therapy
c. include a precordial thump if the patient is asymptomatic and has a pulse
d. include synchronized cardioversion

True or False

24. T   F   First-degree AV block usually does not require treatment unless it is associated with bradycardia and hypotension.

25. Match the following forms of AV block with one or more associated characteristics:

Forms of AV Block

a. Second-degree AV block, Mobitz type I (Wenckebach)
b. Second-degree AV block, Mobitz type II
c. Third-degree AV block

Characteristics

_____ does not require therapy in the absence of hemodynamic compromise

_____ requires a demand pacemaker to maintain heart rate near 60 per minute

_____ uncommon in acute MI, but carries significant risk of progression to complete AV block

_____ treated with atropine

_____ associated with extensive myocardial injury and a grim prognosis

True or False

26. T   F   Intraventricular blocks are more likely to occur with anterior wall MI and require pacemaker control to maintain an adequate heart rate.

27. T   F   Prophylactic lidocaine may reduce the incidence of primary ventricular fibrillation in patients with acute MI.

28. T   F   The length of time a patient is in ventricular fibrillation has no effect on the likelihood of successful restoration of an effective cardiac rhythm.

29. T   F   Electrical countershock should be performed at the earliest possible instant following the onset of ventricular fibrillation.

30. Cardiogenic shock is said to be present when the blood pressure falls because of (circle one):

    a. a relative deficiency in circulating blood volume

    b. the extent of myocardial damage

    c. an inappropriate decrease in systemic vascular resistance

    d. an abrupt slowing of the heart rate

31. Which of the following are signs of a hyperdynamic circulatory state?

    a. poor peripheral perfusion

    b. tachycardia

    c. oliguria

    d. hypertension

    e. bounding pulses

32. Which of the following may result from a hyperdynamic state?

    a. increased myocardial oxygen consumption

    b. relative deficiency in circulating blood volume

    c. decreased systemic vascular resistance

    d. excessive catecholamine influences on the heart

    e. decreased cardiac stroke volume

33. The preferred treatment for excessive catecholamine activity is:

    a. beta adrenergic blockade

    b. vasodilator therapy

    c. intraaortic balloon counterpulsation

    d. colloid IV solutions

    e. IV diuretics

34. T   F   Norepinephrine's alpha stimulating properties cause peripheral vasoconstriction, and its beta stimulating properties increase both heart rate and contractility.

35. Match the conditions described in Figure 8–3 with their respective illustration:

    a. inappropriately reduced systemic vascular resistance or decreased stroke volume

    b. heart rate is too slow or too fast to circulate blood effectively

    c. cardiogenic shock resulting from damage to 35% or more of the heart muscle

    d. inadequate intravascular volume caused by either diminished systemic vascular resistance or low absolute volume

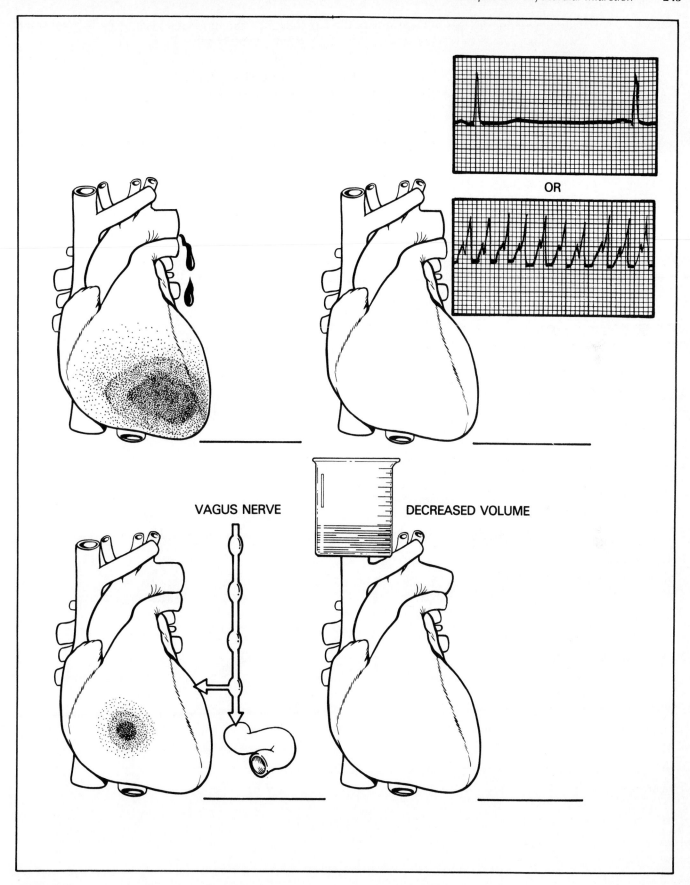

VAGUS NERVE

DECREASED VOLUME

OR

Figure 8-3

36. T   F   Norepinephrine increases myocardial oxygen consumption (MVO$_2$).

37. T   F   Norepinephrine decreases coronary perfusion and seriously compromises ischemic myocardium.

38. T   F   Norepinephrine is used to treat hypotension due to inappropriate reductions of systemic vascular resistance following acute MI.

39. T   F   Norepinephrine is administered in an initial dosage of 10 to 20 mg/minute.

40. List the recommended treatments for persistent mild hypertension.

_____

_____

_____

True or False

41. T   F   The major cause of mortality in hospitalized MI patients is primary ventricular fibrillation.

42. Figure 8–4 is an illustration of the normal filling and contracting of the heart and movement of blood through the heart.

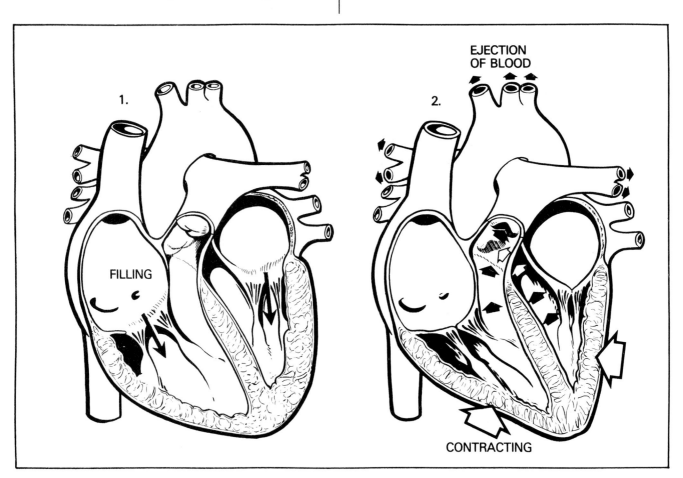

1.   FILLING

2.   EJECTION OF BLOOD

CONTRACTING

Figure 8–4

In Figure 8–5, you will find two illustrations of abnormal contraction and ejection that result in cardiac pump failure. Match the descriptions with these illustrations:

a. There is a decrease in wall motion with a proportionate fall in stroke volume.

b. There may be movement of blood into the bulging or dyssynergic area during systole, thus decreasing the amount of blood ejected into the aorta.

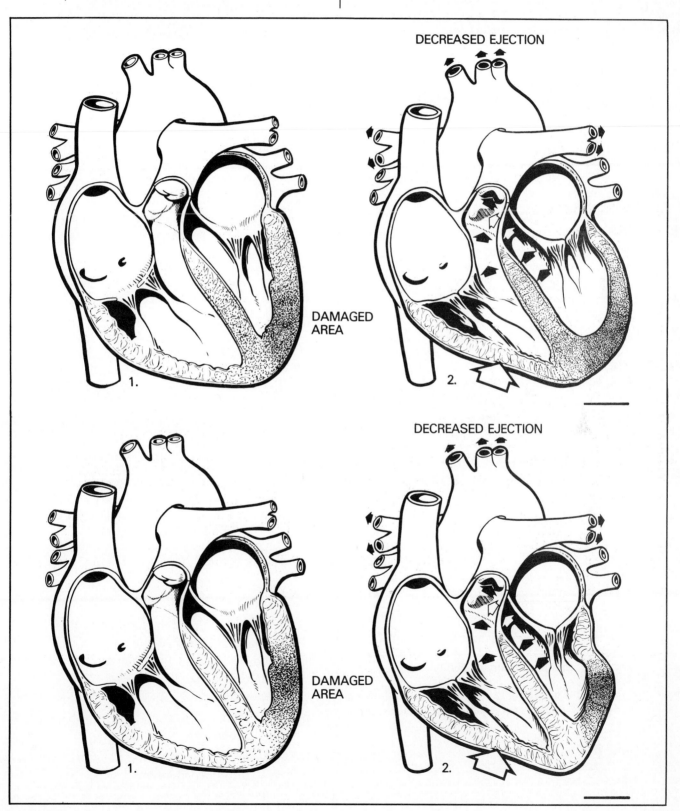

Figure 8–5

43. List the hemodynamic signs of cardiogenic shock.

1) _____

2) _____

3) _____

44. Briefly explain the cause of cardiogenic shock in relation to the concept of "critical mass."

_____

_____

_____

45. Specify six clinical signs associated with cardiogenic shock.

1) _____

2) _____

3) _____

4) _____

5) _____

6) _____

46. T   F   Pulmonary edema is due to an acute increase in the ventricular filling pressures with an abrupt increase in lung water.

47. T   F   Initial management of the patient experiencing acute pulmonary edema includes laying the patient flat and administering oxygen.

48. T   F   Diuretic therapy alone may be adequate in mild cases of pulmonary edema.

49. T   F   Nitroglycerin and morphine sulfate are contraindicated in the presence of acute pulmonary edema.

50. T   F   Occasionally, patients suffering from acute pulmonary edema may require intubation and positive-pressure ventilation.

51. Match the following conditions with their respective characteristics.

Condition

a. massive pulmonary embolism
b. hypovolemic shock
c. septic shock

Characteristic

_____ obstruction of pulmonary arterial system, resulting in pulmonary hypertension and right ventricular failure

_____ treated with crystalloid or colloid solutions or whole blood

_____ increased cardiac output and hypotension due to reduced systemic vascular resistance

_____ chest pain and ECG changes consistent with an acute MI

_____ hypoperfusion and hypotension with normal or low left ventricular filling pressure

True or False

52. T   F   Right ventricular infarction may result in shock secondary to right ventricular failure.

53. T   F   Shock due to right ventricular infarction is suspected when right atrial pressure and right ventricular diastolic pressure are disproportionately low compared to pulmonary capillary wedge pressure.

54. T   F   Treatment of right ventricular infarction consists of augmenting circulating blood volume with or without vasodilators.

55. Which of the following conditions may result in cardiac tamponade?

a. acute rupture of the left ventricle
b. massive pulmonary emboli
c. severe systemic hypertension
d. hypovolemia
e. pericarditis

56. Which of the following signs are indicative of cardiac tamponade?

a. warm, flushed skin
b. systemic hypertension
c. pulsus paradoxus
d. pericardial friction rub
e. enlarging heart shadow on x-ray

57. Which of the following are useful treatments for cardiac tamponade?

    a. agents that accelerate heart rate
    b. blood volume expanders
    c. vasodilators
    d. pericardiocentesis
    e. beta adrenergic blockers

58. Briefly explain how acute mitral regurgitation results in hypotension.

_____

_____

_____

_____

59. List the indicators of acute mitral regurgitation.

1) _____

2) _____

3) _____

60. List three treatments for acute mitral regurgitation.

1) _____

2) _____

3) _____

61. Match the illustrations in Figure 8–6 with the condition that results in reduced cardiac output and hypotension.

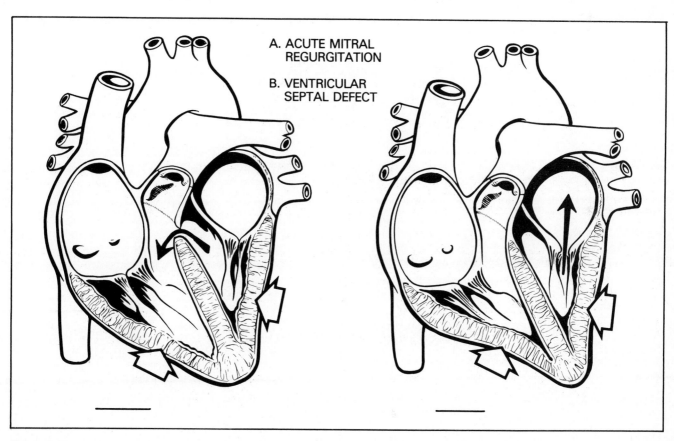

A. ACUTE MITRAL REGURGITATION

B. VENTRICULAR SEPTAL DEFECT

Figure 8–6

62. Briefly explain how a ventricular septal defect can be differentiated from acute mitral regurgitation.

_____

_____

_____

_____

True or False

63. T   F   Initial therapy for a ventricular septal defect is similar to that for acute mitral regurgitation.

ANSWER KEY

1. TRUE: Myocardial infarction occurs when there is necrosis of heart muscle due to an inadequate blood supply to the heart.

2. FALSE: Acute MI may also occur as a result of coronary artery vasospasm with or without thrombosis. Myocardial infarction may also occur when a heart that is already compromised by significant coronary artery disease is subjected to extraordinary circumstances such as tachycardia or hypovolemia and there is insufficient coronary blood flow to meet the myocardial oxygen requirements.

3. FALSE: MI most commonly occurs when the individual is resting or asleep.

4. Location of pain associated with acute MI is shown in Figure 8–7.

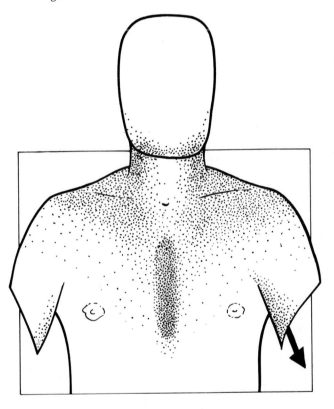

Figure 8–7

5. Time when ventricular fibrillation is most likely following MI (Figure 8–8)

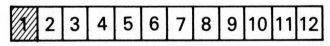

hours

Figure 8–8

6. d: Suspicion of acute myocardial infarction should be based primarily on the patient's history, as everything else may be within normal limits.

7. a, b, d, e: Treatment for patients suspected of experiencing acute myocardial infarction includes monitoring for dysrhythmias, providing continual reassurance, providing supplemental oxygen, and establishing an IV lifeline. Additionally, the health-care provider should consider relieving pain, administering prophylactic antiarrhythmic therapy, employing therapies to limit infarct, and instituting secondary preventions.

8. a, b, c: Stabilization of the cardiac patient outside the medical facility would precede transportation to nearest medical facility, and include pain relief and control of life-threatening dysrhythmias.

9. a, c, e: Nitroglycerin reduces myocardial oxygen demand, decreases susceptibility of ischemic myocardium to ventricular fibrillation and reduces the mean arterial pressure.

10. a, b: Morphine sulfate increases venous capacitance and reduces systemic vascular resistance (thereby reducing preload, afterload, myocardial workload, and myocardial oxygen consumption).

11. TRUE

12. FALSE: Bradydysrhythmias are particularly prevalent during the first hour following MI.

13. TRUE: Most common bradydysrhythmias encountered following myocardial infarction include sinus bradycardia, junctional escape rhythm, and AV block.

14. TRUE: Increased heart rates result in increased myocardial oxygen requirements and may worsen myocardial ischemia/infarction, and thus bradycardias, unless they are accompanied by ventricular ectopy or hypotension; do not usually require drug therapy.

15. FALSE: It is now believed that there is parasympathetic innervation to the ventricles.

16. FALSE: Isoproterenol should maintain the heart rate at about 60 beats per minute.

17. TRUE: Management of sinus tachycardia is directed at identifying and correcting the underlying cause. Rapid supraventricular rhythms such as sinus tachycardia, atrial flutter/fibrillation, and atrial tachycardia are usually due to heart failure. One potential danger of tachycardia is that it may cause an increase in the size of the infarction or an exacerbation of ischemia.

18. TRUE: Analgesia and sedation may be sufficient to relieve sinus tachycardia due to pain and anxiety.

19. TRUE: Young patients having their first acute MI are likely to have sinus tachycardia associated with a hyperdynamic state.

20. TRUE: Excessive catecholamines may increase myocardial ischemia and cardiac workload, increase automaticity, and lower the fibrillation threshold.

21. a. ATRIAL FIBRILLATION OR ATRIAL FLUTTER: common with extensive anterior wall MI; may be associated with increased mortality; may be secondary to left atrial dilatation

     b. HEMODYNAMICALLY COMPROMISING SUPRAVENTRICULAR TACHYCARDIA: cardioversion, verapamil, or rapid atrial pacing is treatment; needs immediate conversion to sinus rhythm

     c. PREMATURE ATRIAL CONTRACTIONS: does not require therapy, but may manifest occult heart failure or excessive adrenergic tone

     d. JUNCTIONAL RHYTHM: sequential AV pacing is treatment; may compromise cardiac output through loss of atrial contribution to ventricular function

22. a, b, c, d: Accelerated idioventricular rhythms may compromise cardiac function, deteriorate into ventricular tachycardia, represent an escape rhythm, and be successfully converted by a precordial thump.

23. b, c, d: Treatment for ventricular tachycardia may include lidocaine bolus therapy (or procainamide therapy if the ventricular tachycardia is refractory to lidocaine), a precordial thump if the patient is asymptomatic and has a pulse, and synchronized cardioversion.

24. TRUE: First-degree AV block usually does not require treatment unless it is associated with bradycardia and hypotension.

25. a. SECOND-DEGREE AV BLOCK, MOBITZ I (WENCKEBACH): does not require therapy in the absence of hemodynamic compromise; treated with atropine (if hemodynamic compromise exists)

     b. SECOND-DEGREE AV BLOCK, MOBITZ II: requires use of demand pacemaker to maintain heart rate near 60 beats per minute; uncommon in acute MI, but carries significant risk of progression to complete AV block; treated with atropine

     c. THIRD-DEGREE AV BLOCK: requires use of demand pacemaker to maintain heart rate near 60 per minute; treated with atropine; is associated with extensive myocardial injury and a grim prognosis

26. TRUE: Intraventricular blocks (bundle branch) are more likely to occur with anterior wall MI and often require pacemaker control to maintain an adequate heart rate.

27. TRUE: Prophylactic lidocaine may reduce the incidence of primary ventricular fibrillation in patients with acute MI. Remember, not all patients display heralding ventricular ectopy prior to episodes of ventricular fibrillation; thus it is best to employ prophylactic measures such as lidocaine.

28. FALSE: The longer the patient is in ventricular fibrillation, the less likely he is to be successfully converted to an effective electromechanical rhythm.

29. TRUE: Electrical countershock should be performed at the earliest possible instant following the onset of ventricular fibrillation, in some cases (especially when the defibrillator is immediately available) defibrillation should precede CPR.

30. b: Cardiogenic shock is said to be present when the blood pressure falls because of the extent of myocardial damage. When hypotension is caused by depression of left ventricular function, inotropic agents may be useful.

31. b, d, e: Tachycardia, hypertension, and bounding pulses are signs of a hyperdynamic state.

32. a, d: Increased myocardial oxygen consumption and excessive catecholamine influences on the heart may result from a hyperdynamic state. Therapy may include the relief of pain and anxiety with morphine sulfate or sublingual nitroglycerin and the use of IV furosemide if pulmonary congestion is present.

33. a: The preferred treatment for excessive catecholamine activity (with associated hyperdynamic state) is beta adrenergic blockade (i.e., 1 to 3 mg of IV propranolol every 5 minutes to a maximum dosage of 0.1 mg/kg or metoprolol, up to three doses of 5 mg each).

34. TRUE: See Figure 8–9. Norepinephrine's alpha stimulating properties cause peripheral vasoconstriction, and its beta stimulating properties increase both heart rate and contractility.

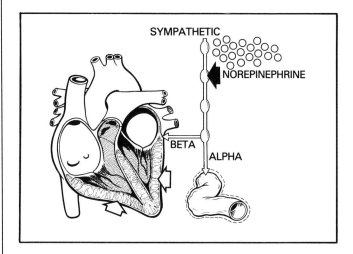

Figure 8–9

35. Conditions resulting in hypotension are shown in Figure 8–10.

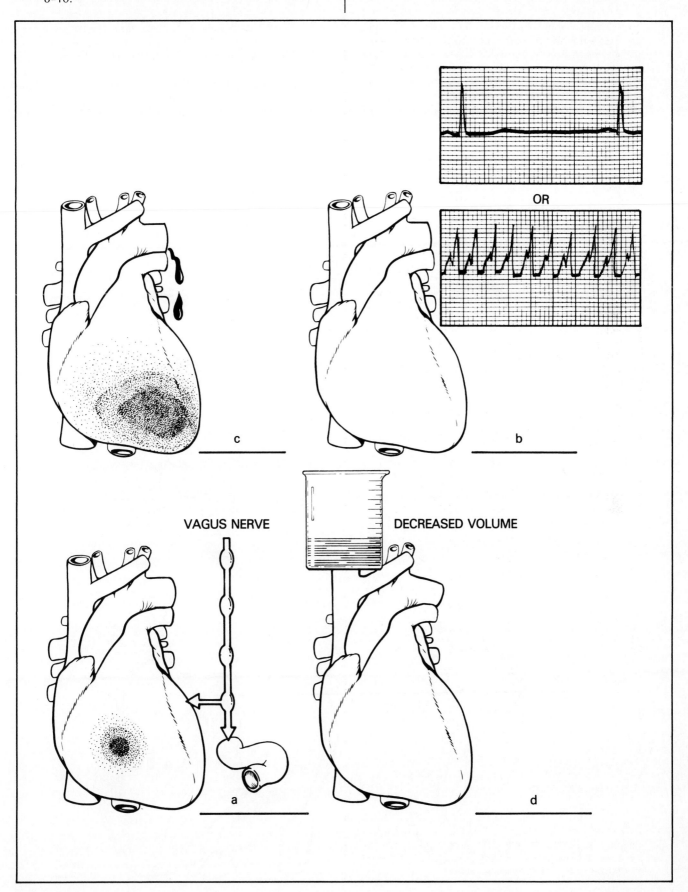

Figure 8–10

36. TRUE: Norepinephrine increases myocardial oxygen consumption (MVO₂)

37. FALSE: Norepinephrine may initially decrease coronary perfusion (due to coronary vasoconstriction), but this is usually a transient response; coronary vasodilation follows as a result of increased coronary metabolic activity and improved coronary perfusion pressures.

38. TRUE: Norepinephrine is used to treat hypotension due to inappropriate reductions of systemic vascular resistance following acute MI.

39. FALSE: Norepinephrine should be administered in an initial dosage of 16 μg/ml titrated to effect.

40. Suggested treatments for persistent mild hypertension are (1) pain relief, (2) oxygen, (3) nitroglycerin sublingually or ointment, and (4) oral nitrates.

41. FALSE: Most hospital deaths from MI are due to pump failure.

42. Abnormal cardiac ejection resulting in pump failure is shown in Figure 8–11.

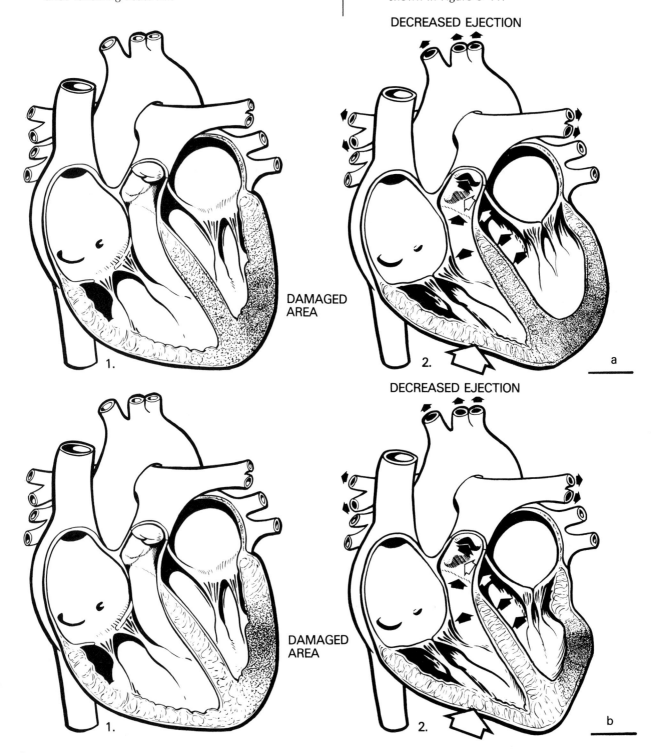

Figure 8–11

43. Hemodynamic indexes of cardiogenic shock are (1) decreased cardiac output, (2) decreased blood pressure, and (3) elevation of pulmonary capillary wedge pressure.

44. Cardiogenic shock is caused by depression of ventricular function resulting from loss of a critical mass (usually 35% or more) of myocardium.

45. Clinical signs of cardiogenic shock include (1) hypotension, (2) oliguria, (3) mental obtundation, (4) pallor, (5) diaphoresis, and (6) tachycardia.

46. TRUE: Pulmonary edema is due to an acute increase in the ventricular filling pressures with an abrupt increase in lung water.

47. FALSE: Initial management of the patient experiencing acute pulmonary edema would include sitting the patient upright and administering oxygen.

48. TRUE: Diuretic therapy alone may be adequate in mild cases of pulmonary edema.

49. FALSE: Nitroglycerin and morphine sulfate may be used in the treatment of acute pulmonary edema. However, morphine would be contraindicated in the presence of hypotension or severe obstructive lung disease. Sodium nitroprusside, IV nitroglycerin, or sublingual nifedipine may assist in providing relief of pulmonary edema by decreasing the pulmonary artery occlusive pressure and decreasing systemic vascular resistance (and afterload). These agents should be used with caution as they may precipitate hypotension and decreased coronary blood flow. Inotropic agents may help in pulmonary edema by improving hemodynamics.

50. TRUE: Occasionally, patients suffering from acute pulmonary edema may require intubation and positive-pressure ventilation.

51.   a. MASSIVE PULMONARY EMBOLISM: obstruction of pulmonary arterial system, resulting in pulmonary hypertension and right ventricular failure; chest pain and ECG changes consistent with acute MI (see Figure 8–12)

   b. HYPOVOLEMIC SHOCK: treated with crystalloid or colloid solutions or whole blood; decreased perfusion with hypotension and normal or low left ventricular filling pressure

   c. SEPTIC SHOCK: increased cardiac output and hypotension due to reduced systemic vascular resistance

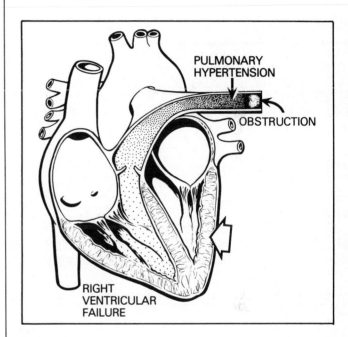

Figure 8–12

52. TRUE (see Figure 8–13)

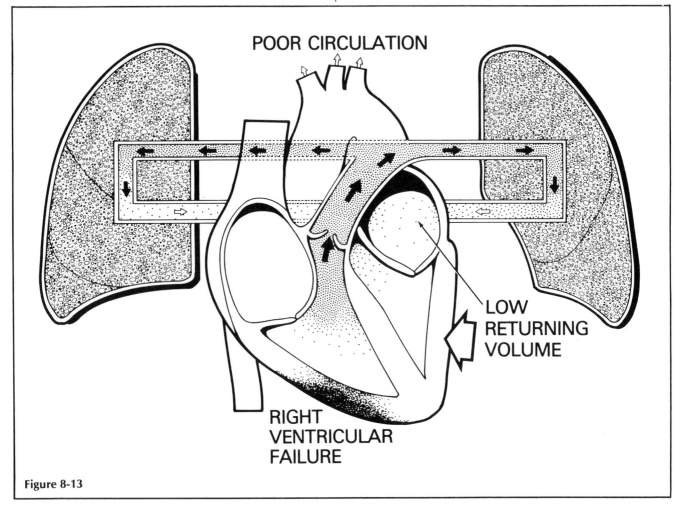

POOR CIRCULATION

LOW RETURNING VOLUME

RIGHT VENTRICULAR FAILURE

Figure 8-13

Figure 8–13

53. TRUE

54. TRUE

55. a, e

56. c, d, e

57. b, d

58. Acute mitral regurgitation results in hypotension because the inability of the mitral valve to close allows left ventricular blood to regurgitate back into the left atrium each time the ventricle contracts; this decreases the volume and pressure of blood leaving the left ventricle and entering the systemic circulation.

59. Indicators of acute mitral regurgitation are shock associated with a (1) holosystolic murmur, (2) large systolic wave on the pulmonary capillary wedge pressure tracing, and (3) pulmonary congestion.

60. Treatments for acute mitral regurgitation include (1) vasodilators, (2) intraaortic balloon counterpulsation, and (3) mitral valve replacement.

61. Conditions resulting in decreased cardiac output and hypotension are shown in Figure 8–14.

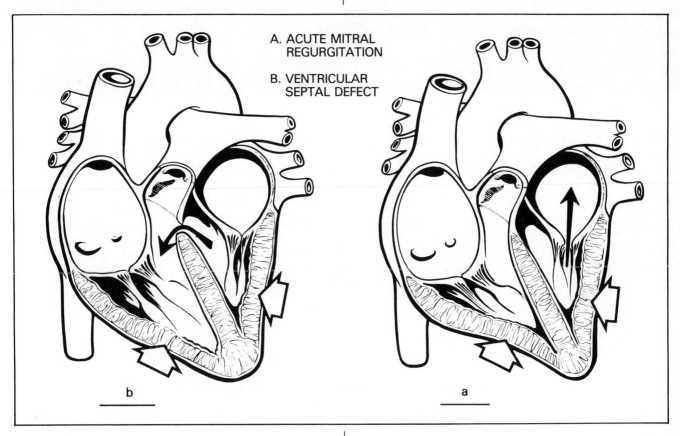

A. ACUTE MITRAL
REGURGITATION

B. VENTRICULAR
SEPTAL DEFECT

b

a

Figure 8–14

62. A ventricular septal defect has a holosystolic murmur that is more pronounced at the lower left sternal border and a ventricular and pulmonary arterial oxygen content at least 1 volume percent greater than the highest sample from the right atrium.

63. TRUE

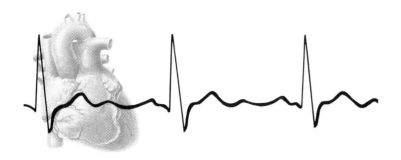

Chapter 9

Sudden Death

OBJECTIVES

Upon completion of this chapter, you will be able to:

- Identify the mechanism and causes of sudden death syndrome.

- Describe the recommended management of sudden death syndrome.

- Specify major elements included in the treatment algorithms for monitored and unmonitored ventricular fibrillation, electromechanical dissociation, asystole, and ventricular tachycardia.

- Recall which treatment modality would be considered the "true definitive treatment" for ventricular fibrillation.

- Recognize factors that enhance the effectiveness of defibrillation.

- Relate the rationale for administration of epinephrine in the initial treatment of cardiac arrest.

- List the clinical conditions that may mimic electromechanical dissociation.

- List the dosage schedules for drugs commonly used in advanced cardiac life support.

- Compare the treatment of victims of near-drowning, electrocution, trauma, and hypothermia to the treatment of victims of sudden death syndrome.

1. When does sudden death due to coronary heart disease usually occur?

    _____

    _____

2. The mechanism of sudden death is usually:

    a. ventricular fibrillation
    b. ventricular tachycardia
    c. asystole
    d. severe bradycardia

3. The initial approach to patient care in an unwitnessed cardiac arrest is to:

    a. administer intracardiac epinephrine
    b. deliver CPR
    c. insert an esophageal airway
    d. establish an IV lifeline

4. For which type of cardiac arrest is immediate defibrillation the most appropriate initial approach?

    a. ventricular asystole (cardiac standstill)
    b. electromechanical dissociation (EMD)
    c. ventricular fibrillation
    d. ventricular tachycardia

5. The most effective way to ventilate and oxygenate a cardiac arrest victim is with:

    a. mouth-to-mouth ventilation
    b. bag-valve-mask device and 60% oxygen
    c. esophageal airway and 80% oxygen
    d. endotracheal intubation, bag-valve-mask device, and 100% oxygen

6. If no vein has been cannulated prior to cardiac arrest a (an) _____ vein would be considered the "site of first choice."

    a. antecubital
    b. subclavian
    c. femoral
    d. distal hand or wrist

7. Circle the correct answers. Sodium bicarbonate administration during cardiac arrest is:

    a. withheld until other more proven treatments have been employed without success
    b. begun without delay in witnessed cardiac arrest
    c. accompanied by effective pulmonary ventilation
    d. withheld if defibrillation is accomplished promptly and easily

8. When employed in cardiac arrest, the initial dosage of sodium bicarbonate is _____ and the repeat dosage is _____

    _____

9. Match the following conditions with their appropriate description:

    Condition

    a. monitored ventricular fibrillation
    b. asystole
    c. electromechanical dissociation
    d. unmonitored ventricular fibrillation
    e. ventricular tachycardia

    Description

    _____ 1. situation in which a chaotic ventricular rhythm can be definitively and immediately treated

    _____ 2. situation in which definitive treatment for a chaotic ventricular rhythm is delayed

    _____ 3. organized cardiac electrical activity (ECG) without a palpable pulse

    _____ 4. absence of all cardiac electrical activity and no palpable pulse

    _____ 5. three or more ventricular beats in succession

10. Which of the following would be considered the "true definitive treatment" for ventricular fibrillation?

    a. lidocaine
    b. defibrillation
    c. endotracheal intubation
    d. epinephrine

11. The correct dosage for the initial defibrillation attempt in the adult patient is _____ joules.

    a. 20
    b. 60
    c. 200
    d. 360

12. Initially, in the treatment of ventricular fibrillation the patient may be consecutively defibrillated up to a total of _____ times.

    a. 2
    b. 3
    c. 4
    d. 5

13. Which of the following medications is used in the treatment of most types of cardiac arrest?

a. atropine
b. lidocaine
c. epinephrine
d. isoproterenol

14. Following successful resuscitation from ventricular fibrillation, all patients should receive:

a. lidocaine, 2 to 4 mg/minute, IV infusion
b. supplemental oxygen
c. atropine, 0.5 to 1.0 mg, IV push
d. sodium bicarbonate, 1 mEq/kg, IV push

15. Which of the following medications may be useful in preparing the heart for defibrillation?

a. oxygen
b. isoproterenol
c. epinephrine
d. atropine
e. verapamil

16. Whenever sinus rhythm is observed on the ECG monitor during the course of resuscitation, the rescuer should:

a. defibrillate immediately
b. administer calcium chloride, IV push
c. assess pulses to determine circulatory status
d. establish an IV lifeline
e. apply MAST trousers

17. Match the following conditions with their recommended treatments. More than one treatment may be used for each condition.

Treatment

a. defibrillation
b. pacemaker
c. synchronized cardioversion
d. atropine
e. lidocaine
f. isoproterenol
g. procainamide
h. sodium bicarbonate
i. epinephrine
j. bretylium
k. oxygen

Condition

_____ ventricular fibrillation

_____ ventricular tachycardia with a pulse

_____ asystole

_____ electromechanical dissociation

18. T   F   In cardiac arrest secondary to near-drowning, resuscitation should be withheld if the victim has been submerged more than 20 minutes.

19. T   F   Extended resuscitation efforts in the field setting are considered acceptable when treating patients who have experienced cardiac arrest secondary to traumatic injury.

20. T   F   Resuscitation of the victim who has experienced cardiac arrest secondary to electrical shock is no different from that of cardiac arrest from any other cause.

21. T   F   In the hypothermic patient who has not yet gone into cardiac arrest, physical manipulations may precipitate ventricular fibrillation.

22. T   F   Management of cardiac arrest due to hypothermia should be the same as management of the normothermic arrest.

Questions 23 through 29 give algorithms for managing different cardiac emergencies. Fill in the missing treatments in the algorithm for each condition.

23.

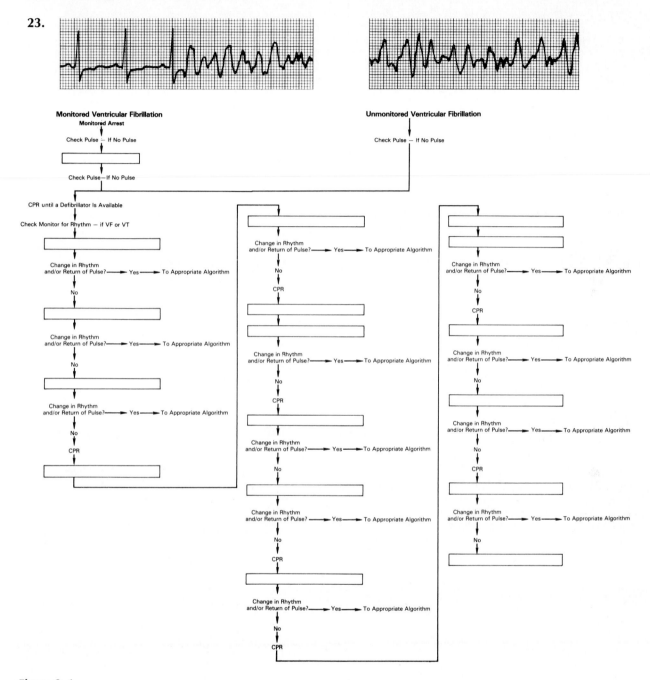

Figure 9–1

24.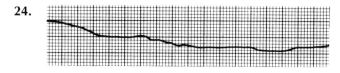

Asystole

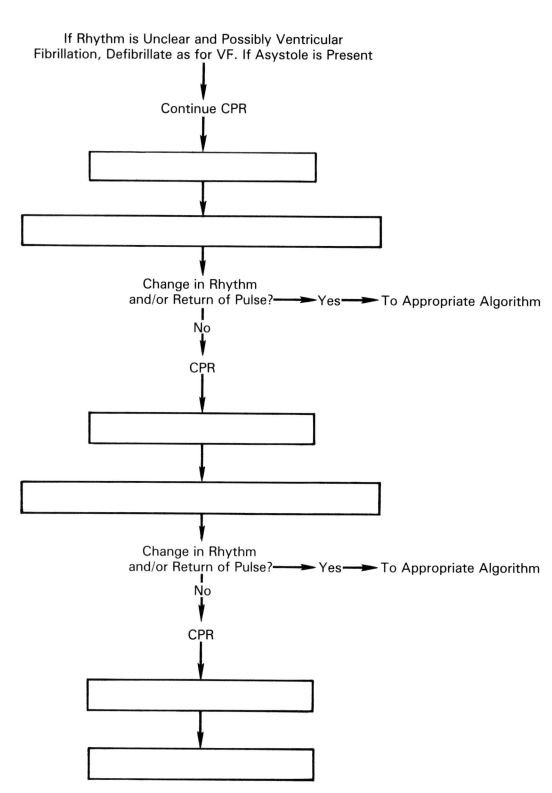

Figure 9–2

25.

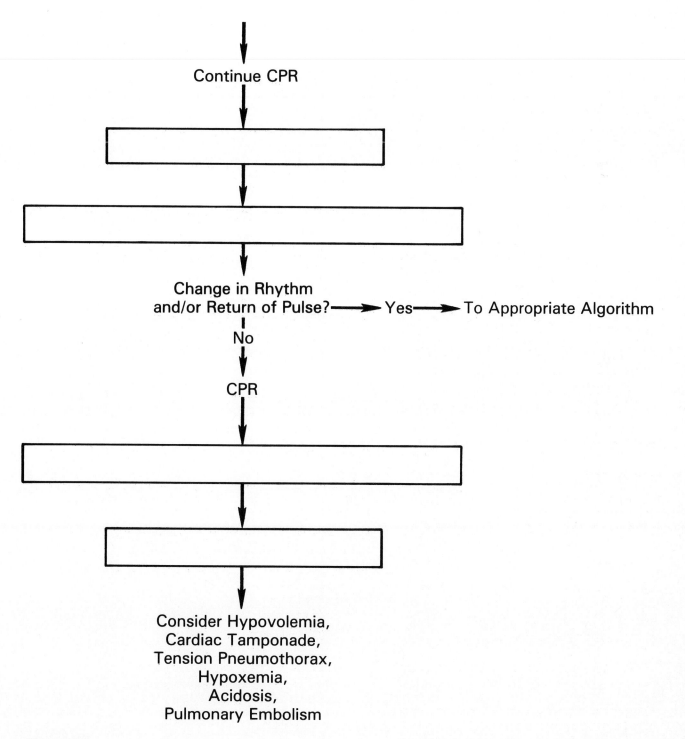

Electromechanical Dissociation

Continue CPR

Change in Rhythm
and/or Return of Pulse? ——▶ Yes ——▶ To Appropriate Algorithm

No

CPR

Consider Hypovolemia,
Cardiac Tamponade,
Tension Pneumothorax,
Hypoxemia,
Acidosis,
Pulmonary Embolism

Figure 9–3

26.

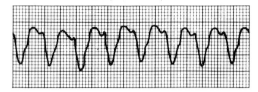

Ventricular Tachycardia

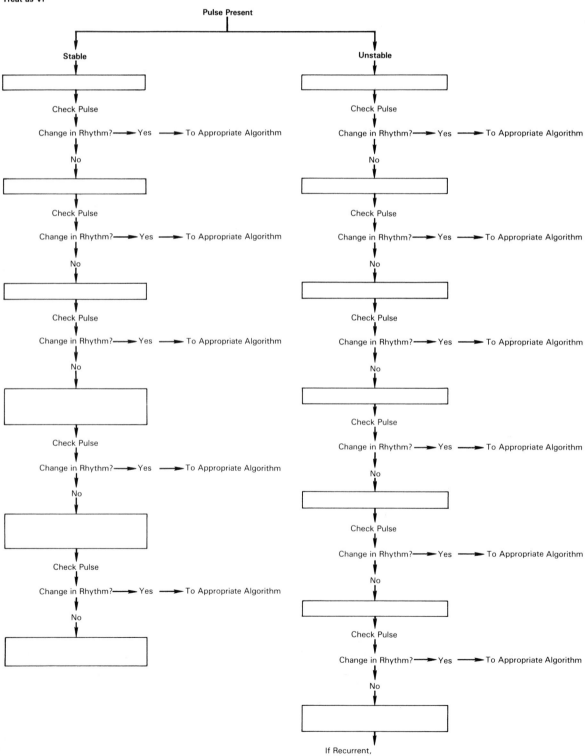

Figure 9–4

27.

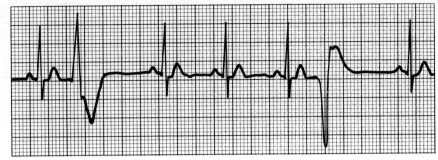

Ventricular Ectopy

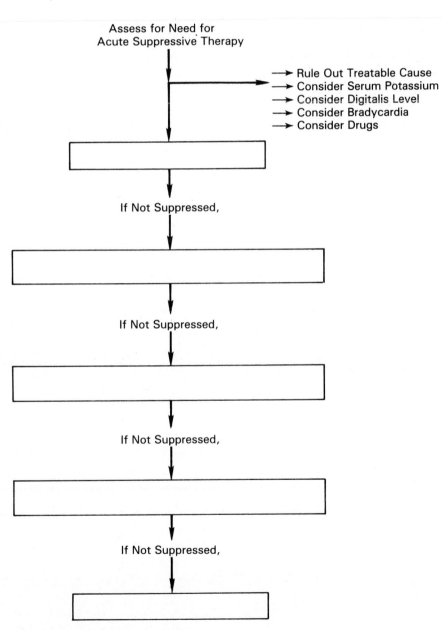

Assess for Need for
Acute Suppressive Therapy

→ Rule Out Treatable Cause
→ Consider Serum Potassium
→ Consider Digitalis Level
→ Consider Bradycardia
→ Consider Drugs

If Not Suppressed,

If Not Suppressed,

If Not Suppressed,

If Not Suppressed,

Once Ectopy Resolved, Maintain as Follows:

Figure 9-5

28.

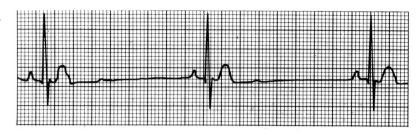

Bradycardia

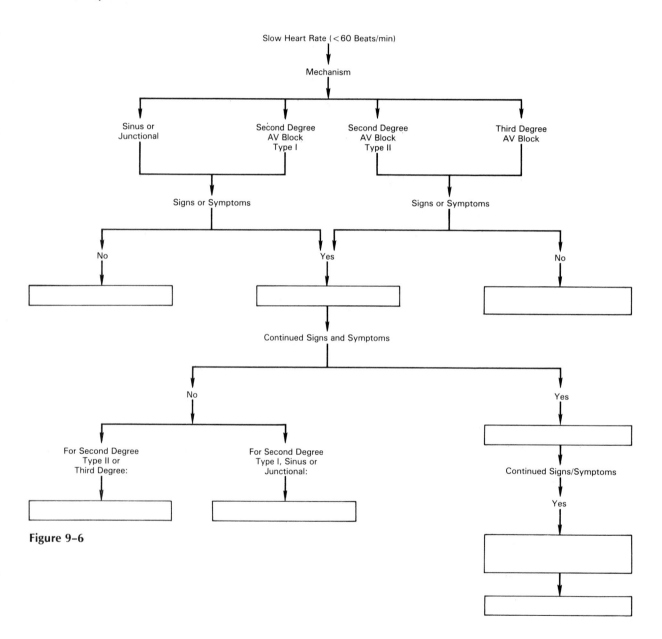

Figure 9–6

29.

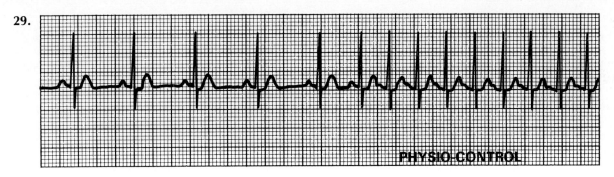

Paroxysmal Supraventricular Tachycardia (PSVT)

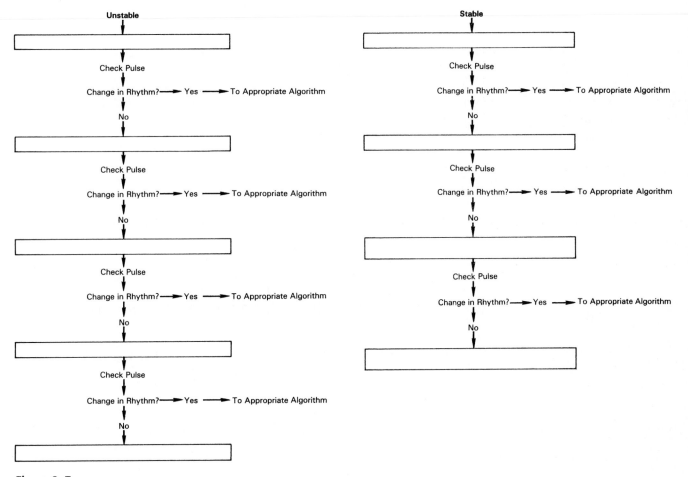

Figure 9–7

30. A 44-year-old newspaper reporter comes into your emergency department complaining of chest pain and shortness of breath. The patient is being monitored (ECG) and you are just preparing to put an IV lifeline in place. Suddenly the patient has a seizure, becomes unconscious, and shows ventricular fibrillation on the monitor; there is a defibrillator readily available. Number each of the treatments below to indicate the order in which you would perform them for this patient. (Assume the patient remains in ventricular fibrillation until the fourth defibrillation, at which time he converts to sinus rhythm with a good pulse and blood pressure. Assume that once CPR is initiated, it is continued whenever appropriate.)

_____ Perform a precordial thump; check for a pulse and rhythm change.

_____ Defibrillate at 200 joules; check for a pulse and rhythm change.

_____ Establish unresponsiveness and pulselessness.

_____ Defibrillate at 360 joules; check for a pulse and rhythm change.

_____ Administer lidocaine, 1 mg/kg bolus, followed by a 2- to 4-mg/minute IV infusion.

_____ Defibrillate at 200 to 300 joules; check for a pulse and rhythm change.

_____ Establish an IV lifeline.

_____ Insert an esophageal airway or endotracheal tube.

_____ Administer epinephrine, 0.5 to 1.0 mg.

_____ Begin CPR.

_____ Repeat defibrillation at 360 joules; check for a pulse and rhythm change.

31. Your rescue squad patient is a 35-year-old businessman who collapsed while standing in line at a local bank. You arrive at the scene to find bystanders performing CPR. The patient is pulseless and a "quick look" with the ECG paddles reveals that the patient is in ventricular fibrillation. Number each of the treatments below to indicate the order in which you would perform them for this patient. (Assume the patient remains in ventricular fibrillation despite treatment and that CPR is being performed as necessary.)

_____ Defibrillate at 200 joules; check for a pulse and rhythm change.

_____ Establish an IV lifeline.

_____ Administer lidocaine, 1 mg/kg.

_____ Defibrillate at 360 joules; check for a pulse and rhythm change.

_____ Repeat defibrillation at 360 joules; check for a pulse and rhythm change.

_____ Insert an esophageal airway or endotracheal tube.

_____ Defibrillate at 360 joules for the fifth time; check for a pulse and rhythm change.

_____ Administer epinephrine, 0.5 to 1.0 mg.

_____ Defibrillate at 200 to 300 joules; check for a pulse and rhythm change.

_____ Administer bretylium, 5 mg/kg, IV push.

_____ Consider bicarbonate, 1 mEq/kg, IV push.

_____ Defibrillate at 360 joules for the third time; check for a pulse and rhythm change.

_____ Defibrillate at 360 joules for the fourth time; check for a pulse and rhythm change.

_____ Administer bretylium, 10 mg/kg, IV push.

32. Explain why a second and third defibrillation are provided immediately after a first unsuccessful defibrillation.

_____

_____

_____

_____

_____

33. A 54-year-old construction worker was admitted to your CCU yesterday for a rule-out MI. The patient is being monitored, is receiving oxygen, and has an IV lifeline in place. The ECG shows sinus rhythm. While you are taking a routine blood pressure, the patient suddenly develops ventricular tachycardia and loses consciousness, but has a weak, palpable pulse. Number each of the treatments below to indicate the order in which you would perform them for this patient. (Assume that the patient remains in this condition until you are advised otherwise.)

_____ Cardiovert with 100 joules; check for a pulse and rhythm change.

_____ Cardiovert with up to 360 joules; check for a pulse and rhythm change; the patient is now in sinus rhythm with a good pulse and blood pressure.

_____ Administer lidocaine, 1-mg/kg bolus, followed by a 2- to 4-mg/minute IV infusion.

_____ Cardiovert with 50 joules; check for a pulse and rhythm change.

_____ Cardiovert with 200 joules; check for a pulse and rhythm change.

34. A 60-year-old female who has been in cardiac arrest for several minutes prior to your arrival is found to be in asystole. CPR has been initiated. Number each of the treatments below to indicate the order in which you would perform them for this patient. (Assume that the patient remains in asystole and that CPR is being provided as indicated.)

_____ Administer epinephrine, 0.5 to 1.0 mg.

_____ Establish an IV lifeline.

_____ Administer atropine, 1.0 mg.

_____ Consider sodium bicarbonate administration, 1 mEq/kg.

_____ Insert an esophageal airway or endotracheal tube.

_____ Consider pacing.

35. Explain why defibrillation in "uncertain asystole" is considered acceptable.

_____

_____

_____

_____

_____

_____

36. Identify mechanisms that may mimic electromechanical dissociation.

_____

_____

_____

_____

37. Your patient is a 75-year-old female who has experienced cardiac arrest while watching television. You have begun CPR and taken a "quick look" at the ECG rhythm; the patient is in a sinus rhythm, but there are no palpable pulses. Number each of the treatments below to indicate the order in which they should be performed for this patient. (Assume that the patient remains in this condition despite treatment and that CPR is continued.)

_____ Establish an IV lifeline.

_____ Consider sodium bicarbonate administration, 1 mEq/kg.

_____ Insert an esophageal airway or endotracheal tube.

_____ Administer epinephrine, 0.5 to 1.0 mg.

38. Match the following medications with their appropriate dosage and time for repeat administration. Answers may be used more than once.

Medication	Dosage	Repeat Time
Atropine	_____	_____
Sodium bicarbonate	_____	_____
Epinephrine	_____	_____
Bretylium	_____	_____
Lidocaine	_____	_____
Procainamide	_____	_____

a. 0.5 to 1.0 mg of a 1:10,000 solution (5 to 10 ml)
b. initial dosage: 1 mEq/kg; repeat dosage: half the initial dosage
c. 20 mg (up to 1000 mg)
d. repeat every 5 minutes
e. every minute until conversion
f. 1 mg/kg IV push followed by a 2- to 4-mg/minute IV infusion
g. repeat every 8 to 10 minutes
h. 1 mg (10 ml)
i. initial dosage: 5 mg/kg; repeat dosage: 10 mg/kg
j. repeat as necessary
k. repeat every 10 minutes
l. repeat at 15- to 30-minute intervals

ANSWER KEY

1. Sudden death usually occurs within 1 hour of symptom onset.

2. a: The mechanism of sudden death is usually ventricular fibrillation.

3. b: CPR should be begun immediately unless it is determined ventricular fibrillation is present and a defibrillator is readily available. In which case, defibrillation should be performed at the earliest possible time.

4. c, d: In ventricular fibrillation, defibrillation should be performed at the earliest possible time. Ventricular tachycardia without a pulse (cardiac arrest) should be treated the same as ventricular fibrillation.

5. d

6. a: An antecubital vein is the site of first choice if no vein has been cannulated prior to cardiac arrest.

7. a, c, d: Sodium bicarbonate is used only after interventions such as defibrillation, CPR, ventilatory support including intubation, and pharmacological therapies such as epinephrine and antiarrhythmics have been employed and have not converted the patient into an effective electromechanical rhythm.

8. When employed in cardiac arrest, the dosage of bicarbonate is 1 mEq/kg initially, and one-half the initial dose every 10 minutes thereafter.

9. 1–a, 2–d, 3–c, 4–b, 5–e

10. b: The "true definitive treatment" for ventricular fibrillation is *defibrillation*. It should be performed as soon as possible in ventricular fibrillation (and ventricular tachycardia without a pulse).

11. c: The dosage for initial defibrillation is 200 joules; if the rhythm does not change, the patient should receive a second immediate defibrillation with 200 to 300 joules. If the rhythm does not change after the second defibrillation attempt, the patient should be immediately defibrillated with 360 joules. Cardiopulmonary resuscitation should be started or restarted if the third defibrillation attempt is unsuccessful.

12. b: Initially, in the treatment of ventricular fibrillation the patient may be consecutively defibrillated up to a total of three times.

13. c: Epinephrine is used in the treatment of most types of cardiac arrest, including ventricular fibrillation, asystole, and EMD (electromechanical dissociation).

14. a, b: following successful resuscitation from ventricular fibrillation, all patients should receive lidocaine, 2- to 4-mg/minute IV infusion. If lidocaine, 1 mg/kg, has not been administered during the resuscitation or if it has been greater than 8 to 10 minutes since the last IV bolus was administered, the patient should receive a loading dose, 0.5 to 1 mg/kg of lidocaine, IV push, prior to the infusion.

15. a, c

16. c: Whenever sinus rhythm is observed during the course of resuscitation, the rescuer should assess pulses.

17. *ventricular fibrillation:* a, e, h*, i, j, k: defibrillation, lidocaine, sodium bicarbonate,* epinephrine, bretylium, oxygen
ventricular tachycardia with pulse: c†, e, g, j, k: synchronized cardioversion, lidocaine, procainamide, bretylium, oxygen
asystole‡: b, d, h*, i, k: pacemaker, atropine, sodium bicarbonate,* epinephrine, oxygen
electromechanical dissociation: h*, i, k: sodium bicarbonate, epinephrine, oxygen

18. FALSE: As there have been reported cases of successful resuscitation with full neurological recovery in prolonged submersion, it is currently believed that rescuers should initiate resuscitation unless there is obvious physical evidence of death. This is different from typical sudden death syndrome, where brain death is thought to occur 4 to 6 minutes following cardiac arrest.

19. FALSE: Currently it is believed that survival from cardiac arrest secondary to traumatic injury is poor and that external cardiac compressions may not provide adequate circulation in the severely hypovolemic patient. When treating the trauma patient, time becomes a critical factor; the patient should be expediently packaged and transported to a trauma center where circulating blood volume can be restored and the underlying vascular injury can be repaired. This is different from sudden death syndrome, where extended time may be spent in the prehospital and/or emergency department setting attempting to stabilize the patient.

20. TRUE: Although associated burn injuries and such must be treated as well, the resuscitation effort is managed similarly to cardiac arrest from most other causes.

21. TRUE: Physical manipulations, such as endotracheal or nasogastric intubation, placement of temporary pacemakers, and/or insertion of pulmonary artery flow-directed catheters, may precipitate ventricular fibrillation in the prearrest hypothermic patient.

22. FALSE: Management of cardiac arrest due to hypothermia is quite different from the management of the normothermic patient. Defibrillation is not likely to be effective in the hypothermic patient until he or she is closer to a normal temperature. The usefulness of bretylium in the resuscitation effort of the hypothermic patient is uncertain. Treatment should be directed toward rapid core rewarming. The patient should not be pronounced dead until he or she is at near "normal core temperature" and still fails to respond to resuscitation efforts.

---

*May be considered.
†If hypotension, pulmonary edema, or unconsciousness is present, unsynchronized cardioversion should be done to avoid delay.
‡If rhythm is unclear and possibly ventricular fibrillation is present, defibrillate as for ventricular fibrillation.

23.

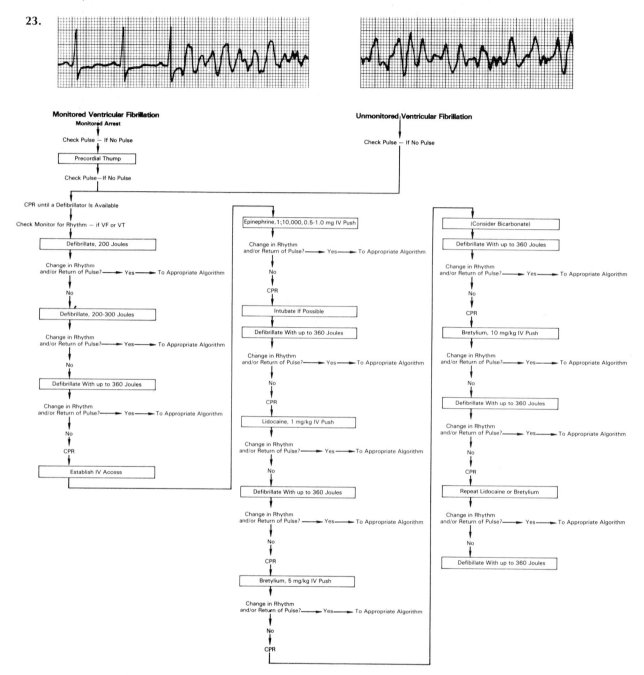

Figure 9–8

24.

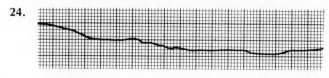

Asystole

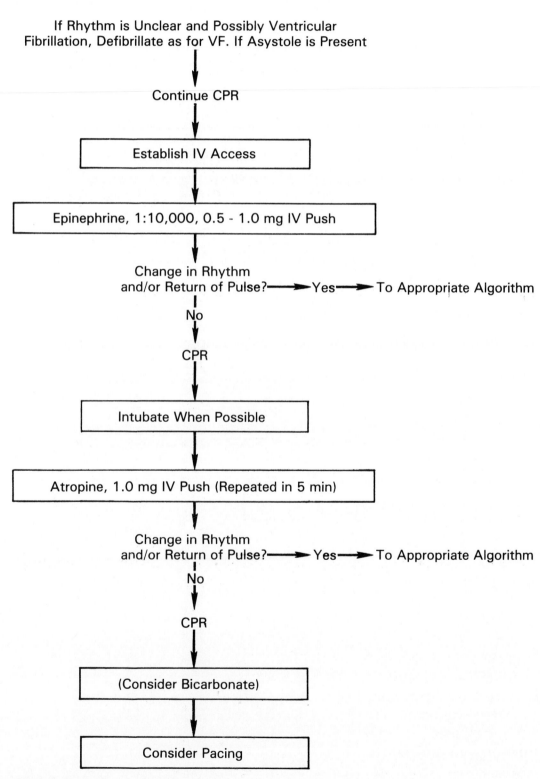

If Rhythm is Unclear and Possibly Ventricular
Fibrillation, Defibrillate as for VF. If Asystole is Present

Continue CPR

Establish IV Access

Epinephrine, 1:10,000, 0.5 - 1.0 mg IV Push

Change in Rhythm
and/or Return of Pulse?———►Yes———►To Appropriate Algorithm

No

CPR

Intubate When Possible

Atropine, 1.0 mg IV Push (Repeated in 5 min)

Change in Rhythm
and/or Return of Pulse?———►Yes———►To Appropriate Algorithm

No

CPR

(Consider Bicarbonate)

Consider Pacing

Figure 9–9

25.

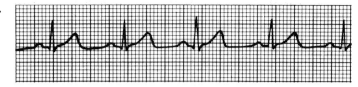

Electromechanical Dissociation

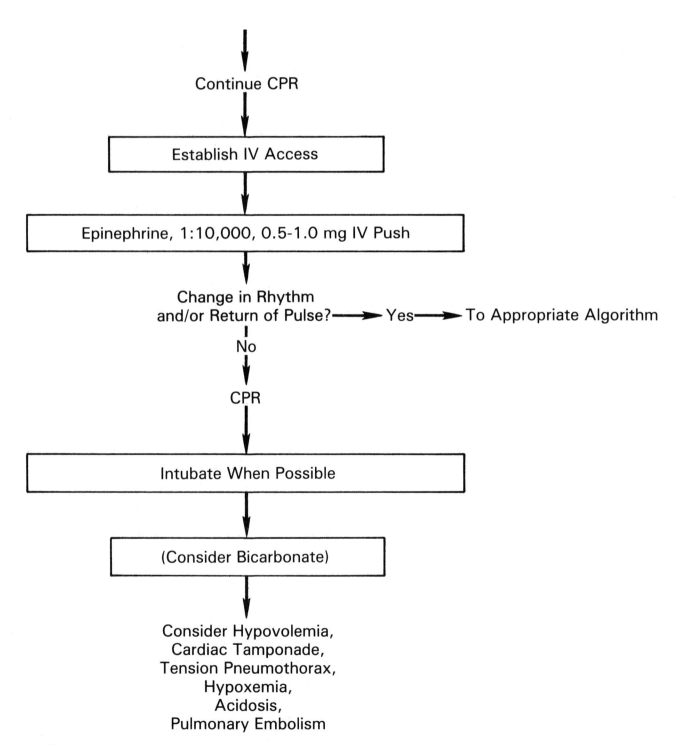

Continue CPR

Establish IV Access

Epinephrine, 1:10,000, 0.5-1.0 mg IV Push

Change in Rhythm
and/or Return of Pulse? ——→ Yes ——→ To Appropriate Algorithm

No

CPR

Intubate When Possible

(Consider Bicarbonate)

Consider Hypovolemia,
Cardiac Tamponade,
Tension Pneumothorax,
Hypoxemia,
Acidosis,
Pulmonary Embolism

Figure 9–10

26.

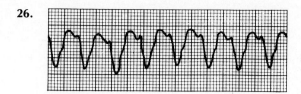

Ventricular Tachycardia

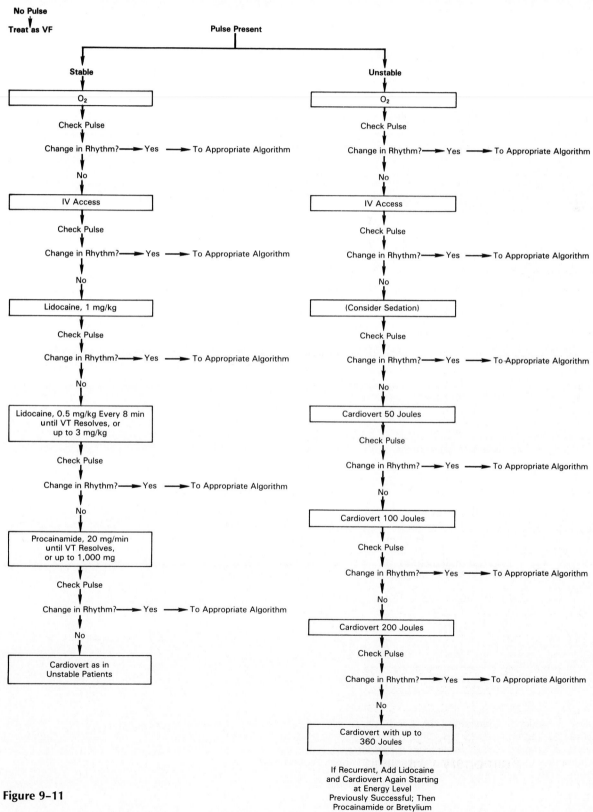

Figure 9–11

27.

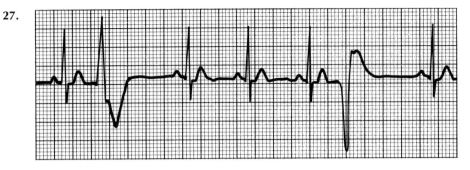

Ventricular Ectopy

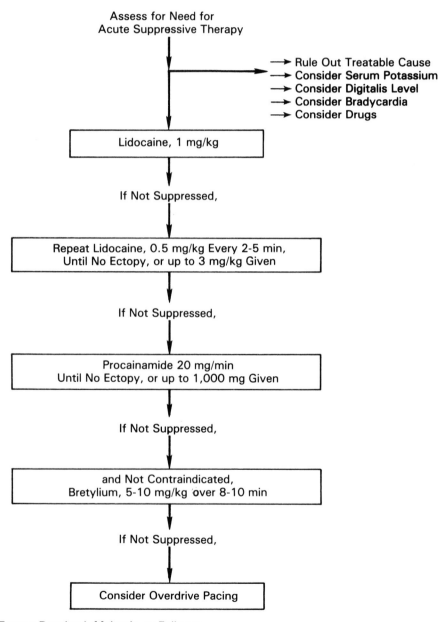

Once Ectopy Resolved, Maintain as Follows:
    After Lidocaine, 1 mg/kg . . . Lidocaine Drip, 2 mg/min
    After Lidocaine, 1-2 mg/kg . . . Lidocaine Drip, 3 mg/min
    After Lidocaine, 2-3 mg/kg . . . Lidocaine Drip, 4 mg/min
    After Procainamide . . . Procainamide Drip, 1-4 mg/min (Check Blood Level)
    After Bretylium . . . Bretylium Drip, 2 mg/min

Figure 9–12

28.

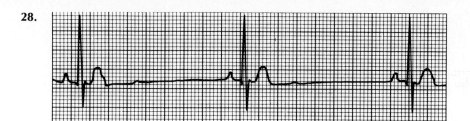

Bradycardia

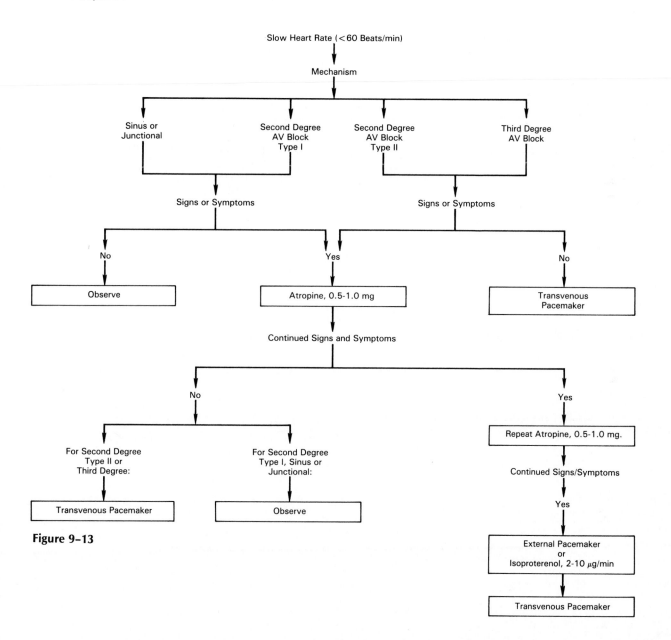

Slow Heart Rate (<60 Beats/min)

↓

Mechanism

Sinus or Junctional　　Second Degree AV Block Type I　　Second Degree AV Block Type II　　Third Degree AV Block

Signs or Symptoms　　　　　　Signs or Symptoms

No → Observe

Yes → Atropine, 0.5-1.0 mg

No → Transvenous Pacemaker

Continued Signs and Symptoms

No → For Second Degree Type II or Third Degree: Transvenous Pacemaker

For Second Degree Type I, Sinus or Junctional: Observe

Yes → Repeat Atropine, 0.5-1.0 mg.

Continued Signs/Symptoms

Yes → External Pacemaker or Isoproterenol, 2-10 µg/min

Transvenous Pacemaker

Figure 9–13

29.

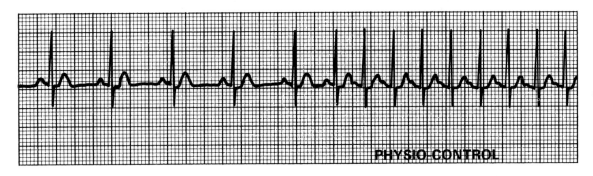

Paroxysmal Supraventricular Tachycardia (PSVT)

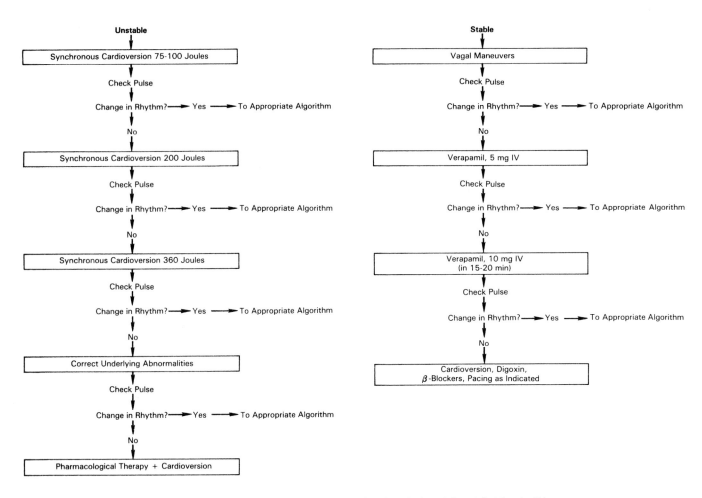

If conversion occurs but PSVT recurs, repeated electrical cardioversion is *not* indicated. Sedation should be used as time permits.

Figure 9–14

30. Monitored ventricular fibrillation:

    1st: Establish unresponsiveness and pulselessness.

    2nd: Perform a precordial thump; check for a pulse and rhythm change.

    3rd: Defibrillate at 200 joules; check for a pulse and rhythm change.

    4th: Defibrillate at 200 to 300 joules; check for a pulse and rhythm change.

    5th: Defibrillate at 360 joules; check for a pulse and rhythm change.

    6th: Begin CPR.

    7th: Establish an IV lifeline.

    8th: Administer epinephrine, 0.5 to 1.0 mg.

    9th: Insert an esophageal airway or endotracheal tube.

    10th: Repeat defibrillation with 360 joules; check for a pulse and rhythm change.

    11th: Administer lidocaine, 1-mg/kg bolus, followed by a 2- to 4-mg/minute IV infusion.

31. Unmonitored ventricular fibrillation:

    1st: Defibrillate at 200 joules; check for a pulse and rhythm change.

    2nd: Defibrillate at 200 to 300 joules; check for a pulse and rhythm change.

    3rd: Defibrillate at 360 joules; check for a pulse and rhythm change.

    4th: Establish an IV lifeline.

    5th: Administer epinephrine, 0.5 to 1.0 mg.

    6th: Insert an esophageal airway or endotracheal tube.

    7th: Repeat defibrillation at 360 joules; check for a pulse and rhythm change.

    8th: Administer lidocaine, 1 mg/kg.

    9th: Defibrillate at 360 joules for the third time; check for a pulse and rhythm change.

    10th: Administer bretylium, 5 mg/kg, IV push.

    11th: Consider sodium bicarbonate, 1 mEq/kg, IV push.

    12th: Defibrillate at 360 joules for the fourth time; check for a pulse and rhythm change.

    13th: Administer bretylium, 10 mg/kg, IV push.

    14th: Defibrillate at 360 joules for the fifth time; check for a pulse and rhythm change.

32. The rationale for attempting defibrillation a second and third time immediately following the first attempt is that the initial defibrillation may reduce the transthoracic resistance, allowing the second and third attempt to deliver more energy to the myocardium.

33. Unstable ventricular tachycardia:

    1st: Cardiovert with 50 joules; check for a pulse and rhythm change.

    2nd: Cardiovert with 100 joules; check for a pulse and rhythm change.

    3rd: Cardiovert with 200 joules; check for a pulse and rhythm change.

    4th: Cardiovert with up to 360 joules; check for a pulse and rhythm change; the patient is now in sinus rhythm with a good pulse and blood pressure.

    5th: Administer lidocaine, 1-mg/kg bolus, followed by a 2- to 4-mg/minute IV infusion.

34. Ventricular asystole:

    1st: Establish an IV lifeline.

    2nd: Administer epinephrine, 0.5 to 1.0 mg.

    3rd: Insert an esophageal airway or endotracheal tube.

    4th: Administer atropine, 1.0 mg.

    5th: Consider sodium bicarbonate administration, 1 mEq/kg.

    6th: Consider pacing.

35. Defibrillation in ''uncertain asystole'' is acceptable because the rhythm may actually be fine ventricular fibrillation that is not apparent on the lead being viewed. In some leads the ECG may not display the usual chaotic baseline, but, rather, just a flat line, which ordinarily would suggest asystole.

36. Mechanisms that may mimic electromechanical dissociation include (1) hypovolemia, (2) cardiac tamponade, and (3) myocardial rupture.

37. Electromechanical dissociation:

    1st: Establish an IV lifeline.

    2nd: Administer epinephrine, 0.5 to 1.0 mg.

    3rd: Insert an esophageal airway or endotracheal tube.

    4th: Consider sodium bicarbonate administration, 1 mEq/kg.

38.

Medication	Dosage	Repeat Time
Atropine	h	d
Sodium bicarbonate	b	k
Epinephrine	a	d
Bretylium	i	l
Lidocaine	f	g
Procainamide	c	e

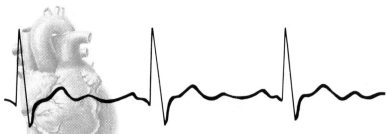

Chapter 10

Neonatal and Pediatric Resuscitation

OBJECTIVES

Upon completion of this chapter, you will be able to:

- Identify the etiology and signs of hypoxia in a neonate.
- Specify considerations in ventilation and resuscitation that are unique to the neonate.
- Describe the Apgar Scoring System for neonates.
- Explain how to cannulate the umbilical vein of a neonate.
- Describe how to effectively ventilate a pediatric CPR victim.
- Compare and contrast the use of oxygen therapy devices for resuscitation of neonates, children, and adults.
- Specify how to defibrillate the pediatric patient.
- Recognize pediatric dosages of drugs commonly employed in emergency cardiac care.

1. Circulatory collapse in infants and children is usually the result of (circle one):

   a. congenital cardiac anomalies
   b. acute myocardial infarction
   c. hypoxia
   d. hyperpyrexia
   e. potassium imbalance

2. Which of the following may lead to hypoxia in the newborn?

   a. high concentrations of supplemental oxygen immediately after delivery
   b. airway obstruction due to mucus, blood, meconium, or displacement of the tongue
   c. respiratory depression from pain medications given to the mother
   d. cardiac, respiratory, or neurologic congenital anomalies
   e. hypovolemic shock due to cord compression or hemorrhage

True or False

3. T F Neither slowing nor speeding of the neonate's heart rate during delivery should be a cause for concern.

4. T F During the first few minutes of life, there is less likelihood of the need for resuscitation than during any other subsequent period.

5. T F All neonates have difficulty tolerating a cold environment.

6. Identify two procedures that can preserve body temperature in the neonate following delivery outside the hospital.

   1) _____

   _____

   2) _____

   _____

7. Fill in the missing elements on the Apgar scoring chart illustrated in Table 10–1.

TABLE 10–1

Sign	Apgar Score		
	0	1	2
Heart rate			
Respirations			
Muscle tone			
Reflex irritability (catheter in nares)			
Color			

8. Explain the importance of suctioning the nostrils of a neonate during and after delivery.

   _____

   _____

9. When suctioning the neonate following delivery:

   a. negative pressures exceeding 100 cm of H_2O can be applied safely
   b. the heart rate should be monitored for bradycardia
   c. negative pressures should be maintained during both insertion and removal of the suction catheter
   d. suctioning duration can exceed 30 seconds

10. The neonate's ventilations should be assisted:

    a. any time the neonate appears cyanotic after delivery
    b. when simple tactile stimuli do not establish spontaneous breathing
    c. as soon as the head is exposed during delivery
    d. when the ventilatory state is not adequate to maintain a heart rate over 100 beats/minute
    e. whenever the Apgar score is less than 2

11. When ventilating neonates with a bag-valve-mask device, the ventilatory rate should be _____ to _____ breaths per minute.

    a. 10 to 16
    b. 20 to 28
    c. 30 to 40
    d. 50 to 60

12. Signs of adequate ventilatory assistance in the neonate include:

    a. bradycardia
    b. full bilateral chest expansion with each delivered breath
    c. improved skin color
    d. normal breath sounds
    e. resistance to assisted ventilation

True or False

13. T   F   To deliver 100% oxygen with a self-inflating bag, a reservoir device must be attached to the intake valve of the bag.

14. T   F   The neonate may not be ventilated adequately during initial ventilations because many self-inflating bags have a pressure-limiting pop-off valve that is preset at 30 cm of H_2O.

15. T   F   The volume of a self-inflating bag to be used for neonates should have a capacity of at least 1600 ml.

16. T   F   Neither anesthesia bags nor pressure face masks are recommended for use with neonates.

17. Explain why endotracheal tubes with a uniform internal diameter are preferable to tapered tubes for neonates.

_____

_____

_____

_____

18. On Figure 10–1, draw an endotracheal tube to indicate the correct tube depth for a neonate.

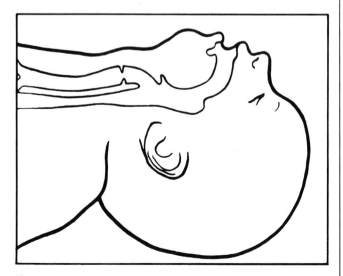

Figure 10–1

19. List three ways to verify correct placement of a neonate's endotracheal tube.

1) _____

_____

2) _____

_____

3) _____

_____

20. When should chest compressions be instituted for the neonate?

_____

_____

_____

21. Describe the technique for cannulating the umbilical vein in the neonate.

_____

_____

_____

_____

_____

True or False

22. T   F   100% oxygen should be used for resuscitating an infant or child.

23. T   F   Infants who develop ventricular fibrillation are usually taking digoxin.

24. Match the following airway devices used for neonates and children with their appropriate description.

Oxygen Device

a. esophageal obturator airway
b. oropharyngeal airway
c. nasopharyngeal airway

Description

_____ 1. useful in the unconscious child, but should not be used if the child is conscious or has a gag reflex

_____ 2. not yet developed for use with infants or children

_____ 3. is better tolerated in the conscious child who is older than 3 to 4 years

25. Why should the pediatric patient's head be prevented from flexing or extending after endotracheal intubation?

_____

_____

_____

_____

26. What should be done if the pediatric patient develops a dysrhythmia during the course of intubation?

_____

_____

_____

27. When administering oxygen to the pediatric patient via simple face mask, the liter flow should

be _____ to _____ liters per minute.

a. 2 to 3
b. 3 to 4
c. 6 to 8
d. 10 to 12

True or False

28. T　F　Oxygen-powered breathing devices should not be used in the infant or child.

29. T　F　Children should receive intravenous solutions through a surgical (regular drip) administration set.

30. Describe defibrillator paddle placement for infants and children.

_____

_____

_____

31. T　F　When defibrillating the infant or child who is on digoxin, the lowest possible energy dose should be used.

32. T　F　When arterial blood gases are not available, the initial dosage of sodium bicarbonate for infants and children is 1 mEq/kg.

33. T　F　When arterial blood gases are not available, the repeat dosage of sodium bicarbonate for infants and children is 1 mEq/kg.

34. T　F　When arterial blood gases are not available, sodium bicarbonate administration may be repeated every five minutes.

35. T　F　When arterial blood gases are available, the dosage of sodium bicarbonate for children and infants should be calculated according to the base deficit.

36. The concentration of epinephrine administered to the pediatric patient is:

a. 1:10
b. 1:100
c. 1:1000
d. 1:10,000

37. The IV push dosage of epinephrine for the pediatric patient is _____ ml/kg.

a. 0.01
b. 0.05
c. 0.10
d. 0.50

38. A continuous infusion of epinephrine may be administered in the pediatric patient at a dose

of _____ μg/kg/minute.

   a. 0.01
   b. 0.05
   c. 0.10
   d. 0.50

39. A continuous infusion of isoproterenol may be administered to the pediatric patient at a dosage

of _____ μg/kg/minute.

   a. 0.01
   b. 0.05
   c. 0.10
   d. 0.50

40. The initial energy dosage for defibrillation in infants and children is _____ joule(s)/kg.

   a. 1
   b. 2
   c. 3
   d. 4

41. If initial defibrillation of the infant or child is not effective, the energy dosage should be:

   a. the same
   b. reduced by one-half
   c. reduced by three-fourths
   d. doubled

42. For a pediatric patient, a bolus of lidocaine should be given at a dosage of _____ mg/kg; a lidocaine infusion should run at a dosage rate

of _____ μg/kg/minute.

   a. 0.1;   1 to 5
   b. 0.1;   5 to 10
   c. 1.0;   20 to 50
   d. 1.0;   50 to 100

ANSWER KEY

1. c

2. b, c, d, e

3. FALSE: Either slowing or speeding of a neonate's heart rate during delivery suggests that the neonate is hypoxic.

4. FALSE: The first few minutes of life have the greatest likelihood of the need for resuscitation than at any other subsequent period.

5. TRUE

6. To preserve body temperature in the neonate (1) dry the neonate completely and place the child under a radiant heater or (2) dry, cover, and place the child next to the mother.

7. Apgar Scoring System (see Table 10–2)

TABLE 10–2

	Apgar Score		
Sign	0	1	2
Heart rate	Absent	Slow (< 100/min)	> 100/min
Respirations	Absent	Slow, irregular	Good, crying
Muscle tone	Limp	Some flexion	Active motion
Reflex irritability (catheter in nares)	No response	Grimace	Cough or sneeze
Color	Blue or pale	Pink body with blue extremities	Completely pink

8. It is important to suction the nostrils of a neonate during and after delivery because neonates are obligate nose breathers.

9. b

10. b, d

11. c

12. b, c, d

13. TRUE (see Figure 10–2)

When the bag of the device is squeezed (forcing the air out) and then released, ambient (room) air will be drawn in to fill the bag. This ambient air contains 21% oxygen. If the bag is being used without a supplemental oxygen source, 21% oxygen is delivered to the patient.

When a supplemental oxygen source is added (10 to 15 liters, direct oxygen tubing) the patient will receive approximately 60% oxygen. This is because ambient air is still being drawn in to fill the bag thus diluting the concentration of the incoming oxygen.

To deliver 100% oxygen, a reservoir device is added. This allows the 100% oxygen to accumulate in the reservoir and when the bag is released (after being squeezed) the contents of the reservoir device will be drawn into the bag.

Figure 10–2

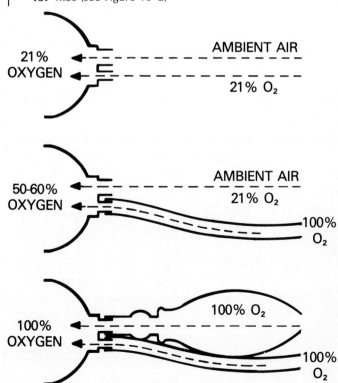

14. TRUE: It may require pressures as high as 40 to 60 cm of H_2O to overcome the resistance of a neonate's nonaerated lung. A pop-off valve usually does not allow pressures of higher than 30 to 35 cm of H_2O to be used.

15. FALSE: The volume of a self-inflating bag to be used for neonates should be no greater than 750 ml.

16. TRUE

17. Endotracheal tubes with uniform diameters are preferable to tapered tubes for neonates because the small end of the tapered tube becomes obstructed easily, provides a high resistance to airflow, makes passage of a suction catheter difficult, and tends to kink at the shoulder (see Figure 10–3).

TWO TYPES OF ENDOTRACHEAL TUBE:

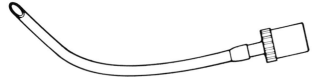

A. Uniform diameter endotracheal tube.

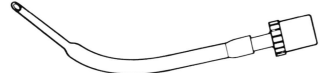

B. "Cole-type" shouldered endotracheal tube.

Figure 10–3

18. The correct depth for an endotracheal tube in the neonate is illustrated in Figure 10–4.

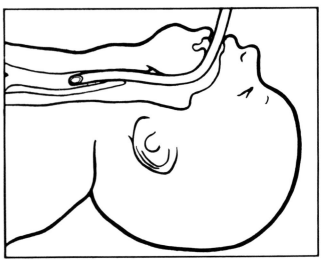

Endotracheal tube in proper position midway in the trachea.

Figure 10–4

19. Ways to verify the correct location of a neonate's endotracheal tube include (1) mark the tube to reflect the distance of the tip from the glottic opening, (2) observe symmetrical movement of the chest wall and auscultate bilateral breath sounds, and (3) a chest roentgenogram.

20. Chest compressions should be instituted when (1) the pulse is absent or (2) the heart rate is less than 80 per minute and does not respond immediately to effective ventilation with oxygen.

21. Wash the umbilical stump and the surrounding tissue with an antiseptic solution and cover the lower legs and abdomen with a sterile drape. Trim the cord with a scalpel 1 cm above the skin and hold the umbilical cord firm to prevent bleeding. Insert a saline-filled 3.5 to 5.0 French catheter (to prevent air embolism) with a three-way stopcock attached 5 to 8 cm or until free blood return is obtained. See Figure 10–5.

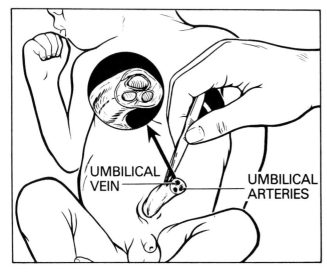

UMBILICAL VEIN

UMBILICAL ARTERIES

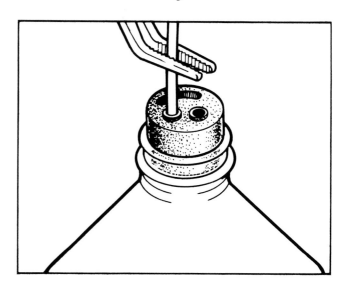

Figure 10–5

22. TRUE

23. TRUE: The important point to understand about this is that defibrillation potentiates the effects of digoxin and may cause irreversible cardiac arrest in the pediatric patient when delivered at the usual dosage. When defibrillating the patient on digoxin, the lowest possible dosage should be used.

24. 1–b, 2–a, 3–c

25. Flexion may advance the endotracheal tube toward the carina or into the right mainstem brochus, whereas extension may result in accidental extubation.

26. The intubation attempt should be interrupted and the patient should be ventilated again with 100% oxygen using a bag-valve-mask device.

27. c

28. TRUE

29. FALSE: IV solutions for children should be administered with an infusion pump; if not available, a microdrip must be used and the infusion rate carefully controlled.

30. Defibrillator paddle placement for infants and children: one paddle to the right of the sternum at the second rib and the other in the left midclavicular line at the xyphoid level (see Figure 10–6).

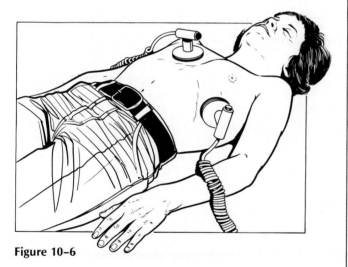

Figure 10–6

31. TRUE: If initial attempts are unsuccessful, energy levels should be increased slowly and cautiously.

32. TRUE: When blood gases are not available, the initial dosage of bicarbonate for children is 1.0 mEq/kg. A dilute solution (0.5 mEq/ml) should be used in infants.

33. TRUE

34. FALSE: Bicarbonate may be administered every 10 minutes.

35. TRUE

36. d

37. c

38. c

39. c

40. b

41. d

42. c

Chapter 11

Perspectives and Legal Aspects in ACLS

OBJECTIVES

Upon completion of this chapter, you will be able to:

- Identify the epidemiological risk factors and causes of sudden cardiac death.
- Distinguish conditions that alter the predisposition to sudden cardiac death.
- Describe known influences on mortality associated with acute myocardial infarction and sudden death.
- Explain the importance of public education and training in reducing mortality associated with cardiac arrest.
- Differentiate among the various components of the EMS–emergency cardiac care system and their roles in resuscitative efforts.
- List the features necessary for stabilization of cardiac patients before transport to a definitive care facility.
- Specify the role of telemetry in prehospital cardiac care.
- Define the components needed by a health-care facility to stabilize cardiac patients.
- List the responsibilities of an EMS medical director.
- Explain the major legal implications of ACLS for physicians and other members of the resuscitation team.
- Identify the AHA guidelines for initiating and terminating CPR and ACLS.
- Specify the elements necessary for malpractice and negligence claims in relation to resuscitative efforts.
- Explain the physician's legal responsibilities in providing ACLS.

1. Utilize Figure 11–1 to match the following disease categories with their incidence as a cause of sudden death:

   a. cardiovascular disease
   b. miscellaneous diseases
   c. digestive and urogenital diseases
   d. respiratory disease
   e. central nervous system disease

CAUSES OF SUDDEN DEATH

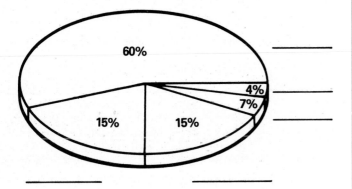

Figure 11–1

2. Match the following factors with their effect on community mortality from coronary heart disease.

Effect

   a. increases mortality
   b. decreases mortality

Factors

_____ increased cigarette smoking

_____ decreased use of saturated fats

_____ increase in health awareness

_____ decrease in individual fitness

_____ decrease in hypertension

True or False

3. T   F   PVCs that follow acute myocardial infarction are associated with an increased incidence of sudden death.

4. T   F   Frequent PVCs in middle-aged men are an independent predictor of coronary artery disease.

5. T   F   PVCs have little or no relationship to sudden death in patients with known heart disease.

6. T   F   Even in the absence of heart disease, PVCs have an adverse prognostic significance.

7. T   F   Research studies indicate that the presence of dysrhythmias alone is a sufficient determinant of poor prognosis in cardiac arrest; ischemia and other abnormalities need not be present to predispose these individuals to cardiac arrest.

8. T   F   To prevent sudden death, treatment should be directed toward the "triggering factors" rather than toward dysrhythmia control per se.

9. Match the following conditions with their appropriate description.

Condition

   a. coronary artery thrombosis
   b. acute myocardial infarction
   c. hemorrhage into an atheromatous plaque
   d. ventricular function abnormalities
   e. coronary artery spasm

Description

_____ predisposes the heart to ventricular fibrillation

_____ event seen with 16% of patients who die within one hour and 54% of those who survive 24 hours; may follow rather than precede myocardial ischemia

_____ associated with sudden death in 10% to 47% of cases

_____ more recently considered as a possible mechanism for myocardial infarction and sudden death

_____ plays a relatively small role in causing sudden cardiac death

10. Which of the following statements may be true concerning the causes of sudden death?

   a. The number one cause of sudden death in both men and women is coronary heart disease.
   b. More women than men experience sudden death due to coronary heart disease.
   c. Acute myocardial infarction is almost universally associated with sudden death.
   d. Diffuse coronary atherosclerosis and previous myocardial infarction are common with sudden death.
   e. Intracerebral hemorrhage and liquid protein diets are associated with sudden death.

11. Match the likelihood of sudden death for *women* with the following factors:

Likelihood of Sudden Death

a. women *more* likely to experience sudden death
b. women *less* likely to experience sudden death

Factor

_____ heavy cigarette smoking

_____ absence of psychiatric history

_____ married

_____ history of hypertension

_____ history of diabetes mellitus

_____ educational incongruity with spouse

12. What percentage of deaths due to myocardial infarction occur before the patient reaches the hospital?

a. 5%
b. 10%
c. 33%
d. 40%
e. over 50%

13. List four reasons why patients with acute myocardial infarction who reach the coronary care unit have a decreased mortality rate.

1) _____

_____

2) _____

_____

3) _____

_____

4) _____

_____

True or False

14. T F Mortality from cardiovascular disease can be lessened by a reduction in the incidence and severity of coronary heart disease.

15. T F CPR programs include education in primary and secondary prevention of heart disease because it is important to educate the public about the risk factors of heart disease.

16. T F Patients who become symptomatic with coronary artery disease often deny or ignore their symptoms, thus delaying care.

17. T F A universal access number such as 911 provides the public with a means to reach a physician or hospital promptly in medical emergencies.

18. T F Public education regarding cardiac symptoms and the need for basic and advanced life support can assist in reducing the length of notification times.

19. T F Myocardial infarction patients who receive care from paramedical personnel within one hour of symptom onset have a higher survival percentage than those who do not receive such care.

20. T F Stabilization of the acute MI patient in the field prior to transport does not appear to have a significant impact on the prevention of cardiac arrest en route to the hospital.

21. T F Cardiac arrest victims have a greater chance of survival in communities where there are large numbers of lay persons trained in CPR and where there are rapidly responsive basic life support EMS units that are complemented by advanced life support units.

22. T F Basic life support alone is usually sufficient to maintain viability and restore effective spontaneous circulation in the cardiac arrest victim.

23. T F ACLS efforts tend to be less effective if they are not properly complemented by prompt initiation of basic life support.

24. Match the results that correspond to mechanisms for reducing deaths due to prehospital cardiac arrests.

Mechanisms

a. field stabilization of acute MI patients
b. ACLS training for emergency department personnel
c. areas serviced by EMS systems with large numbers of laypersons trained in CPR and paramedics who deliver ACLS
d. reduction of risk factors through aggressive CPR training
e. victims who receive bystander CPR within one minute

Result

_____ a five-fold reduction in cardiac arrests enroute to the hospital

_____ successful resuscitation (neurologically intact) of 60% of prehospital cardiac arrest victims

_____ overall survival-to-discharge rate of 15% to 30% for cardiac arrest

25. List the procedures important for stabilization of the cardiac patient prior to transport.

1) _____

2) _____

3) _____

4) _____

5) _____

6) _____

26. You are teaching a group of paramedic students the proper procedures for transporting cardiac patients. Explain why cardiac patients should be transported to the hospital gently, rather than using a red light and siren transport.

_____

_____

_____

_____

_____

27. Figure 11–2 contains illustrations of two response systems. Which of these most closely resembles a two-tiered response system?

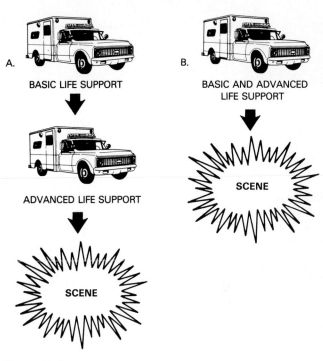

A. BASIC LIFE SUPPORT

ADVANCED LIFE SUPPORT

SCENE

B. BASIC AND ADVANCED LIFE SUPPORT

SCENE

Figure 11–2

True or False

28. T F When delivering advanced life support, paramedical personnel must be in voice communication with the supervising medical authority.

29. T F Telemetry is absolutely necessary in the prehospital care setting.

30. T F Telemetry tends to be extremely expensive and cumbersome for prehospital use.

31. T F Telemetry is useful to the paramedic when treating complex dysrhythmias, particularly those that follow the termination of ventricular fibrillation.

32. T F To achieve the best medical control of cardiac emergencies, a medical director and a single regional hospital should be designated.

33. Which of the following statements are true regarding the transportation of emergency cardiac care patients?

  a. The patient should be immediately transported to an appropriate medical facility when the prehospital personnel cannot deliver ACLS at the scene.

  b. Long delays at the scene are acceptable in situations where the patient fails to respond to ACLS treatments.

  c. It is too cumbersome to continue CPR while transporting, loading, and unloading the patient.

  d. Although chest compressors tend to reduce operator fatigue, they often make the stretcher excessively heavy and difficult to maneuver.

  e. Small station wagon vehicles are considered acceptable for transporting cardiac arrest victims to the hospital.

34. You are the administrator of a small community hospital. Your board of trustees has instructed you to update the facility so that it provides adequate stabilization for any cardiac patient. Which of the following must be accomplished to reach the necessary level of care?

  a. Replace all paramedic ambulance personnel with physicians.

  b. Provide direct radio communication with the local EMS system.

  c. Train all emergency department personnel in CPR and ACLS.

  d. Provide ECG monitoring in the coronary care unit for all suspected myocardial infarction patients.

  e. Develop the capability for cardiac catheterization and cardiopulmonary bypass.

35. You have just been appointed medical director of a local EMS system. List the nine responsibilities of this position.

1) _____

  _____

2) _____

  _____

3) _____

  _____

4) _____

  _____

5) _____

  _____

6) _____

  _____

7) _____

  _____

8) _____

  _____

9) _____

  _____

36. T   F   Advanced Cardiac Life Support certification implies that the provider has the licensure to perform the procedures that were taught in the ACLS course.

37. T   F   It is usually medically and legally acceptable to terminate CPR when 20 minutes have passed and resuscitation efforts have been ineffective.

38. T   F   Even in the hospital emergency facility, the doctor–patient relationship, which establishes the physician's duty to provide care conforming to accepted standards of medical care, becomes effective only after the physician accepts the individual as a patient.

39. T   F   For the health-care provider to be found negligent in the delivery of care to a patient, it must be demonstrated that injury to the patient resulted and that this injury was due to an act or omission on the part of the health-care provider.

40. T   F   When evaluating care delivered for ACLS, the physician's actions may be measured against national performance standards.

41. List four elements that must be established if a malpractice claim is to be successful.

1) _____

_____

2) _____

_____

3) _____

_____

4) _____

_____

42. List the two conditions that should be present when a health-care provider is determining whether to initiate CPR.

1) _____

_____

2) _____

_____

43. Match the following terms with their appropriate definition. (Definitions may have more than one correct response.)

Term

a. negligence
b. accepted standards of medical practice
c. doctor–patient relationship
d. due diligence
e. injury

Definition

_____ establishes the duty to provide care

_____ failure to provide reasonable care

_____ physician must deliver patient care to this level

_____ must exist for a malpractice suit to be successful

44. Which of the following are true regarding the physician's responsibility to provide care to a patient?

a. The physician is obligated to obtain a good result in every instance.
b. The physician must take reasonable steps to protect the patient when there is danger of serious injury or death.
c. The physician is *not* obligated to begin resuscitation efforts if the victim's pupils are nonreactive.
d. The physician should always initiate life support measures, even if "do not resuscitate" orders exist.

ANSWER KEY

1. Causes of sudden death:
   cardiovascular disease: 60%
   miscellaneous diseases: 4%
   digestive and urogenital diseases: 7%
   respiratory disease: 15%
   central nervous system disease: 15%

2. a. INCREASED mortality: increased cigarette smoking
                            decrease in individual fitness
   b. DECREASED mortality: decreased use of saturated fats
                            increase in health awareness
                            decrease in hypertension

3. TRUE

4. TRUE

5. FALSE: There is a relationship between PVCs and sudden death in patients with known heart disease.

6. FALSE: In the absence of heart disease, PVCs are generally considered insignificant.

7. FALSE: Dysrhythmias alone do not typically herald a poor prognosis in cardiac arrest; ischemia and other predispositions must usually be present before the prognosis is adversely influenced.

8. TRUE

9. a. coronary artery thrombosis: event seen with 16% of patients who die within 1 hour and 54% of those who survive 24 hours; may follow rather than precede myocardial ischemia
   b. acute myocardial infarction: is associated with sudden death in 10% to 47% of cases
   c. hemorrhage into an atheromatous plaque: plays a relatively small role in causing sudden cardiac death
   d. ventricular function abnormalities: predispose the heart to ventricular fibrillation
   e. coronary artery spasm: more recently considered as a possible mechanism for myocardial infarction and sudden death

10. True statements concerning the causes of sudden death:
    a. The number one cause of sudden death in both men and women is coronary heart disease.
    d. Diffuse coronary atherosclerosis and previous myocardial infarction are common with sudden death.
    e. Intracerebral hemorrhage and liquid protein diets are associated with sudden death.

11. a. women *more* likely to experience sudden death:
    heavy cigarette smoking
    history of hypertension
    history of diabetes mellitus
    educational incongruity with spouse
    b. women *less* likely to experience sudden death:
    absence of psychiatric history
    married

12. e

13. Reasons why MI patients who reach CCU have decreased mortality:
    1) They are provided with early therapy that is specifically aimed at preventing life-threatening dysrhythmias.
    2) They are resuscitated immediately if they experience cardiac arrest.
    3) They are ECG monitored continuously.
    4) They are provided with other forms of aggressive therapy designed to maintain adequate cardiac output and tissue perfusion.

14. TRUE

15. TRUE

16. TRUE

17. FALSE: A universal access number such as 911 provides the public with ready access to an emergency medical system rather than to a physician or hospital per se.

18. TRUE: When the public fails to recognize cardiac emergencies, is unable to provide immediate care to the victim, or is unable to access medical assistance, a significant delay may be incurred in getting help to the scene.

19. TRUE

20. FALSE: Stabilization of the acute MI patient prior to transport plays a significant role in the prevention of cardiac arrest en route to the hospital.

21. TRUE

22. FALSE: Basic life support alone is rarely sufficient to maintain viability and restore effective spontaneous circulation in the cardiac arrest victim; definitive therapy is usually needed to restore adequate circulation and ventilation.

23. TRUE: Without prompt initiation (usually bystander) of basic life support, victims are typically so severely hypoxic and acidotic that they fail to respond to ACLS therapies.

24. a. field stabilization of acute MI patients: a fivefold reduction in cardiac arrest en route to the hospital

 c. areas serviced by EMS systems with large numbers of laypersons trained in CPR and paramedics who deliver ACLS: overall survival-to-discharge rate of 15% to 30% for cardiac arrest victims

 e. patients who receive bystander CPR within 1 minute and then receive ACLS: successful resuscitation (neurologically intact) of over 60% of the prehospital cardiac arrest victims

25. Procedures important for stabilization of the cardiac patient prior to transport.
 1) pain relief
 2) control of cardiac rhythm
 3) support of blood pressure
 4) assurance of adequate ventilation
 5) continuous ECG monitoring
 6) establishment of an IV lifeline

26. Cardiac patients should be transported to the hospital ''gently'' because a red light and siren transport tend to increase the patient's anxiety level. Anxiety increases catecholamine activity and myocardial oxygen consumption. Both of these factors can increase the severity of the infarction and lower the fibrillation threshold, thereby precipitating ventricular fibrillation.

27. Illustrations of a two-tiered response system: a

28. TRUE

29. FALSE: Telemetry is useful, but not absolutely necessary in the prehospital care setting.

30. FALSE: Telemetry equipment is usually affordable and easy to use.

31. TRUE

32. TRUE

33. a and d

34. b, c, d, e

35. Nine responsibilities of a medical director are to:
 1) obtain necessary certifications for the system
 2) assume medical responsibility for the system
 3) supervise and actively participate in training and certification programs for the EMT and paramedical personnel
 4) approve medical equipment and supplies used by the system
 5) approve treatment and training protocols used by the system
 6) prepare a written yearly evaluation of the system's personnel
 7) provide a liaison from the system to the medical community
 8) ensure a uniform data collection mechanism for the system
 9) develop an ongoing quality assurance program for the system.

36. FALSE: Advanced Cardiac Life Support certification implies only that the provider has successfully completed the ACLS course of instruction according to the cognitive and performance standards of the American Heart Association.

37. FALSE: Time is generally not considered a valid criterion for terminating resuscitation. It is usually medically and legally acceptable to terminate CPR when the cardiovascular system has failed to respond to properly performed basic and advanced life support efforts.

38. FALSE: The duty to provide care is not a legal obligation because in most situations the physician does not establish a patient–doctor relationship until after the individual is accepted as a patient. An example would be when the physician is confronted by an unknown individual who collapsed on the street. Although morally and ethically obligated to provide care, the physician is under no legal obligation. Once the physician begins patient care, however, care must conform to accepted standards.

39. TRUE

40. TRUE

41. Four elements that must be established for a successful malpractice claim include the following:
 1) that the duty to provide care existed
 2) that a breach of duty to provide reasonable care was committed
 3) that the patient suffered an injury
 4) that there was a cause-and-effect relationship between the breach of medical practice or duty and the injury that the patient sustained

42. The two conditions that should be present when a health-care provider is determining whether to initiate CPR are:
 1) the possibility that the brain is viable
 2) no legal or medically legitimate reason to withhold CPR

43. establishes the duty to provide care: c
 failure to provide reasonable care: a
 physician must deliver patient care to this level: b
 must exist for a malpractice suit to be successful: a, c, e

44. b

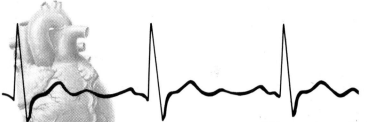

Chapter 12

Case History Scenarios

DIRECTIONS

This chapter consists of 10 case scenarios. They are designed to prepare you for the Mega Code testing station. They integrate the information contained in the preceding chapters and give you the chance to apply your knowledge. Approach this exercise as a realistic situation so that each response simulates performance in an actual resuscitation. As in the Mega Code station, participants must indicate appropriate treatments and dosages as well as supervise other members of the resuscitation team. Scenarios are located in both field and hospital situations. Though a variety of resuscitation roles are portrayed, use the team leader role for answering the questions and completing the exercises.

Begin by reading the opening scenario so that you understand the situation presented. Complete each review item, using additional information regarding patient status and the results of therapies to guide decisions. Designate correct answers by a check mark; fill in dosages for medications and defibrillation when requested. Some questions require only a "yes" or "no" response or the interpretation of an ECG rhythm. As in earlier chapters, answers may be examined individually or collectively at the end of each scenario.

Once you can answer all questions correctly, prepare more fully for the Mega Code station by imposing a very restricted time limit on your completion of the scenario. Repeat the scenarios until you can attain near-perfect accuracy under these time restrictions. This will help to reinforce the ACLS algorithms as you will be expected to provide them during the actual Mega Code testing station.

SCENARIO 1

It is 1:43 p.m. on a Sunday afternoon and you are working the day shift on your community emergency medical service unit. You receive a call for a male having chest pain and arrive on the scene at 1:45 p.m. to find a 41-year-old, 300-pound ex-football player lying in front of the television set in his living room. Apparently he was yelling at the players in the football game when he suddenly began having chest pain and passed out. Family members state that he has no previous medical history and is taking no medications. The patient is unconscious, apneic, and pulseless. Basic life support has not yet been started.

1.01 The first task that your team should do is to

establish an IV lifeline

intubate the trachea

defibrillate using _____ joules

begin CPR

1.02 The next task that your team should do is to

establish an IV lifeline

intubate the trachea

defibrillate using _____ joules

identify the ECG rhythm

1.03 You see the following rhythm (Figure 12–1) on the ECG monitor. The patient's ECG shows

_____

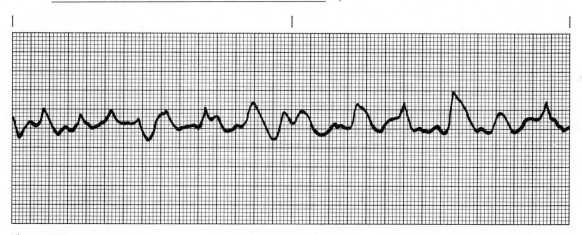

Figure 12–1

1.04 Should you continue or temporarily withhold CPR? _____

1.05 The rescuers should now

defibrillate using _____ joules

intubate the trachea

administer sodium bicarbonate,

_____ IV push

establish an IV lifeline

administer atropine, _____ IV push

Following the above treatment, the ECG rhythm is shown in Figure 12-2.

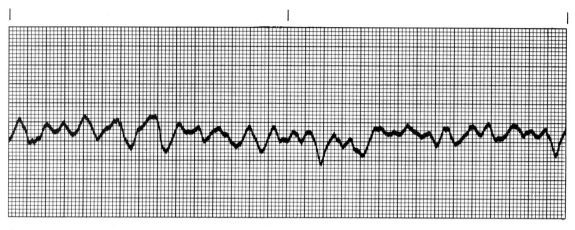

Figure 12-2

1.06 The rescue team should now

check for a pulse

defibrillate using _____ joules

administer epinephrine, _____ IV push

administer dopamine, _____ IV infusion

insert a pacemaker

The patient is still apneic and pulseless.

1.07 Should you continue or temporarily withhold CPR? _____

1.08 The next task your team needs to do is to

administer epinephrine, _____ IV push

administer atropine, _____ IV push

defibrillate using _____ joules

administer sodium bicarbonate,

_____ IV push

intubate the trachea

Following the above treatment, the ECG monitor reveals (Figure 12-3):

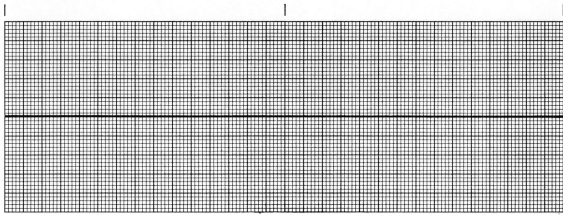

Figure 12-3

1.09 Now you should

check for a pulse

defibrillate using _____ joules

administer epinephrine, _____ IV push

administer dopamine, _____ IV infusion

insert a pacemaker

The patient remains apneic and pulseless.

1.10 The ECG rhythm above is _____

1.11 Should you continue or discontinue CPR?

_____

1.12 It is now 1:47; the next task your team should do is to

administer epinephrine, _____ IV push

intubate the trachea

administer calcium chloride, _____ IV push

establish an IV lifeline

defibrillate using _____ joules

1.13 Following the above treatments, the patient's condition remains the same. It is now 1:48. The next task that your team should do is:

administer sodium bicarbonate,

_____ IV push

defibrillate using _____ joules

administer epinephrine, _____ IV

    push

administer atropine, _____ IV push

administer bretylium, _____ IV push

Following the above treatments, the patient remains pulseless and apneic; his ECG monitor reveals the rhythm in Figure 12–4.

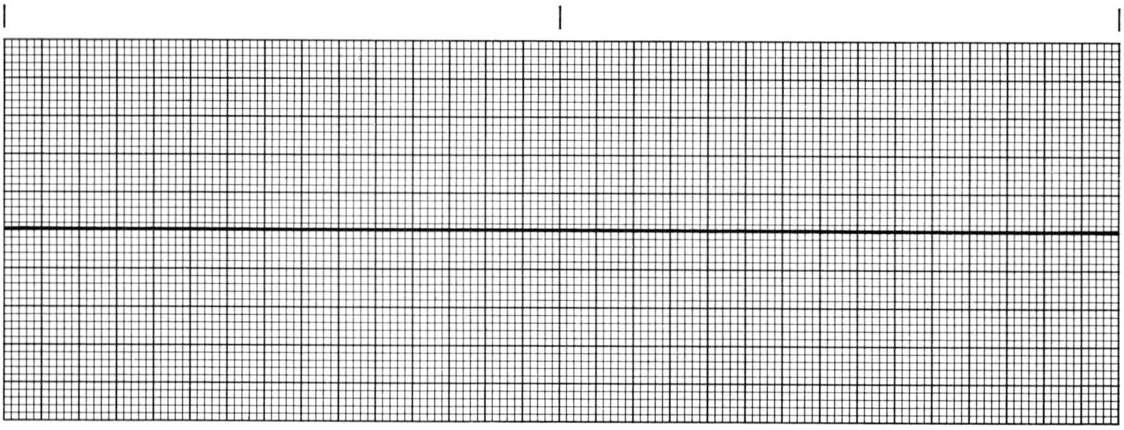

Figure 12–4

1.14 Should you continue or discontinue CPR?

_____

1.15 It is 1:49 p.m. Your team should next

administer atropine, _____ IV push

defibrillate using _____ joules

perform endotracheal intubation

administer isoproterenol, _____ IV in-

    fusion

insert a pacemaker

Following the above treatment, the patient is still apneic and pulseless. His ECG monitor shows (Figure 12-5):

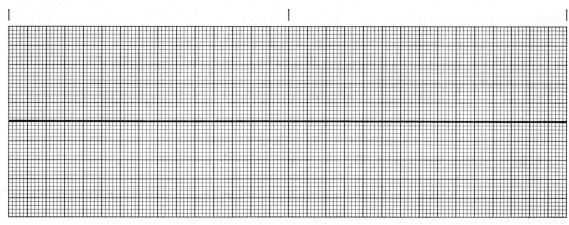

Figure 12-5

You decide to continue CPR.

1.16 It is 1:51. Now your rescue team should

administer epinephrine, _____ IV push

administer atropine, _____ IV push

defibrillate using _____ joules

administer calcium chloride, _____ IV push

administer isoproterenol, _____ IV infusion

Following the above treatment, the ECG monitor shows (Figure 12-6):

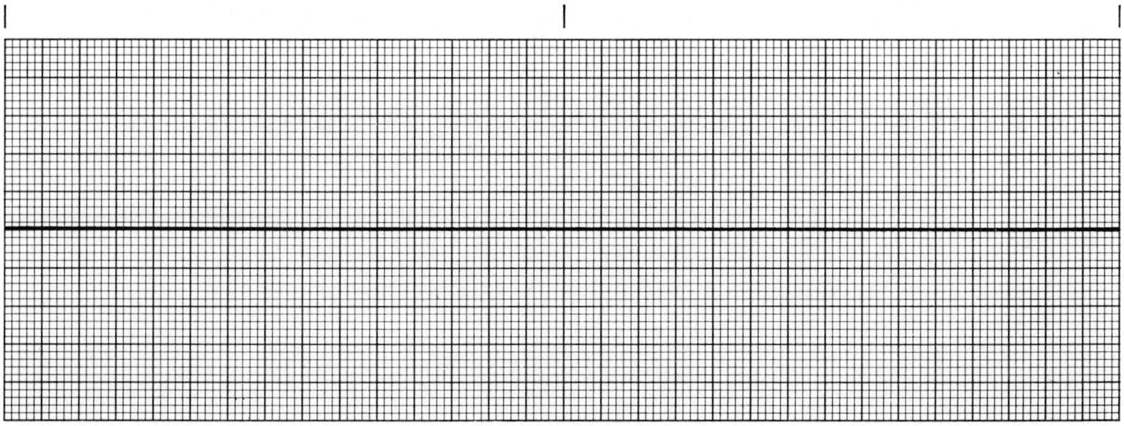

Figure 12-6

1.17 The next task your team should do is

check for a pulse

defibrillate using _____ joules

administer epinephrine, _____ IV
push

administer dopamine, _____ IV
infusion

insert a pacemaker

You resume CPR because the patient is still apneic and pulseless.

1.18 It is 1:53 now; the rescue team should

administer bretylium, _____ IV push

defibrillate using _____ joules

administer sodium bicarbonate,

_____ IV push

administer isoproterenol, _____ IV infusion

administer epinephrine, _____ IV
push

Following this treatment, the patient is still pulseless and apneic, but his ECG monitor now shows the rhythm in Figure 12–7.

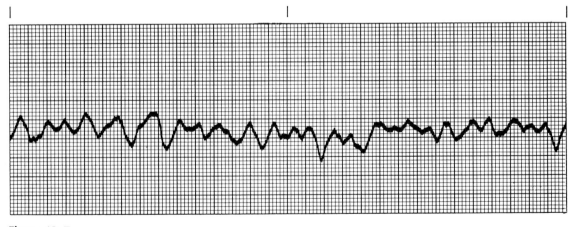

Figure 12–7

1.19 This dysrhythmia is called _____

_____

1.20 Should you continue or temporarily withhold

CPR? _____

1.21 The next task your team should do is:

administer sodium bicarbonate,

_____ IV push

defibrillate using _____ joules

perform carotid sinus massage

insert a pacemaker

administer calcium chloride, _____ IV

push

1.22 Following the above treatment, the ECG (Figure 12–8) reveals the following rhythm. This is called

_____

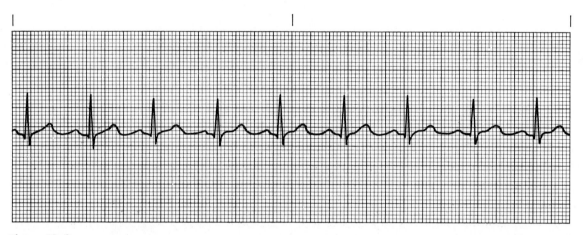

Figure 12–8

1.23 Your next task is to

check for a pulse

defibrillate using _____ joules

administer epinephrine, _____ IV

push

administer dopamine, _____ IV infu-

sion

insert a pacemaker

The patient is still apneic but has a strong pulse and a blood pressure of 136/100.

1.24 Should you continue or discontinue CPR?

_____

1.25 The patient should now receive

epinephrine, _____IV push

atropine, _____, IV push

sodium bicarbonate, _____IV push

lidocaine, _____ IV push

1.26 Rescuers should now

administer sodium bicarbonate,

_____ IV push

administer lidocaine, _____ IV infu-

sion

administer dopamine, _____ IV

infusion

administer norepinephrine, _____ IV

infusion

discontinue ventilatory assistance

Enroute to the hospital, the patient displays the ECG rhythm in Figure 12–9.

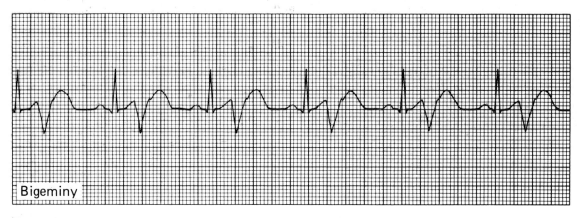

Bigeminy

Figure 12–9

1.27 This dysrhythmia is called _____

_____

The patient's vital signs remain unchanged.

1.28 At this time, treatment for the dysrhythmia consists of

isoproterenol, _____ IV infusion

increasing the lidocaine infusion rate

atropine, _____ IV push

lidocaine, _____ IV push

bretylium, _____ IV push

1.29 Following the above treatment the ECG in Figure 12–10 is observed; this ECG reveals _____ _____

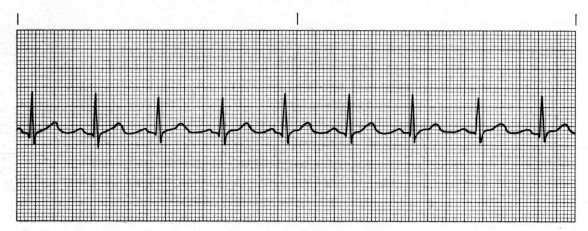

Figure 12–10

The patient's vital signs and ECG remain unchanged. No other problems develop en route to the hospital. The patient's stay in the emergency department is uneventful, and he is admitted to the coronary care unit in stable condition.

SCENARIO 2

It is 9:11 p.m. on a Monday evening. You are working at a suburban hospital emergency department. A 53-year-old, 120-pound saleswoman in cardiac arrest has just been brought in by the local rescue squad. CPR has been provided but has been halted to transfer the patient onto the ED treatment table. It is not known if the patient has any previous medical history; she apparently collapsed at work. The patient is unconscious, apneic, and pulseless.

2.01 The first task the ED staff should do is to

establish an IV lifeline

intubate the trachea

defibrillate using _____ joules

begin CPR

administer epinephrine, _____ intra-
  cardiac

2.02 The next task that your staff should do is

establish an IV lifeline

intubate the trachea

defibrillate using _____ joules

identify the ECG rhythm

2.03 The patient is still pulseless and apneic. You see the rhythm on the ECG monitor (Figure 12–11).

The patient's ECG shows _____

_____

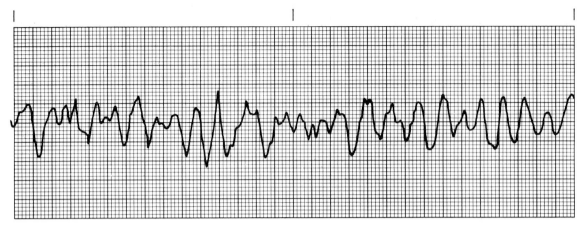

Figure 12–11

2.04 Should you continue or temporarily withhold

CPR? _____

2.05 The staff should now

defibrillate using _____ joules

intubate the trachea

administer sodium bicarbonate,

_____ IV push

establish an IV lifeline

administer atropine, _____ IV push

Following the above treatment, the ECG monitor reveals (Figure 12–12):

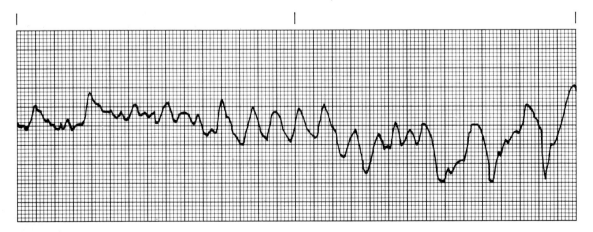

Figure 12–12

2.06 The ED staff should now

check for a pulse

defibrillate using _____ joules

administer epinephrine, _____ IV
push

administer dopamine, _____ IV
infusion

insert a pacemaker

The patient is still apneic and pulseless.

2.07 Should you continue or temporarily withhold

CPR? _____

2.08 The next task your staff needs to do is to

administer epinephrine, _____ IV
push

administer atropine, _____ IV push

defibrillate using _____ joules

administer sodium bicarbonate,

_____ IV push

intubate the trachea

Following the above treatment, the ECG monitor (Figure 12–13) reveals:

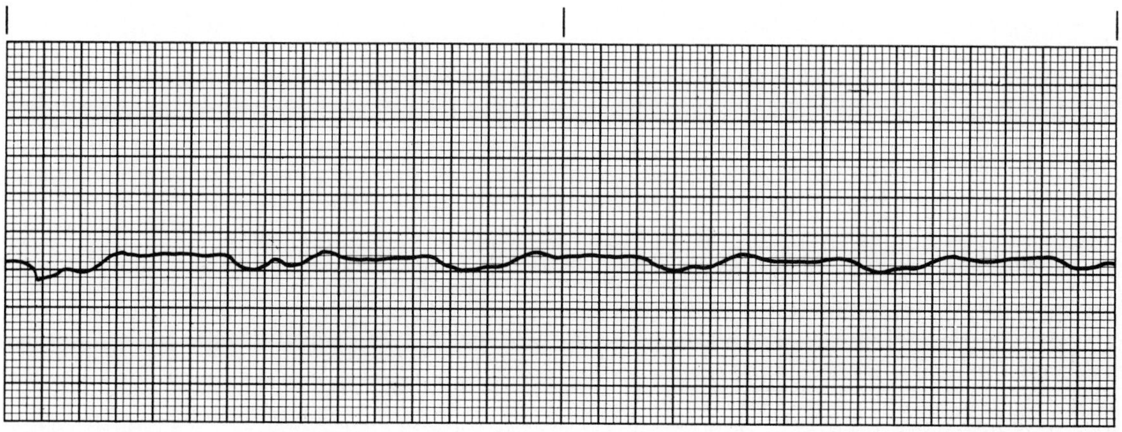

Figure 12–13

2.09 Now you should

check for a pulse

defibrillate using _____ joules

administer epinephrine, _____ IV

push

administer dopamine, _____ IV

infusion

insert a pacemaker

The patient remains apneic and pulseless.

2.10 The next thing you should do is to

defibrillate using _____ joules

administer epinephrine, _____ IV

push

administer dopamine, _____ IV

infusion

insert a pacemaker

2.11 The patient remains pulseless and apneic. Should you continue or discontinue CPR?

_____

2.12 It is now 9:12; the next task your team should do is

administer epinephrine, _____ IV

push

intubate the trachea

administer calcium chloride, _____ IV

push

establish an IV lifeline

defibrillate using _____ joules

2.13 Following the above treatment, the patient's condition remains the same. It is now 9:13. The next task that your staff should do is

administer sodium bicarbonate,

_____ IV push

defibrillate using _____ joules

administer epinephrine, _____ IV

push

administer atropine, _____ IV push

administer bretylium, _____ IV push

check for a pulse

Following the above treatment, the patient remains pulseless and apneic; you have placed an endotracheal tube; the ECG monitor reveals the rhythm in Figure 12–14.

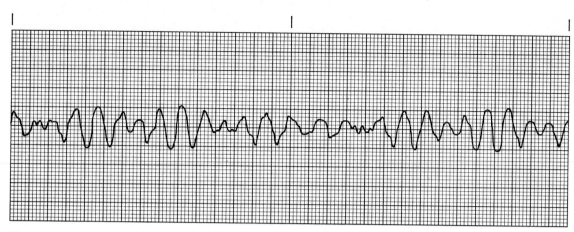

Figure 12–14

2.14 Should you continue or temporarily withhold CPR? _____

2.15 It is 9:14. Your team should next

administer atropine, _____ IV push

defibrillate using _____ joules

administer calcium chloride, _____ IV push

administer isoproterenol, _____ IV infusion

administer epinephrine, _____ IV push

The patient has no palpable pulses and is still apneic. After the above treatment, the ECG monitor shows the rhythm in Figure 12–15.

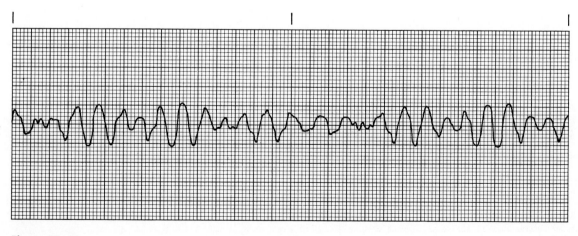

Figure 12–15

You continue CPR while other staff obtain an arterial blood gas (ABG) sample and deliver it to the laboratory.

2.16 It is 9:15 p.m. The CPR team should now

administer atropine, _____ IV push

defibrillate using _____ joules

administer lidocaine, _____ IV push

administer bretylium, _____ IV push

administer epinephrine, _____ IV
    push

Following the above treatment, the ECG monitor reveals the rhythm in Figure 12–16.

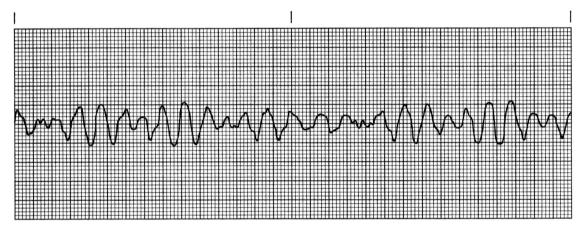

Figure 12–16

2.17 The patient is still pulseless and apneic at 9:16 p.m. The next task your staff should do is

administer bretylium, _____ IV push

defibrillate using _____ joules

administer sodium bicarbonate,

_____ IV push

administer isoproterenol, _____ IV
    infusion

administer epinephrine, _____ IV
    push

There is no change in the patient's condition. Her ECG now shows the rhythm in Figure 12-17.

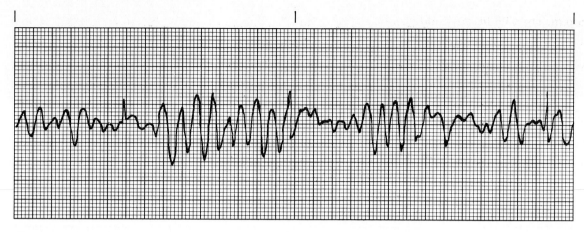

Figure 12-17

2.18 Should you continue or discontinue CPR?

_____

2.19 The next thing you should do is to

check for a pulse

defibrillate using _____ joules

administer epinephrine, _____ IV push

administer bretylium, _____ IV push

insert a pacemaker

The patient remains pulseless and apneic and the rhythm remains unchanged.

2.20 Upon auscultation of the patient's chest, you find there are clear sounds on the right side but no breath sounds on the left side. Which of the following are the most likely causes of this finding?

inadvertent esophageal intubation

pneumothorax

right mainstem bronchus intubation

bag-valve-mask device malfunction

2.21 Which of the following should be done immediately?

emergency chest decompression

remove the endotracheal tube and insert an esophageal airway

remove the bag-valve-mask device and ventilate by mouth

withdraw the endotracheal tube until breath sounds are heard bilaterally

order a chest x-ray

Your treatment has solved the problem; bilateral breath sounds are present.

2.22 The patient should now receive 100% oxygen and

bretylium, _____ IV push

sodium bicarbonate, _____ IV push

atropine, _____ IV push

epinephrine, _____ IV push

Following the above treatments, the ECG reveals (Figure 12–18):

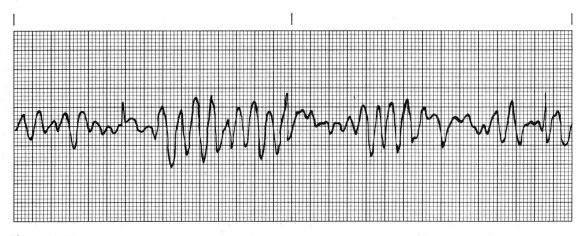

Figure 12–18

2.23 You temporarily withhold CPR in order to

defibrillate using _____ joules

insert a pacemaker

administer lidocaine, _____ IV infusion

administer atropine, _____ IV push

administer epinephrine, _____ IV push

The patient remains apneic and pulseless. Her ECG shows the rhythm in Figure 12–19.

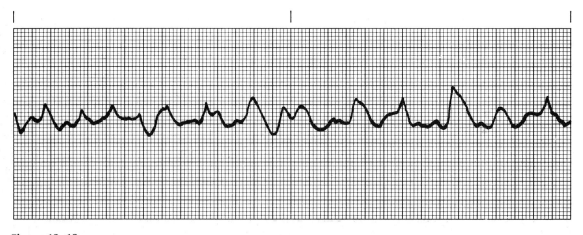

Figure 12–19

2.24 Your staff continues CPR. It is now 9:18 p.m. The next task your staff should do is to

defibrillate using _____ joules

insert a pacemaker

administer lidocaine, _____ IV infusion

administer bretylium, _____ IV push

administer epinephrine, _____ IV push

Following the above treatment, the ECG monitor shows (Figure 12–20):

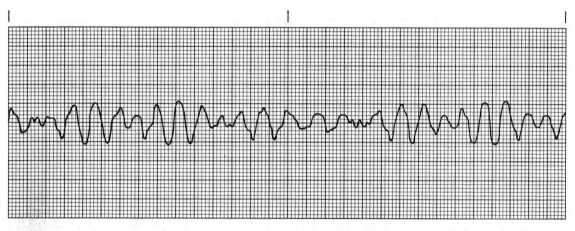

Figure 12–20

2.25 You should now

defibrillate using _____ joules

check for a pulse

administer lidocaine, _____ IV push

administer atropine, _____ IV push

administer calcium chloride, _____ IV push

2.26 You resume CPR because the patient's condition is unchanged but temporarily stop CPR to

defibrillate using _____ joules

insert a pacemaker

administer lidocaine, _____ IV infusion

administer bretylium, _____ IV push

administer epinephrine, _____ IV push

The ECG in Figure 12–21 appears after this last treatment.

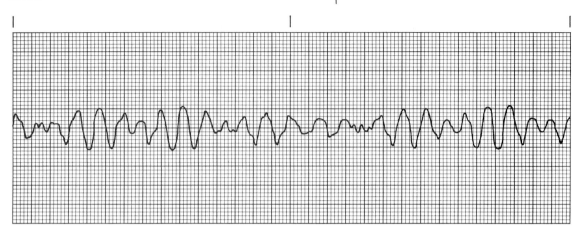

Figure 12–21

There is no change in the patient's status, so your staff continues CPR.

2.27 Now it is 9:20 p.m. The next task that should be done is to

defibrillate using _____ joules

administer sodium bicarbonate,

_____ IV push

administer lidocaine, _____ IV infu-

sion

administer bretylium, _____ IV push

administer epinephrine, _____ IV

push

The ECG monitor then shows the rhythm in Figure 12–22.

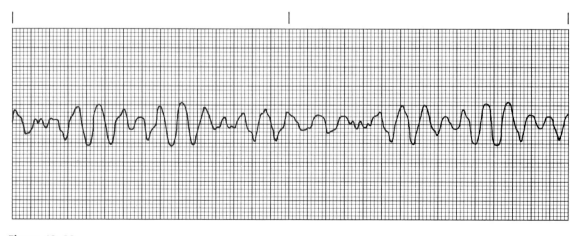

Figure 12–22

2.28 The patient's condition remains the same. Should you continue or temporarily withhold CPR?

_____

2.29 It is now 9:22 p.m. The next task for the staff to do is to

defibrillate using _____ joules

insert a pacemaker

administer lidocaine, _____ IV infusion

administer bretylium, _____ IV push

administer epinephrine, _____ IV push

2.30 Following this treatment, the ECG in Figure 12–23 is seen on the monitor; this ECG shows

_____

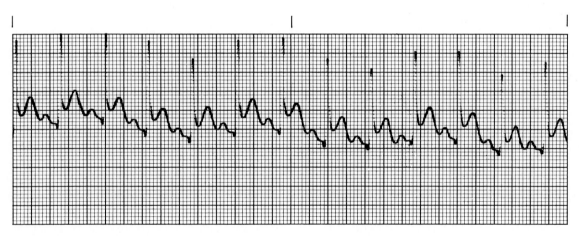

Figure 12–23

2.31 You should now

defibrillate using _____ joules

insert a pacemaker

check for a pulse

administer dopamine, _____ IV infusion

administer epinephrine, _____ IV push

The patient is still apneic but now has a palpable pulse of 130 per minute and a blood pressure of 112/72.

2.32 Should you continue or discontinue CPR?

_____

2.33 At this time your staff should administer

sodium bicarbonate, _____ IV push

lidocaine, _____ IV push

atropine, _____ IV push

epinephrine, _____ IV push

2.34 The next treatment should be to

discontinue ventilatory assistance

administer dopamine, _____ IV infu-

sion

administer lidocaine, _____ IV infu-

sion

administer sodium bicarbonate,

_____ IV push

administer norepinephrine, _____ IV

infusion

The patient's condition remains unchanged, and she is admitted to coronary care. She later experienced several bouts of ventricular tachycardia during the next day but now is stable.

SCENARIO 3

It is 9:45 a.m. on a Sunday morning. You are working in the emergency department of a large urban hospital. An 80-year-old, 100-pound female was complaining of shortness of breath at home this morning and her family brought her to the hospital when she fainted. According to family members, the patient has been unresponsive for about five minutes; she has a history of two previous heart attacks and hypertension. Assessment reveals an unconscious, apneic, and pulseless victim. Basic life support has not been started as yet.

3.01 The first task to do is to

establish an IV lifeline

intubate the trachea

begin CPR

administer epinephrine, _____ intra-

cardiac

3.02 The second task your staff should do is to

establish an IV lifeline

intubate the trachea

begin CPR

identify the ECG rhythm

defibrillate using _____ joules

3.03 This patient's ECG presently shows the rhythm in Figure 12–24; this is _____

_____

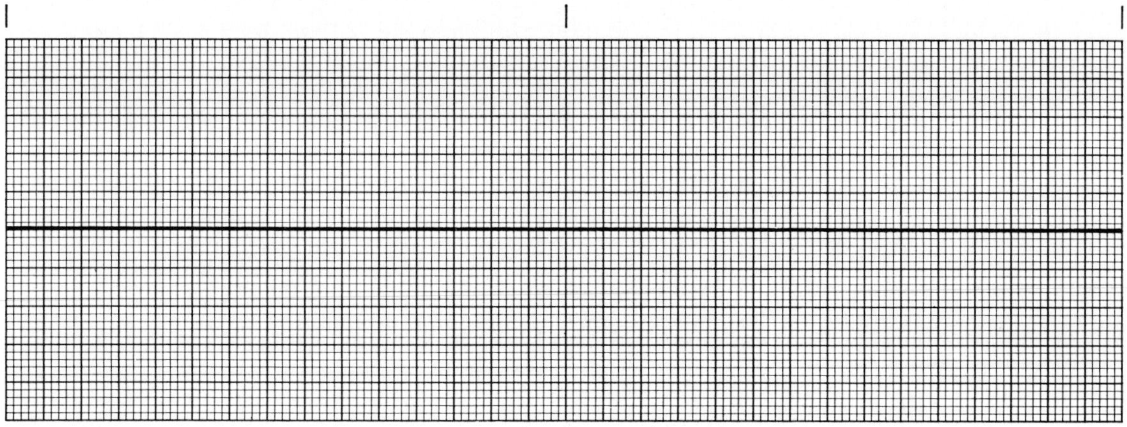

Figure 12–24

3.04 Should you continue or discontinue CPR?

_____

3.05 It is 9:46 a.m. The next task your staff should do is to

establish an IV lifeline

intubate the trachea

administer calcium chloride, _____ IV push

administer epinephrine, _____ intra-cardiac

defibrillate using _____ joules

3.06 The patient's condition remains unchanged. It is now 9:47. The next task to do is to

administer bretylium, _____ IV push

administer atropine, _____ IV push

administer sodium bicarbonate, _____ IV push

administer epinephrine, _____ IV push

defibrillate using _____ joules

Following the above treatment, the ECG monitor shows (Figure 12–25):

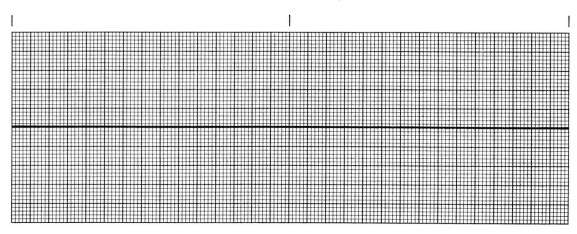

Figure 12–25

Because the patient is still apneic and pulseless, you re-institute CPR.

3.07 It is 9:49. The next task your team should do is to administer

epinephrine, _____ IV push

atropine, _____ IV push

calcium chloride, _____ IV push

isoproterenol, _____ IV infusion

perform an endotracheal intubation

ABGs are being drawn and sent to the laboratory. There is no change in the patient's condition or ECG following this treatment, so you continue CPR.

3.08 It is 9:50. Your team should now

administer   epinephrine, _____ IV push

administer atropine, _____ IV push

administer calcium chloride, _____ IV push

perform endotracheal intubation

administer defibrillation using

_____ joules

This patient's ECG now shows the rhythm in Figure 12–26.

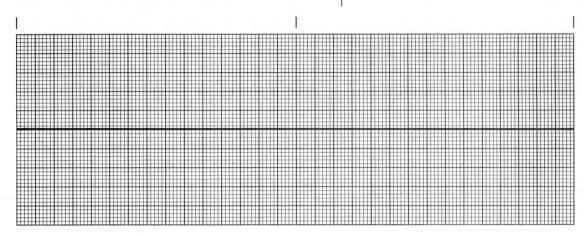

Figure 12–26

There is no change in the patient's status; CPR is resumed.

3.09 It is 9:52; your staff should now administer

epinephrine, _____ IV push

sodium bicarbonate, _____ IV push

bretylium, _____ IV push

isoproterenol, _____ IV infusion

There is no change in the ECG, no spontaneous breathing, and no pulse; your staff continues CPR. The ABG report is now available: PaO$_2$ is 56 mm of Hg, PaCO$_2$ is 60 mm of Hg, pH is 7.17, and base deficit is −5. As you begin investigating causes for these ABG values, you note that the person ventilating is delivering one ventilation every five or six seconds and that there is no oxygen supply line or reservoir device attached to the bag-valve-mask unit. Breath sounds are normal bilaterally.

3.10 To correct the ventilation problem, you direct the person delivering ventilations to

reposition the endotracheal tube

remove the endotracheal tube and insert an esophageal obturator airway

increase the rate of ventilation

attach an oxygen supply line and reservoir device to the bag-valve-mask unit

suction the endotracheal tube

3.11 Your staff should now

administer sodium bicarbonate, _____ IV push

defibrillate using _____ joules

insert a pacemaker

administer calcium chloride, _____ IV push

perform carotid sinus massage

3.12 After the above treatment, the ECG shows the rhythm in Figure 12–27, which is _____

_____

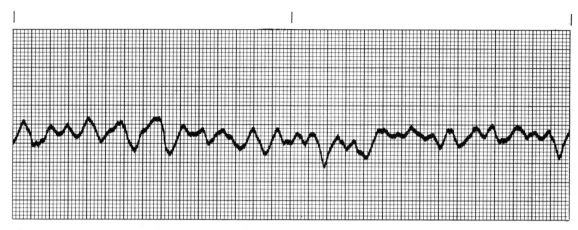

Figure 12–27

3.13 The patient remains pulseless and apneic. Should you continue or temporarily withhold CPR?

_____

3.14 Your staff now needs to administer

epinephrine, _____ IV push

bretylium, _____ IV push

sodium bicarbonate, _____ IV push

isoproterenol, _____ IV infusion

defibrillation using _____ joules

3.15 Now the patient's ECG monitor shows the following; this rhythm in Figure 12–28 is, _____

_____

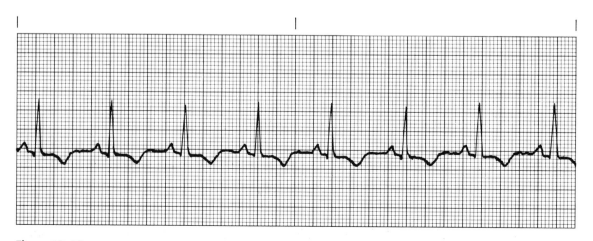

Figure 12–28

3.16 The next task your staff should do is to

administer epinephrine, _____ IV push

administer dopamine, _____ IV infusion

defibrillate using _____ joules

check for a pulse

The patient now has spontaneous respirations at six per minute, a palpable pulse, and a blood pressure of 120/60.

3.17 Should you continue or discontinue CPR?

_____

3.18 Staff should now administer

epinephrine, _____ IV push

atropine, _____ IV push

sodium bicarbonate, _____ IV push

lidocaine, _____ IV push

3.19 A final action your staff should provide would be to administer

norepinephrine, _____ IV infusion

dopamine, _____ IV infusion

sodium bicarbonate, _____ IV push

lidocaine, _____ IV infusion

SCENARIO 4

It is 3:43 p.m. on a Tuesday afternoon and you are working in the coronary care unit at a local community hospital. You are a member of the hospital's cardiac arrest team, which has just received a call for a female who fainted in an elevator. You arrive at 3:45 to find a 48-year-old, 150-pound nursing supervisor lying unconscious, apneic, and pulseless in the rear of the elevator. She had been complaining of dizziness and nausea before she collapsed. Her co-workers state that she has no previous medical history and is taking no medications. Basic life support has not been started.

4.01 The first task the CPR team should do is to

establish an IV lifeline

intubate the trachea

defibrillate using _____ joules

begin CPR

administer epinephrine _____ intracardiac

4.02 You attach the patient to an ECG monitor and observe the rhythm in Figure 12–29 this condition is;

_____

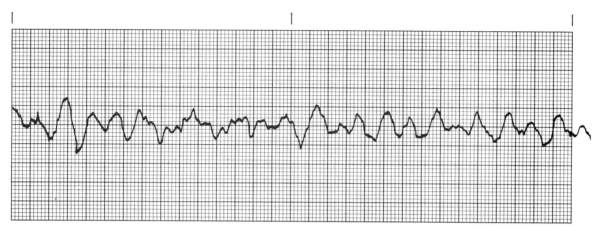

Figure 12–29

Since the patient is still pulseless and apneic, the team resumes CPR.

4.03 The next task the team should do is to

establish an IV lifeline

intubate the trachea

administer sodium bicarbonate,

_____ IV push

administer atropine, _____ IV push

defibrillate using _____ joules

The patient's condition remains the same; her ECG rhythm appears in Figure 12–30.

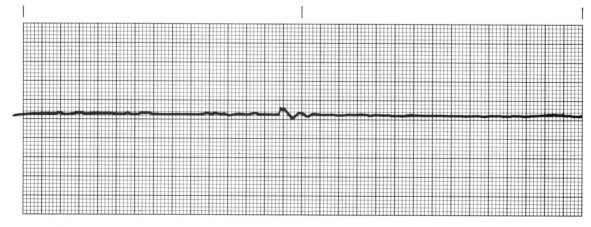

Figure 12–30

You continue CPR.

4.04 It is 3:47 p.m. The next task your team should do is

establish an IV lifeline

intubate the trachea

administer calcium chloride, _____ IV
   push

administer epinephrine, _____ IV
   push

defibrillate using _____ joules

4.05 The patient's condition remains unchanged. It is now 3:48 p.m. The next task to do is

administer bretylium, _____ IV push

administer atropine, _____ IV push

administer sodium bicarbonate,

_____ IV push

administer epinephrine, _____ IV
   push

defibrillate using _____ joules

Following the above treatment, the patient is still apneic and pulseless and the ECG monitor shows the rhythm in Figure 12–31.

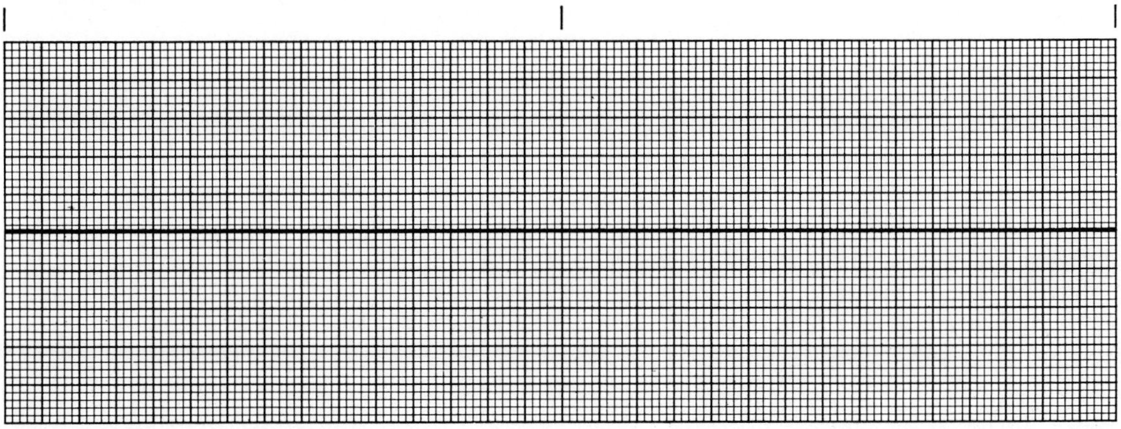

Figure 12–31

Because the patient is still apneic and pulseless, you resume CPR.

4.06 It is 3:50. You have successfully placed an endo-tracheal tube. The next task your team should do is to administer

epinephrine, _____ IV push

atropine, _____ IV push

calcium chloride, _____ IV push

isoproterenol, _____ IV infusion

defibrillation using _____ joules

There is no change in the patient's vital signs, but the ECG following this treatment now shows the rhythm in Figure 12–32.

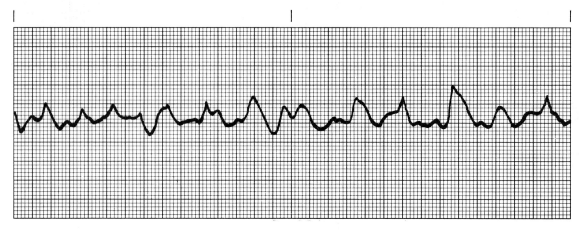

Figure 12–32

4.07 The next task for your team to do is to

check for a pulse

administer epinephrine, _____ IV push

administer dopamine, _____ IV infusion

insert a pacemaker

defibrillate using _____ joules

The patient remains pulseless; CPR is withheld.

4.08 Your team now prepares to administer

epinephrine, _____ IV push

sodium bicarbonate, _____ IV push

atropine, _____ IV push

defibrillation using _____ joules

Following administration of the above treatment, the ECG monitor now reveals the rhythm in Figure 12–33.

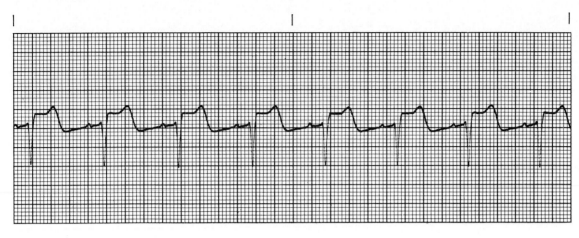

Figure 12–33

4.09 The next action to take is to _____

_____

4.10 This patient is both apneic and pulseless, yet has the ECG rhythm above; this condition is called

_____

4.11 Should you continue or discontinue CPR?

_____

4.12 It is 3:53. Now the team should administer

epinephrine, _____ IV push

atropine, _____ IV push

isoproterenol, _____ IV infusion

administer calcium chloride, _____
     IV push

After the above treatment, the ECG shows the rhythm in Figure 12–34.

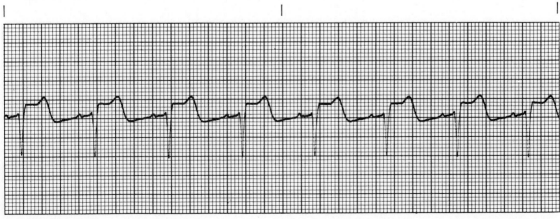

Figure 12–34

4.13 Next the CPR team should

check for a pulse

defibrillate using _____ joules

administer   epinephrine,   _____   IV

push

administer dopamine, _____ IV infu-

sion

insert a pacemaker

You find that the patient is still apneic and pulseless; you continue CPR.

4.14 Now it is 3:54; the team needs to consider administering

epinephrine, _____ IV push

bretylium, _____ IV push

sodium bicarbonate, _____ IV push

calcium chloride, _____ IV push

4.15 Now   the   patient's   ECG   monitor   shows   the

rhythm in Figure 12–35; this rhythm is _____

_____

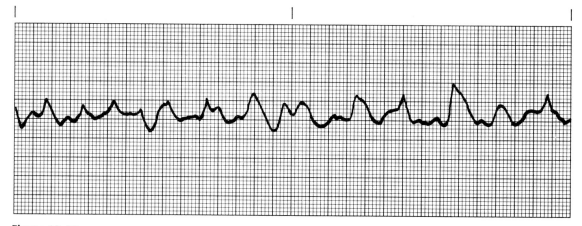

Figure 12–35

The patient's condition is unchanged.

4.16 CPR should now be withheld temporarily to

administer   epinephrine,   _____   intra-

cardiac

administer calcium chloride, _____ IV

push

defibrillate using _____ joules

insert a pacemaker

administer   procainamide,   _____   IV

push

4.17 Following the above treatment, the ECG reveals the rhythm in Figure 12–36; this rhythm is

_____

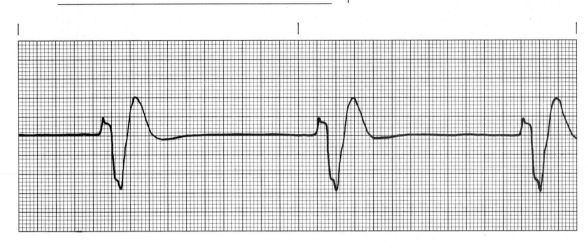

Figure 12–36

There is still no palpable pulse or spontaneous breathing; CPR continues.

4.18 It is now 3:58. The staff needs to administer

epinephrine, _____ IV push

atropine, _____ IV push

sodium bicarbonate, _____ IV push

lidocaine, _____ IV push

4.19 Following this treatment, the ECG reveals (Figure 12–37) _____

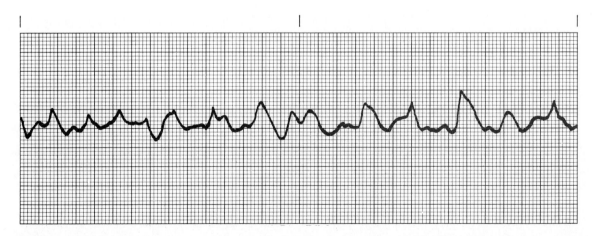

Figure 12–37

4.20 The patient's status is unchanged, so the team prepares to administer

norepinephrine, _____ IV infusion

dopamine, _____ IV infusion

sodium bicarbonate, _____ IV push

lidocaine, _____ IV infusion

defibrillation using _____ joules

4.21 After this treatment, the patient's ECG appears as in Figure 12–38; this dysrhythmia is called _____

_____

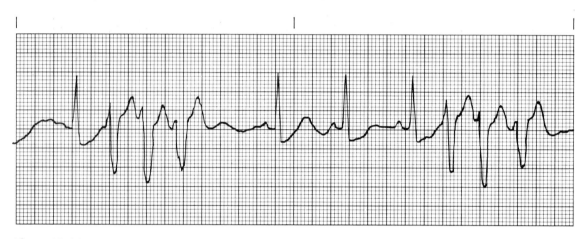

Figure 12–38

4.22 The patient is still apneic but now has a weak carotid pulse. Should you continue or discontinue CPR? _____

4.23 Before you are able to provide any other therapy, you see the rhythm in Figure 12–39 on the ECG monitor. This dysrhythmia is called _____

_____

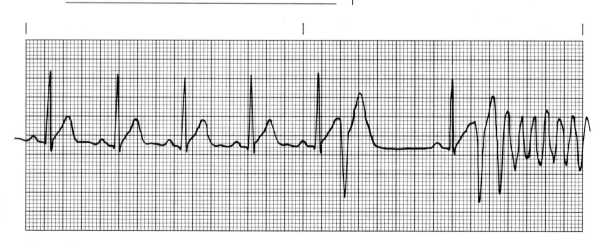

Figure 12–39

4.24 The patient is now apneic and pulseless. The next thing you should do is to

deliver a precordial thump

administer lidocaine, _____ IV push

administer dopamine, _____ IV infusion

administer norepinephrine, _____ IV infusion

defibrillate using _____ joules

4.25 Following this treatment, the ECG reveals the rhythm in Figure 12–40; this dysrhythmia is called _____

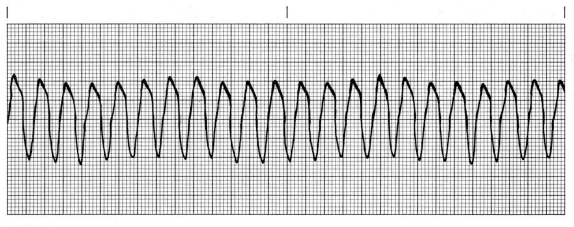

Figure 12–40

The patient is still apneic and pulseless.

4.26 The CPR team should now

deliver a precordial thump

administer lidocaine, _____ IV push

administer bretylium, _____ IV push

deliver a synchronized countershock

defibrillate using _____ joules

4.27 After the above therapy, the ECG shows the rhythm in Figure 12–41, which is called _____

_____

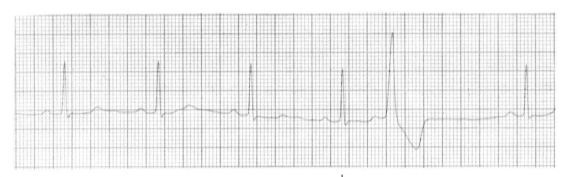

Figure 12–41

4.28 The next task the team should do is to

check for a pulse

defibrillate using _____ joules

administer epinephrine, _____ IV push

administer dopamine, _____ IV infusion

insert a pacemaker

The patient is apneic but has a weak pulse and a blood pressure of 100/70. You discontinue chest compressions and continue providing assisted ventilations.

4.29 The next task to do is to administer

epinephrine, _____ IV push

atropine, _____ IV push

sodium bicarbonate, _____ IV push

lidocaine, _____ IV push

4.30 This treatment should be followed by administration of

norepinephrine, _____ IV infusion

dopamine, _____ IV infusion

sodium bicarbonate, _____ IV push

lidocaine, _____ IV infusion

4.31 After this therapy, the ECG reveals the rhythm in

Figure 12–42; this is _____

_____

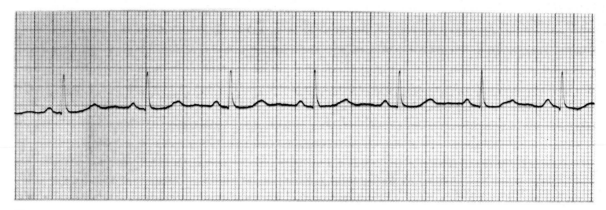

Figure 12–42

Following the above treatments, the patient has occasional spontaneous respirations and begins to display nonpurposeful movement of both arms. Following transfer to CCU, her blood pressure improves.

SCENARIO 5

It is 7:30 a.m. on a Friday morning, and you are working in a small rural hospital coronary care unit. You have just completed rounds when the ECG alarm sounds in the room of a recently admitted 160-pound male patient. You find the patient unconscious, pulseless, and apneic. His ECG monitor shows the rhythm in Figure 12–43; an IV lifeline is in place. You have the defibrillator with you.

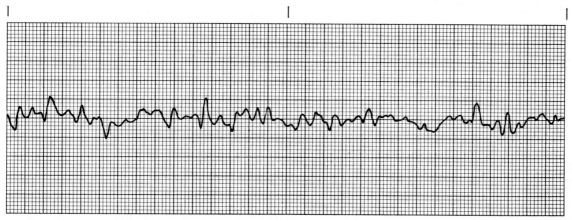

Figure 12–43

5.01 This type of cardiac arrest is called _____

_____

5.02 The first task you should do is to

deliver a precordial thump

intubate the trachea

defibrillate using _____ joules

begin CPR

Following this treatment, the patient is still apneic and pulseless; his ECG monitor shows (Figure 12–44):

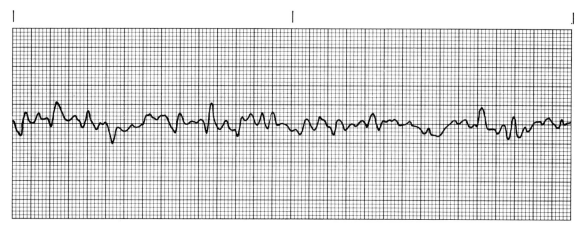

Figure 12–44

5.03 You should now

administer lidocaine _____ IM

intubate the trachea

defibrillate using _____ joules

deliver a synchronized countershock

administer epinephrine, _____ endo-

    tracheally

5.04 After the above treatment, you see the rhythm in Figure 12–45 on the ECG monitor, but the patient is still pulseless and apneic. This condition

is called _____

_____

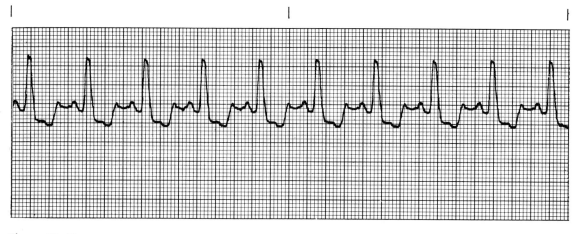

Figure 12–45

5.05 It is now 7:31. The next thing to do is to

administer sodium bicarbonate,

_____ IV push

intubate the trachea

defibrillate using _____ joules

begin CPR

administer atropine, _____ IV push

5.06 Now it is 7:32. The CPR team arrives; ABGs have been drawn and sent to the lab. The next thing the CPR team should do is to

insert a pacemaker

intubate the trachea

defibrillate using _____ joules

deliver a synchronized countershock

administer epinephrine, _____ IV push

5.07 The patient remains pulseless; the next task the team should do is to

administer epinephrine, _____ IV push

administer atropine, _____ IV push

administer sodium bicarbonate,

_____ IV push

administer isoproterenol, _____ IV infusion

intubate the trachea

After this, the monitor shows the rhythm in Figure 12–46, but the patient remains pulseless and apneic.

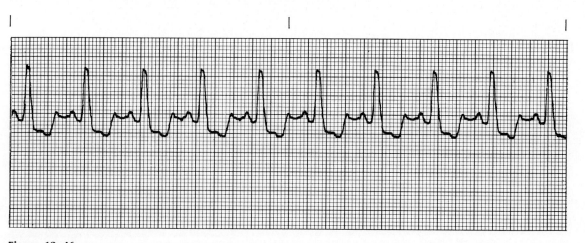

Figure 12–46

5.08 CPR is reinstituted. It is 7:36 a.m. Now the CPR team should

administer epinephrine, _____ IV

   push

administer calcium chloride, _____ IV

   push

administer sodium bicarbonate,

   _____ IV push

The patient's condition is unchanged, so CPR is resumed.

5.09 It is now 7:37. The CPR team should now administer

epinephrine, _____ IV push

bretylium, _____ IV push

sodium bicarbonate, _____ IV push

isoproterenol, _____ IV infusion

5.10 The patient's ECG in Figure 12–47 now reveals

_____

The patient is still apneic and pulseless.

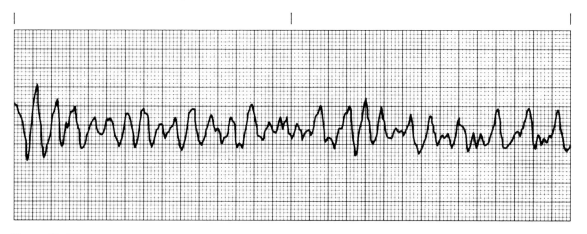

Figure 12–47

5.11 It is now 7:39. You should immediately administer

calcium chloride, _____ IV push

defibrillation using _____ joules

sodium bicarbonate, _____ IV push

isoproterenol, _____ IV infusion

5.12 Following the above treatment, the patient has a strong pulse, a blood pressure of 150/106, and has spontaneous ventilations. His ECG in Figure

12–48 shows _____

_____

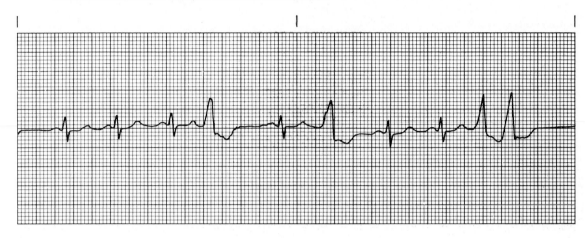

Figure 12–48

5.13 The next task the team should do is to

administer propranolol, _____ IV

push

administer sodium bicarbonate,

_____ IV push

administer lidocaine, _____ IV push

5.14 After this treatment the team should administer

norepinephrine, _____ IV infusion

dopamine, _____ IV infusion

sodium bicarbonate, _____ IV push

lidocaine, _____ IV infusion

At 7:45 the patient's condition is stable, but his ECG shows the rhythm in Figure 12–49.

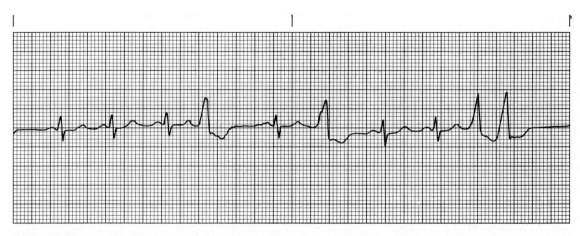

Figure 12–49

5.15 You should now administer

epinephrine, _____ IV push

dopamine, _____ IV infusion

procainamide, _____ IV push

lidocaine, _____ IV push

5.16 Following this treatment the ECG in Figure 12–

50 reveals _____

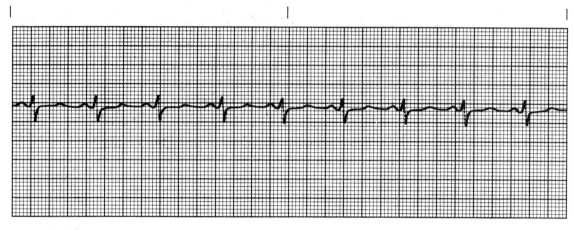

Figure 12–50

The patient now has a blood pressure of 140/90; he is still unconscious and is being ventilated by a ventilator.

SCENARIO 6

It is 2:43 on a Saturday morning in the emergency department of a large community hospital. The rescue squad calls to say they are on the scene with a 38-year-old, 190-pound male who was in cardiac arrest when they arrived at 2:41. Prior to their arrival, the patient reportedly complained of acute dyspnea. Family members state that the patient has no previous medical history and takes no medications. The patient is unconscious, pulseless, and apneic. Basic life support is being provided by the paramedics. The patient's ECG is being transmitted (see Figure 12–51).

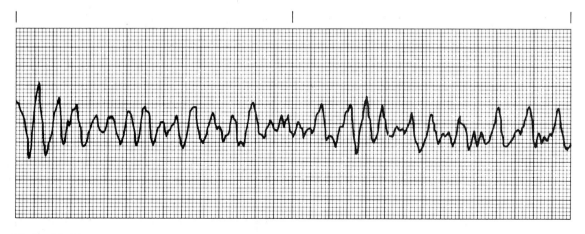

Figure 12–51

6.01 This dysrhythmia is called _____

_____

6.02 Should you have the paramedics continue or temporarily withhold CPR? _____

6.03 You should now direct the paramedics to

defibrillate using _____ joules

administer atropine, _____ IV push

administer sodium bicarbonate,

_____ IV push

intubate the trachea

establish an IV lifeline

After this treatment, the ECG (Figure 12–52) reveals:

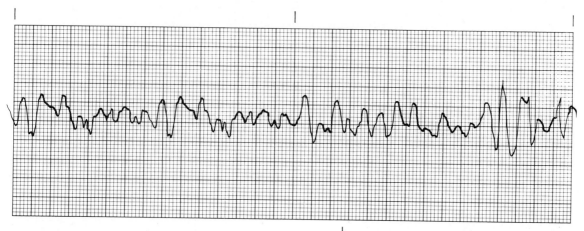

Figure 12–52

6.04 The paramedics continue CPR; you then direct them to

defibrillate using _____ joules

administer atropine, _____ IV push

administer sodium bicarbonate,

_____ IV push

intubate the trachea

administer epinephrine, _____ IV push

6.05 The patient remains apneic and pulseless. His ECG shows the rhythm in Figure 12–53. The paramedics continue CPR; you should direct them to

defibrillate using _____ joules

administer atropine, _____ IV push

administer sodium bicarbonate,

_____ IV push

intubate the trachea

administer epinephrine, _____ IV push

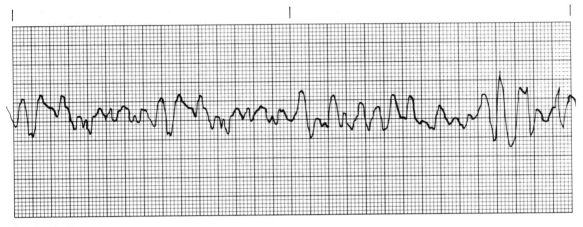

Figure 12–53

6.06 The patient remains apneic and pulseless. His ECG shows the rhythm in 12–54; this dysrhythmia is called _____

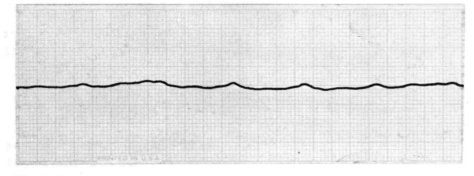

Figure 12–54

6.07 It is now 2:46. The next task you should have the paramedics do is to

defibrillate using _____ joules

administer epinephrine, _____ IV push

administer calcium chloride, _____ IV push

intubate the trachea

establish an IV lifeline

6.08 There is no change in the patient's condition. It is now 2:48. The next thing the paramedics should do is to administer

defibrillation using _____ joules

epinephrine, _____ IV push

sodium bicarbonate, _____ IV push

bretylium, _____ IV push

atropine, _____ IV push

The monitor shows the rhythm in Figure 12–55 as the paramedics report no change in the patient's condition; they resume CPR. They advise you that they have endotracheally intubated the patient.

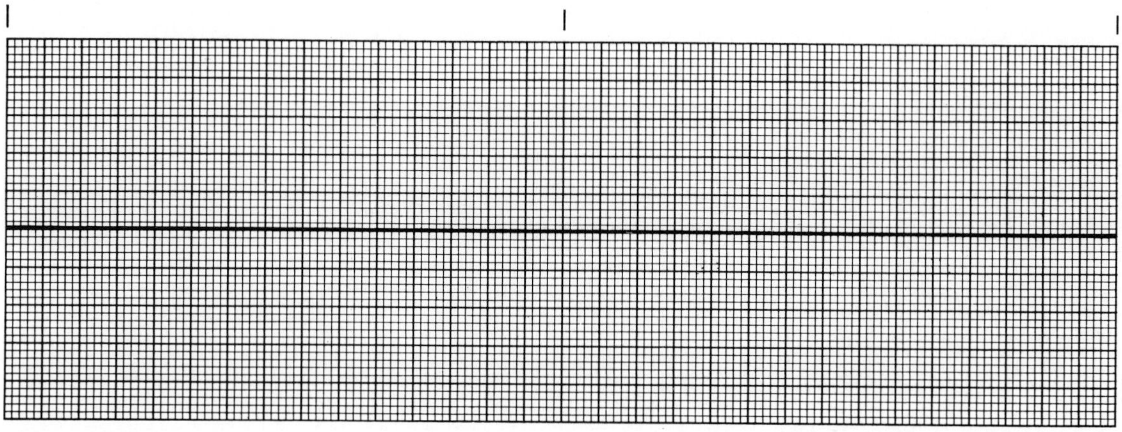

Figure 12–55

6.09 At 2:50 you should have the paramedics administer

epinephrine, _____ IV push

atropine, _____ IV push

calcium chloride, _____ IV push

isoproterenol, _____ IV infusion

There is no change in the patient's status. CPR resumes.

6.10 It is 2:52 when you ask the paramedics to now administer

epinephrine, _____ IV push

atropine, _____ IV push

calcium chloride, _____ IV push

sodium bicarbonate, _____ IV push

6.11 After this treatment, the patient has a feeble pulse, but is still apneic; his ECG monitor (Figure 12–56) shows _____

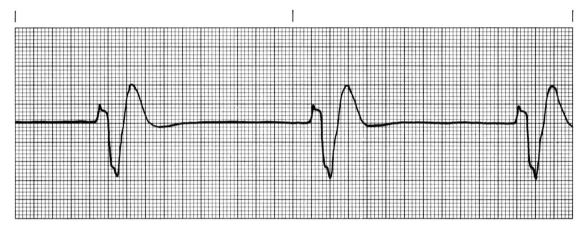

Figure 12–56

6.12 The next drug the paramedics should be asked to administer is

epinephrine, _____ IV push

bretylium, _____ IV push

sodium bicarbonate, _____ IV push

isoproterenol, _____ IV infusion

atropine, _____ IV push

The patient is now pulseless again and his ECG shows the rhythm in Figure 12–57.

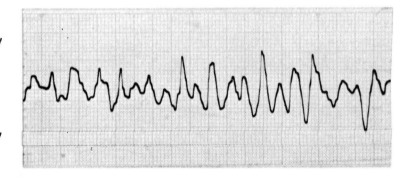

Figure 12–57

6.13 It is now 2:54. Now you should have the paramedics administer

epinephrine, _____ IV push

atropine, _____ IV push

calcium chloride, _____ IV push

isoproterenol, _____ IV infusion

defibrillation using _____ joules

Following the above therapy the ECG monitor shows the rhythm in Figure 12–58; the patient remains apneic and pulseless.

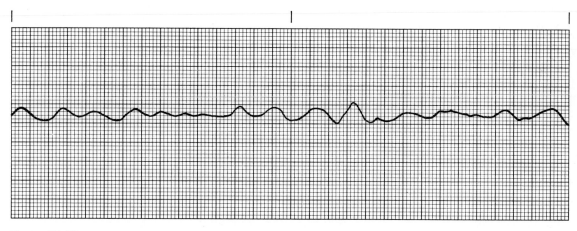

Figure 12–58

6.14 The dysrhythmia above is called _____

_____

6.15 It is now 2:55. At this point you should have the paramedics administer

epinephrine, _____ IV push

bretylium, _____ IV push

sodium bicarbonate, _____ IV push

isoproterenol, _____ IV infusion

lidocaine, _____ IV push

After this treatment, the ECG shows the rhythm in Figure 12–59.

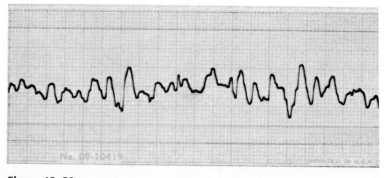

Figure 12–59

The paramedics report that the patient's condition is unchanged.

6.16 It is 2:57. Now the paramedics should be directed to administer

epinephrine, _____ IV push

bretylium, _____ IV push

sodium bicarbonate, _____ IV push

isoproterenol, _____ IV infusion

defibrillation using _____ joules

6.17 There is no change in the patient's status over the next minute. The next drug the paramedics should administer is

epinephrine, _____ IV push

bretylium, _____ IV push

sodium bicarbonate, _____ IV push

procainamide, _____ IV infusion

Following this therapy, the ECG in Figure 12–60 shows:

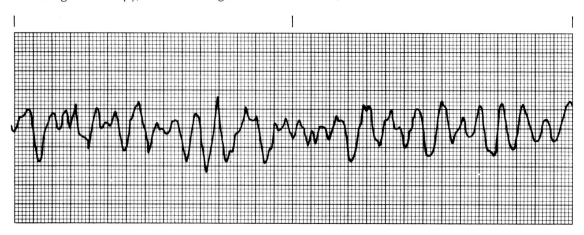

Figure 12–60

The patient's condition is unchanged; CPR is reinstituted for the next minute.

6.18 Now the paramedics should administer

epinephrine, _____ IV push

bretylium, _____ IV push

sodium bicarbonate, _____ IV push

procainamide, _____ IV infusion

defibrillation using _____ joules

6.19 After this treatment, the patient is still apneic but now has a weak pulse and a blood pressure of 90/60. The ECG in Figure 12–61 reveals that the cardiac rhythm is now _____

_____

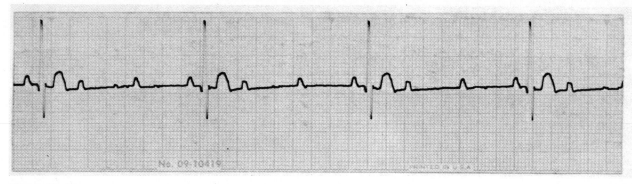

Figure 12–61

The paramedics discontinue chest compressions but maintain ventilations.

6.20 It is now 3:01. To treat the dysrhythmia above, you should have the paramedics administer*

epinephrine, _____ IV push

atropine, _____ IV push

sodium bicarbonate, _____ IV push

lidocaine, _____ IV push

Following this treatment, the ECG shows the rhythm below. The patient still has a pulse and blood pressure of 90/60, but the ECG is the same.

6.21 It is now 3:06 and the paramedics are enroute to the hospital. The next task the paramedics should do is to administer

norepinephrine, _____ IV infusion

atropine, _____ IV push

lidocaine, _____ IV infusion

dopamine, _____ IV infusion

The patient's ECG, blood pressure, and pulse are not affected by this treatment.

6.22 It is now 3:08 and the paramedics should be directed to administer

norepinephrine, _____ IV infusion

dopamine, _____ IV infusion

lidocaine, _____ IV infusion

isoproterenol, _____ IV infusion

*If you elected to administer atropine in question 6.12, proceed directly to question 6.22.

Following this treatment, the ECG reveals the rhythm in Figure 12–62.

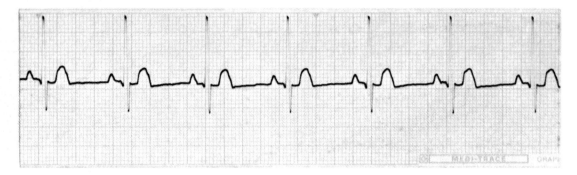

Figure 12–62

6.23 The patient is still apneic, but has a strong pulse and blood pressure of 142/100. The ECG in Figure 12–62 shows _____

When the patient arrives at the hospital, his condition is stable. Several minutes after his transfer, however, you see the rhythm in Figure 12–63 on his ECG monitor.

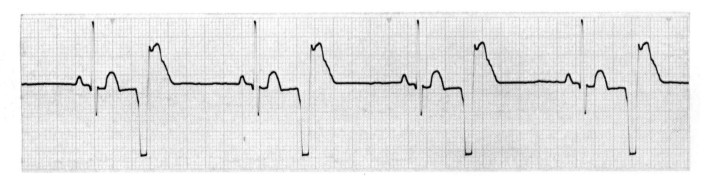

Figure 12–63

6.24 This dysrhythmia is called _____

_____

6.25 The next two tasks your staff should do are to

administer epinephrine, _____ IV push

discontinue the isoproterenol infusion

administer sodium bicarbonate,

_____ IV push

administer lidocaine, _____ IV push

defibrillate using _____ joules

6.26 Now the patient should receive

norepinephrine, _____ IV infusion

dopamine, _____ IV infusion

sodium bicarbonate, _____ IV push

lidocaine, _____ IV infusion

6.27 After the above treatment, the ECG in Figure 12–64 shows _____

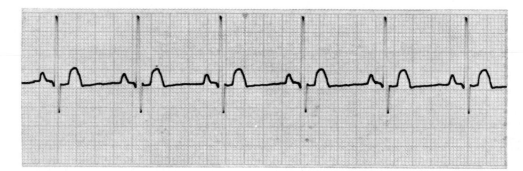

Figure 12–64

The patient is still apneic, but has a strong pulse and blood pressure of 142/100. He is transferred to the coronary care unit.

SCENARIO 7

It is 11:46 p.m. on a Monday night. You are working in the CCU step-down unit of a large urban hospital. A 56-year-old, 145-pound male patient who is recovering from a heart attack is now complaining of chest pain and shortness of breath. The patient has an IV lifeline in place and is receiving oxygen. You are taking his blood pressure when his ECG monitor shows the rhythm in Figure 12–65.

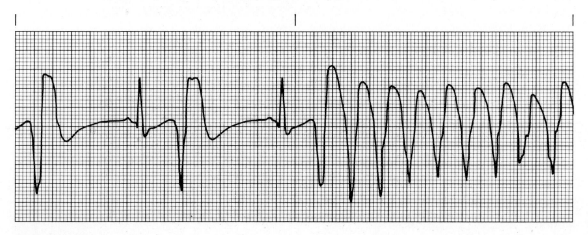

Figure 12–65

7.01 This rhythm is _____

_____

7.02 The first thing you should do is to

check for a pulse

intubate the trachea

defibrillate using _____ joules

begin CPR

The patient has a pulse and is breathing; his blood pressure is 60/40; he is still unconscious.

7.03 The next task you should do is to

deliver a synchronized countershock

begin CPR

deliver unsynchronized cardioversion,

_____ joules

deliver a precordial thump

Following this treatment, you see the rhythm in Figure 12–66 on the ECG monitor.

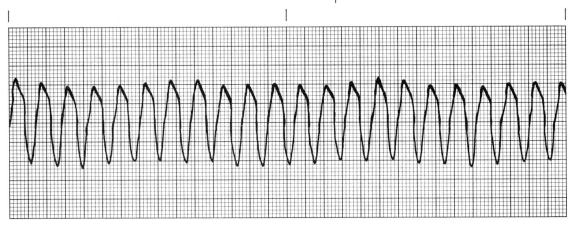

Figure 12–66

7.04 The patient's vital signs remain unchanged; he has a palpable pulse, but is still unconscious. The

ECG above shows this patient has _____

_____

7.05 It is 11:47. The next task you should do is to administer

epinephrine, _____ IV push

lidocaine, _____ IV push

calcium chloride, _____ IV push

bretylium, _____ IV push

a synchronized countershock

an unsynchronized countershock,

_____ joules

The patient's condition remains the same.

7.06 It is now 11:48 p.m. You should now administer

atropine, _____ IV push

isoproterenol, _____ IV infusion

calcium chloride, _____ IV push

bretylium, _____ IV push

an unsynchronized countershock,

_____ joules

The patient's status is unchanged following this treatment.

7.07 The next task you should do is to administer

epinephrine, _____ IV push

lidocaine, _____ IV push

calcium chloride, _____ IV push

isoproterenol, _____ IV infusion

an unsynchronized countershock,

_____ joules

Following this therapy, the ECG monitor (Figure 12–67) reveals:

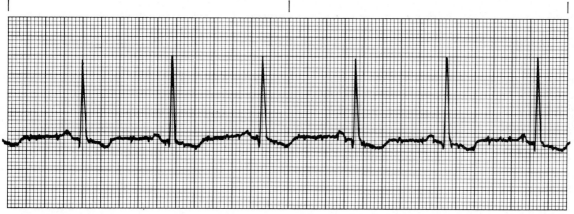

Figure 12–67

The patient now has a strong pulse and a blood pressure of 110/70. He has also regained consciousness.

7.08 The remaining treatment is to administer

epinephrine, _____ IV push

lidocaine, _____ IV infusion

calcium chloride, _____ IV push

sodium bicarbonate, _____ IV push

lidocaine, _____ IV push

The patient's condition remains stable throughout the remainder of your shift.

SCENARIO 8

You work for a local EMS. It is 5:30 p.m. when you receive a call for a 65-year-old, 220-pound male having chest pain. You arrive at the scene to find the patient alert and well-oriented. He says the chest pain started while he was watching television; it is a dull, aching, substernal pain, which is not affected by breathing or movement. The patient has a history of hypertension and takes Aldomet® daily. Examination reveals a respiratory rate of 30/minute, blood pressure 180/100, and cold, clammy, diaphoretic skin. Breath sounds are clear bilaterally; there is no peripheral edema or jugular venous distention. The ECG monitor shows the rhythm in Figure 12–68.

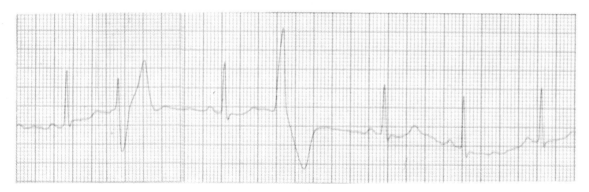

Figure 12–68

8.01 The patient's ECG shows _____

_____

8.02 This patient is most likely suffering from a (an)

acute myocardial infarction

congestive heart failure episode

cerebral vascular accident

aortic aneurysm

pulmonary embolism

8.03 Treatment of this patient should be directed toward which of the following:

relieving pain

eliminating ventricular ectopy

increasing heart rate

relieving hypoxia

raising the fibrillation threshold

8.04 This ECG rhythm may deteriorate into _____

_____

8.05 You are preparing to start an IV lifeline. Which of the following solutions should be used for this patient?

lactated Ringer's

normal (0.9%0) saline

D5/normal saline

Dextran

D5/water

8.06 Which two drugs should now be administered to this patient?

epinephrine, _____IV infusion

lidocaine, _____ IV push

sodium bicarbonate, _____ IV push

furosemide, _____ IV push

morphine sulfate, _____ slow IV push

8.07 Which of the above medications will need supplemental continuous IV infusion in order to maintain its therapeutic blood level? _____

_____

8.08 Following the above treatments, the patient's ECG (Figure 12–69) shows _____

_____

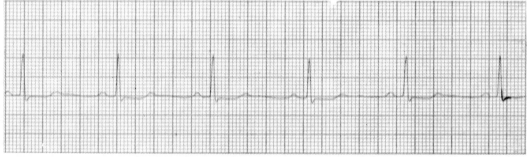

Figure 12–69

The patient's condition remains stable aside from the blood pressure, which lowers to 150/90; he is admitted to the CCU.

SCENARIO 9

You are the emergency department physician in an urban hospital. It is 10:30 a.m. on a Sunday morning when a 43-year-old male complaining of chest pain and shortness of breath is brought in. The pain is described as "crushing"; it is substernal and does not radiate; it began during church services while the patient was sitting quietly. The patient denies previous medical history and medications. He has a respiratory rate of 24 per minute, a blood pressure of 66/40, and cold, clammy, diaphoretic skin. Breath sounds are clear bilaterally. Oxygen administration and an IV lifeline were started. The ECG is shown in Figure 12–70.

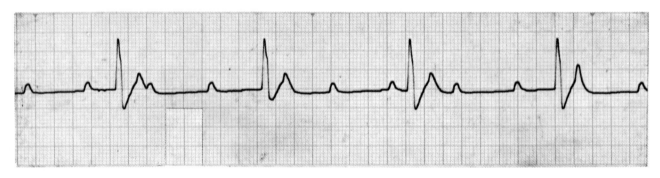

Figure 12–70

9.01 This ECG shows _____

_____

9.02 Treatment of this patient should be directed at which two areas:

decreasing automaticity

eliminating ventricular ectopy

increasing heart rate

eliminating hypoxia

raising the fibrillation threshold

9.03 This rhythm may deteriorate into _____

_____

9.04 It is now 10:31. Which of the following should be administered to this patient?

epinephrine, _____ IV push

lidocaine, _____ IV push

sodium bicarbonate, _____ IV push

atropine, _____ IV push

morphine sulfate, _____ IV push

9.05 The patient's condition is unchanged, and it is now 10:36. Which of the following should now be administered?

epinephrine, _____ IV push

lidocaine, _____ IV push

sodium bicarbonate, _____ IV push

atropine, _____ IV push

morphine sulfate, _____ IV push

9.06 Following the maximum dosage of the above medication, the patient's status is the same. Which of the following medications should now be used to improve the patient's condition?

epinephrine, _____ IV push

lidocaine, _____ IV push

isoproterenol, _____ IV infusion

calcium chloride, _____ IV push

morphine sulfate, _____ IV push

Following this therapy the ECG in Figure 12–71 reveals:

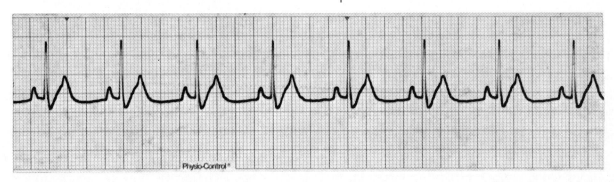

Figure 12–71

9.07 This rhythm is called _____

_____

The patient's blood pressure is now 126/80; his skin color improves, but he is still complaining of severe substernal chest pain.

9.08 Which of the following should now be administered to this patient?

epinephrine, _____ IV push

lidocaine, _____ IV push

sodium bicarbonate, _____ IV push

atropine, _____ IV push

morphine sulfate, _____ slow IV push

9.09 Which of the following will eventually be required to assure maintenance of an adequate cardiac output for this patient?

a permanent pacemaker

medical antishock trousers

dopamine, _____ IV infusion

dobutamine, _____ IV infusion

The patient's condition remains stable and he is admitted to the coronary care unit.

SCENARIO 10

It is 8:10 p.m. and you are working in a community-based EMS. You have just been called to the scene of a 57-year-old, 175-pound male city council member who suddenly collapsed during a council meeting. A nurse in attendance administered oxygen after he collapsed. You find the patient conscious and oriented. The patient's only complaint is that he feels dizzy. His pulses are palpable, and the blood pressure is 124/80.

10.01 The ECG in Figure 12–72 shows that this patient's

cardiac rhythm is _____

_____

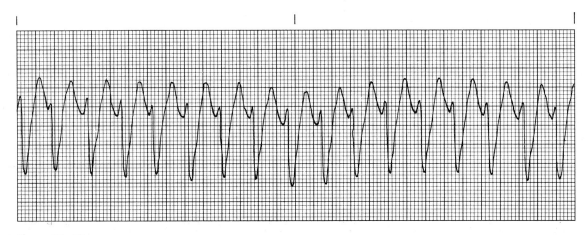

Figure 12–72

10.02 The first task you should do is to

deliver a synchronized countershock

begin CPR

defibrillate using _____ joules

deliver a precordial thump

establish an IV lifeline

The patient's ECG, pulse, and neurologic status remain the same.

10.03 It is now 8:12 p.m. Next you should administer

epinephrine, _____ IV push

lidocaine, _____ IV push

bretylium, _____ IV push

calcium chloride, _____ IV push

synchronized countershock

There is no change in the patient's ECG.

10.04 At 8:14 you should administer

isoproterenol, _____ IV infusion

calcium chloride, _____ IV push

bretylium, _____ IV push

synchronized countershock at

_____ joules

lidocaine, _____ IV push

The ECG monitor now shows the rhythm in Figure 12–73.

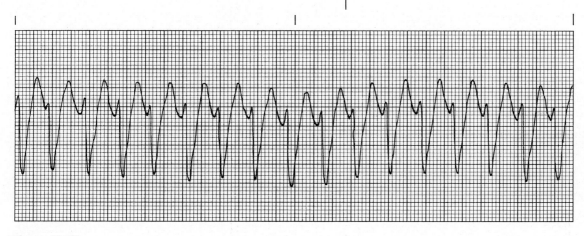

Figure 12–73

10.05 It is 8:16. Your team should now administer

procainamide, _____ slow IV push

lidocaine, _____ IV push

bretylium, _____ IV push

isoproterenol, _____ IV infusion

synchronized countershock

Following this therapy, the ECG rhythm is shown in Figure 12–74.

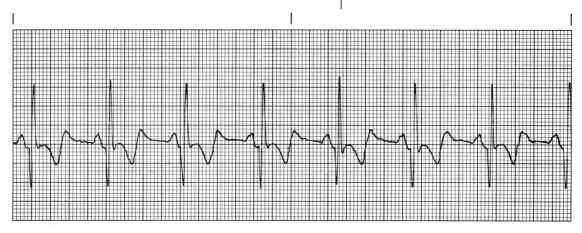

Figure 12–74

10.06 The next task you should do is to

administer epinephrine, _____ IV

push

check for a pulse

administer dopamine, _____ IV infu-

sion

insert a pacemaker

The patient now has a strong pulse and a blood pressure of 140/66. The chest pain has subsided and his condition remains stable for transport. You have begun a continuous procainamide infusion.

ANSWER KEY

SCENARIO 1

1.01 *Begin CPR:* Because the patient has been in cardiac arrest for several minutes, it is important to reestablish breathing and circulation to maintain patient viability. CPR will provide oxygen enriched blood to maintain function of the vital organs.

1.02 *Identify the ECG rhythm:* Treatment protocols vary depending upon the condition. Dysrhythmias such as ventricular tachycardia or ventricular fibrillation can be treated at once with defibrillation, whereas other conditions such as asystole or electromechanical dissociation (EMD) require pharmacological intervention. Obtain an ECG reading as soon as possible. It can be determined by either the "quick-look" paddles of the defibrillator or by attaching the patient to the ECG monitor leads. Some prefer the expediency of the paddles; others prefer to monitor the patient continuously using the monitor leads.

1.03 *Ventricular fibrillation:* This chaotic ventricular rhythm occurs when multiple areas of the ventricles depolarize and repolarize in a totally uncoordinated fashion. Since there is no organized depolarization of the ventricles as a chamber, the ventricles do not contract in a uniform fashion. There is no cardiac output with this dysrhythmia because the ventricles are quivering rather than contracting. Ventricular fibrillation is the most common mechanism of cardiac arrest that results from myocardial ischemia or infarction.

1.04 *Temporarily withhold CPR:* CPR should be temporarily stopped to defibrillate the patient. This should only be a short delay as the patient will be without circulation and breathing during this time period. If unnecessary delays are encountered in preparing for defibrillation, CPR should be reinitiated until defibrillation can be readily performed.

1.05 *Defibrillate using 200 joules:* Since the only definitive treatment for ventricular fibrillation is defibrillation, the patient should be defibrillated as soon as possible. Previously it was taught that CPR should be performed for at least 2 minutes before defibrillation, while medications such as epinephrine and bicarbonate were given and circulated. It is now thought that defibrillation is more likely to be successful the sooner it is provided following the onset of ventricular fibrillation.

1.06 *Check for a pulse:* Each time definitive therapy is instituted, the pulse should be checked. This should be done regardless of the ECG rhythm because many factors such as loose ECG electrodes influence the rhythm seen. The pulse is a true evaluation of circulation, whereas the ECG shows only the electrical activity of the heart.

1.07 *Temporarily withhold CPR:* CPR should be temporarily stopped to defibrillate the patient. This should only be a short delay as the patient will be without circulation and breathing during this time period. If unnecessary delays are encountered in preparing for defibrillation, CPR should be reinitiated until defibrillation can be readily performed.

1.08 *Defibrillate again using 200 to 300 joules:* The reason for a second immediate countershock is because there is a reduction of transthoracic resistance with repeated countershock. Reduced electrical resistance allows more energy to reach the fibrillating myocardium and increases the likelihood of successful defibrillation. The second countershock can be delivered immediately following the first countershock and pulse check. CPR need not be reinstituted during this period unless a significant delay results in delivery of the second countershock.

1.09 *Check for a pulse:* Each time definitive therapy is instituted, the pulse should be checked. This should be done regardless of the ECG rhythm because many factors such as loose ECG electrodes influence the rhythm seen. The pulse is a true evaluation of circulation, whereas the ECG shows only the electrical activity of the heart.

1.10 *Asystole:* Asystole is the total absence of cardiac electrical activity. Since there is no depolarization of the myocardial cells, the heart does not contract, and there is no cardiac output. Asystole may occur in cardiac arrest as a primary event or it may follow ventricular fibrillation; in the latter instance, it is usually due to a hypoxic and acidotic myocardium. Asystole may also be seen with complete AV block when there is no escape pacemaker. Treatment of asystole is directed at stimulating electrical and mechanical activity of the heart as well as eliminating hypoxia and acidosis.

Apparent asystole: It should be remembered that ventricular fibrillation can masquerade as asystole; thus the health professional should confirm that this is asystole by checking the rhythm with at least two different ECG leads. Whenever the rhythm is unclear and could possibly be ventricular fibrillation, one should treat the dysrhythmia as ventricular fibrillation. In this scenario, if the health professional suspected that the rhythm in Figure 12–3 might be ventricular fibrillation, defibrillation with 360 joules would be the next treatment as the patient has already been defibrillated twice. The revised standards now recommend a third immediate defibrillation when the first two attempts are unsuccessful. Energy levels up to 360 joules may be used.

1.11 *Continue CPR:* Since there is no cardiac output, CPR should be performed. This will provide oxygenated blood to the cells and circulate medications that are administered. The effectiveness of CPR should be checked periodically by determining if a pulse is generated with cardiac compressions. If no pulse is generated, the depth of compression should be increased and the hand position of the rescuer doing compressions should be checked.

1.12 *Establish an IV lifeline:* In general, an IV lifeline provides the most effective route for medication administration in cardiac arrest. Lidocaine, epinephrine, and atropine can, however, be effectively administered via an endotracheal tube.

1.13 *Administer epinephrine, 0.5 to 1.0 mg:* Epinephrine is used to elevate perfusion pressures generated during chest compression, to improve myocardial contractility, stimulate spontaneous contractions, and to make ventricular fibrillation more susceptible to cardioversion.

Because sodium bicarbonate is of questionable value in cardiac arrest, it is no longer recommended in the early cardiac arrest sequence. More recent data suggest that bicarbonate does not enhance the outcomes of defibrillation and may produce undesirable shifts in acid–base balance and in the oxyhemoglobin dissociation curve. If used at all, bicarbonate should only be used after more proven interventions have been employed. Remember that acidosis in cardiac arrest is often at least partly due to hypoxia. As long as the patient is hypoxic, he will continue to have anaerobic metabolism and acidosis. This further emphasizes the need to deliver the highest possible concentrations of oxygen to patients in cardiac arrest.

1.14 *Continue CPR:* Since there is no cardiac output, CPR should be performed. This will provide oxygenated blood to the cells and circulate administered medications. The effectiveness of CPR should be checked periodically by determining if a pulse is generated with cardiac compressions. If no pulse is generated, the depth of compression should be increased and the hand position of the rescuer doing compressions should be checked.

1.15 *Intubate the trachea:* An endotracheal tube should be placed for optimal patient ventilation and oxygenation. This allows direct access to the trachea for medication administration and suctioning and seals the airway to prevent aspiration. It is also the easiest device to maintain once it is in place.

1.16 *Administer atropine, 1.0 mg IV push:* Since asystole may be caused by high levels of parasympathetic tone, atropine may be an effective treatment. Its vagolytic action blocks the effects of acetylcholine and may allow the heart to return to its intrinsic rate or allow the sympathetic nervous system to accelerate heart rate. Higher dosages are used to treat asystole because it shortens the time required for achieving a therapeutic response. Atropine can also be administered via endotracheal route. Atropine administration (1.0 mg) can be repeated in five minutes.

1.17 *Check for a pulse:* Each time definitive therapy is instituted, the pulse should be checked. This should be done regardless of the ECG rhythm because many factors such as loose ECG electrodes influence the rhythm seen. The pulse is a true evaluation of circulation, whereas the ECG shows only the electrical activity of the heart.

1.18 *Administer epinephrine, 0.5 to 1.0 mg IV push:* Epinephrine is used to elevate perfusion pressures generated during chest compression, to improve myocardial contractility, stimulate spontaneous contractions, and to make ventricular fibrillation more susceptible to cardioversion. Epinephrine administration may be repeated once every 5 minutes. Epinephrine can also be administered via endotracheal route.

1.19 *Ventricular fibrillation:* This chaotic ventricular rhythm occurs when multiple areas of the ventricles depolarize and repolarize in a totally uncoordinated fashion. Since there is no organized depolarization of the ven-

tricles as a chamber, the ventricles do not contract in a uniform fashion. There is no cardiac output with this dysrhythmia because the ventricles are quivering rather than contracting. Ventricular fibrillation is the most common mechanism of cardiac arrest that results from myocardial ischemia or infarction.

1.20 *Temporarily withhold CPR:* CPR should be temporarily stopped to defibrillate the patient. This should only be a short delay as the patient will be without circulation and breathing during this time period. If unnecessary delays are encountered in preparing for defibrillation, CPR should be reinitiated until defibrillation can be readily performed.

1.21 *Defibrillate using 360 joules:* Defibrillation is the only definitive therapy for ventricular fibrillation. It should be performed as soon as possible because successful resuscitation is more likely the sooner defibrillation is performed following the onset of ventricular fibrillation. A higher dosage is indicated here to improve chances for successful defibrillation. When a lower dosage is successful in converting ventricular fibrillation, but the patient reverts to this dysrhythmia, the lower dosage may be employed. When lower dosages have not been successful, a higher dosage may be applied.

1.22 *(Normal) sinus rhythm:* This rhythm has P waves of normal configuration and contour preceding each QRS complex and the rate is between 60 and 100 per minute. QRS complexes have a normal duration and configuration. This rhythm is generally associated with a palpable pulse and usually provides adequate cardiac output.

1.23 *Check for a pulse:* Each time definitive therapy is instituted, the pulse should be checked. This should be done regardless of the ECG rhythm because many factors such as loose ECG electrodes influence the rhythm seen. The pulse is a true evaluation of circulation, whereas the ECG shows only the electrical activity of the heart.

1.24 *Discontinue CPR:* Because the patient now has a palpable pulse and satisfactory blood pressure, it can be assumed that vital organs are being perfused adequately. Chest compressions may, therefore, be discontinued. If the victim is still apneic or has an insufficient ventilatory rate, however, continue assisted ventilations (rescue breathing).

1.25 *Lidocaine, 1-mg/kg bolus IV push:* This patient would need a dose of 135 mg. Since the patient was in ventricular fibrillation, the fibrillation threshold of the myocardium is probably lower. Additionally, many medications administered during resuscitation stimulate cardiac electrical activity and may lower the fibrillation threshold. Lidocaine raises the fibrillation threshold and discourages reentry; its use may prevent the patient from slipping back into ventricular tachycardia or fibrillation. Lidocaine should be administered routinely following successful termination of ventricular fibrillation. Do not wait for ventricular ectopic activity such as PVCs to develop before giving lidocaine.

1.26 *Lidocaine infusion at 2 to 4 mg/minute:* Since the half-life of lidocaine in the central compartment is less than

10 minutes, a single bolus of lidocaine will maintain therapeutic levels for only a short time. To sustain adequate levels of lidocaine in the central compartment, a continuous IV infusion must be administered after the bolus dose(s).

1.27 *Ventricular bigeminy:* Sinus beats alternate with premature ventricular contractions (PVCs). The ectopic beats have QRS complexes which are wide (over 0.12 second), bizarre, not preceded by P waves, and associated with T waves oriented in an opposite direction; these are followed by a (full) compensatory pause. When ectopic beats alternate with normal beats, the rhythm is referred to as a bigeminy; this is ventricular bigeminy because the premature beats are of ventricular origin.

1.28 *Lidocaine, 0.5 mg/kg or a 50 to 100 mg IV bolus:* This patient would require a 70-mg bolus. With breakthrough ventricular ectopy, an additional lidocaine bolus is administered. The rate of lidocaine infusion may also be increased. If the ventricular ectopy persists after the above therapy, additional boluses of lidocaine can be administered up to a total dose of 225 mg.

1.29 *(Normal) sinus rhythm:* This rhythm has P waves of normal configuration and contour preceding each QRS complex and the rate is between 60 and 100 per minute. QRS complexes have a normal duration and configuration. This rhythm is generally associated with a palpable pulse and usually provides adequate cardiac output.

SCENARIO 2

2.01 *Begin CPR:* Because the patient has been in cardiac arrest for several minutes, it is important to reestablish breathing and circulation to maintain patient viability. CPR will provide oxygen enriched blood to maintain function of the vital organs.

2.02 *Identify the ECG rhythm:* Treatment protocols vary depending on the condition. Dysrhythmias such as ventricular tachycardia or ventricular fibrillation can be treated at once with defibrillation, whereas other conditions such as asystole or electromechanical dissociation (EMD) require pharmacological intervention. Obtain an ECG reading as soon as possible. It can be determined by either the "quick-look" paddles of the defibrillator or by attaching the patient to the ECG monitor leads. Some prefer the expediency of the paddles; others prefer to monitor the patient continuously using the monitor leads.

2.03 *Ventricular fibrillation:* This chaotic ventricular rhythm occurs when multiple areas of the ventricles depolarize and repolarize in a totally uncoordinated fashion. Since there is no organized depolarization of the ventricles as a chamber, the ventricles do not contract in a uniform fashion. There is no cardiac output with this dysrhythmia because the ventricles are quivering rather than contracting. Ventricular fibrillation is the most common mechanism of cardiac arrest that results from myocardial ischemia or infarction.

2.04 *Temporarily withhold CPR:* CPR should be temporarily stopped to defibrillate the patient. This should only be a short delay as the patient will be without circulation and breathing during this time period. If unnecessary delays are encountered in preparing for defibrillation, CPR should be reinitiated until defibrillation can be readily performed.

2.05 *Defibrillate using 200 joules:* Since the only definitive treatment for ventricular fibrillation is defibrillation, the patient should be defibrillated as soon as possible. Previously it was taught that CPR should be performed for at least 2 minutes before defibrillation, while medications such as epinephrine and bicarbonate were given and circulated. It is now thought that defibrillation is more likely to be successful the sooner it is provided following the onset of ventricular fibrillation.

2.06 *Check for a pulse:* Each time definitive therapy is instituted, the pulse should be checked. This should be done regardless of the ECG rhythm because many factors such as loose ECG electrodes influence the rhythm seen. The pulse is a true evaluation of circulation, whereas the ECG shows only the electrical activity of the heart.

2.07 *Temporarily withhold CPR:* CPR should be temporarily stopped to defibrillate the patient. This should only be a short delay as the patient will be without circulation and breathing during this time period. If unnecessary delays are encountered in preparing for defibrillation, CPR should be reinitiated until defibrillation can be readily performed.

2.08 *Defibrillate again using 200 to 300 joules:* The reason for a second immediate countershock is because there is a reduction of transthoracic resistance with repeated countershock. Reduced electrical resistance allows more energy to reach the fibrillating myocardium and increases the likelihood of successful defibrillation. The second countershock can be delivered immediately following the first countershock and pulse check. CPR need not be reinstituted during this period unless a significant delay results in delivery of the second countershock.

2.09 *Check for a pulse:* Each time definitive therapy is instituted, the pulse should be checked. This should be done regardless of the ECG rhythm because many factors such as loose ECG electrodes influence the rhythm seen. The pulse is a true evaluation of circulation, whereas the ECG shows only the electrical activity of the heart.

2.10 *Defibrillation using up to 360 joules:* This condition appears to be find ventricular fibrillation. Defibrillation with 360 joules would be the next treatment as the patient has already been defibrillated twice. The revised standards now recommend a third immediate defibrillation when the first two attempts are unsuccessful. Energy levels up to 360 joules may be used.

2.11 *Continue CPR:* Since there is no cardiac output, CPR should be performed. This will provide oxygenated blood to the cells and circulate medications which are administered. The effectiveness of CPR should be checked periodically by determining if a pulse is generated with cardiac compressions. If no pulse is generated, the depth of compression should be increased and the hand position of the rescuer doing compressions should be checked.

2.12 *Establish an IV lifeline:* In general, an IV lifeline provides the most effective route for medication administration in cardiac arrest. Lidocaine, epinephrine, and atropine can, however, be effectively administered via an endotracheal tube.

2.13 *Administer epinephrine 0.5 to 1.0 mg:* Epinephrine is used to elevate perfusion pressures generated during chest compression, to improve myocardial contractility, stimulate spontaneous contractions, and to make ventricular fibrillation more susceptible to cardioversion.

Because sodium bicarbonate is of questionable value in cardiac arrest, it is no longer recommended in the early cardiac arrest sequence. More recent data suggest that bicarbonate does not enhance the outcomes of defibrillation and may produce undesirable shifts in acid–base balance and in the oxyhemoglobin dissociation curve. If used at all, bicarbonate should only be used after more proven interventions have been employed. Remember that acidosis in cardiac arrest is often at least partly due to hypoxia. As long as the patient is hypoxic, she will continue to have anaerobic metabolism and acidosis. This further emphasizes the need to deliver the highest possible concentrations of oxygen to patients in cardiac arrest.

2.14 *Temporarily withhold CPR:* CPR should be temporarily stopped to defibrillate the patient. This should only be a short delay as the patient will be without circulation and breathing during this time period. If unnecessary delays are encountered in preparing for defibrillation, CPR should be reinitiated until defibrillation can be readily performed.

2.15 *Defibrillate using 360 joules:* Defibrillation is the only definitive therapy for ventricular fibrillation. It should be performed as soon as possible because successful resuscitation is more likely the sooner defibrillation is performed following the onset of ventricular fibrillation. A higher dosage is indicated here to improve chances for successful defibrillation. When a lower dosage is successful in converting ventricular fibrillation, but the patient reverts into this dysrhythmia, the lower dosage may be employed. When lower dosages have not been successful, a higher dosage may be applied.

2.16 *Lidocaine, 1 mg/kg:* This patient would need 55 mg. Lidocaine is now recommended for ventricular fibrillation that is resistant to defibrillation, since it may improve the response to electrical therapy. Among the positive effects of lidocaine in ventricular fibrillation is that it raises the fibrillation threshold and blocks reentry. Lidocaine can also be administered via endotracheal route.

2.17 *Defibrillate using 360 joules:* Defibrillation is the only definitive therapy for ventricular fibrillation. It should be performed as soon as possible because successful resuscitation is more likely the sooner defibrillation is performed following the onset of ventricular fibrillation. A higher dosage is indicated here to improve chances for successful defibrillation. When a lower

dosage is successful in converting ventricular fibrillation, but the patient reverts into this dysrhythmia, the lower dosage may be employed. When lower dosages have not been successful, a higher dosage may be applied.

2.18 *Continue CPR:* Since there is no cardiac output, CPR should be performed. This will provide oxygenated blood to the cells and circulate medications that are administered. The effectiveness of CPR should be checked periodically by determining if a pulse is generated with cardiac compressions. If no pulse is generated, the depth of compression should be increased and the hand position of the rescuer doing compressions should be checked.

2.19 *Administer bretylium, 5 mg/kg IV bolus:* This patient would require a dose of about 275 mg. Bretylium and lidocaine are used for refractory ventricular fibrillation. These medications may be effective in raising the fibrillation threshold and preventing reentry. Epicardial mapping studies indicate that ventricular fibrillation may result from the presence of more than one activation line passing across the myocardium at the same time. This event may result from a conduction delay of the normal wavefront such as that which occurs through ischemic and infarcted areas. Bretylium causes an initial transient release of catecholamines, which may improve the phase 0 characteristics of the depressed Purkinje fibers of infarcted tissues, reducing the difference in conduction times between normal and infarcted tissues. If 5 mg/kg is not effective, the dose may be increased to 10 mg/kg. Some may prefer repeated doses of lidocaine, which may be given in 0.5-mg/kg boluses every 8 minutes to a total dose of 3 mg/kg.

2.20 *Pneumothorax or right mainstem bronchus intubation:* When breath sounds can be heard on only one side of the chest, one of these two problems should be suspected. Inserting an endotracheal tube too far into the trachea or pushing it down into the right mainstem bronchus during resuscitation is not uncommon. To avoid this, secure the tube in place with tape or ties and auscultate breath sounds frequently; use one hand to ventilate the patient and the other to hold the tube in place until it has been secured.

Pneumothorax can result from vigorous resuscitation, improper hand position that fractures ribs, or improper placement of central IV lines. A chest x-ray can confirm this suspicion.

2.21 *Withdraw the endotracheal tube until breath sounds are heard bilaterally:* Other treatments may be indicated if the problem is actually a pneumothorax, but it is best to start by treating the most likely and most readily resolved problem first.

2.22 *Sodium bicarbonate (1 mEq/kg):* Sodium bicarbonate is used to treat metabolis acidosis. This patient would require a dose of 55 mEq. Many medications do not work in an acidotic medium. Remember that acidosis in cardiac arrest is often at least partly due to hypoxia. As long as the patient is hypoxic, he will continue to have anaerobic metabolism and acidosis. This further emphasizes the need to deliver the highest possible concentration of oxygen to patients in cardiac arrest.

2.23 *Defibrillate using 360 joules:* Defibrillation is the only definitive therapy for ventricular fibrillation. It should be performed as soon as possible because successful resuscitation is more likely the sooner defibrillation is performed following the onset of ventricular fibrillation. A higher dosage is indicated here to improve chances for successful defibrillation. When a lower dosage is successful in converting ventricular fibrillation, but the patient reverts into this dysrhythmia, the lower dosage may be employed. When lower dosages have not been successful, a higher dosage may be applied.

2.24 *Administer epinephrine, 0.5 to 1.0 mg IV push:* Epinephrine is used to elevate perfusion pressures generated during chest compression, to improve myocardial contractility, stimulate spontaneous contractions, and to make ventricular fibrillation more susceptible to cardioversion. Epinephrine administration may be repeated once every 5 minutes. Epinephrine can also be administered via endotracheal route.

2.25 *Check for a pulse:* Each time definitive therapy is instituted, the pulse should be checked. This should be done regardless of the ECG rhythm because many factors such as loose ECG electrodes influence the rhythm seen. The pulse is a true evaluation of circulation, whereas the ECG shows only the electrical activity of the heart.

2.26 *Defibrillate using 360 joules:* Defibrillation is the only definitive therapy for ventricular fibrillation. It should be performed as soon as possible because successful resuscitation is more likely the sooner defibrillation is performed following the onset of ventricular fibrillation. A higher dosage is indicated here to improve chances for successful defibrillation. When a lower dosage is successful in converting ventricular fibrillation, but the patient reverts into this dysrhythmia, the lower dosage may be employed. When lower dosages have not been successful, a higher dosage may be applied.

2.27 *Administer bretylium, 10 mg/kg IV bolus:* This patient would require a dose of about 550 mg. Bretylium and lidocaine may be used to treat refractory ventricular fibrillation. These medications may be effective in raising the fibrillation threshold and preventing reentry. Epicardial mapping studies indicate that ventricular fibrillation may result from the presence of more than one activation wave passing across the myocardium at the same time. This event may result from a conduction delay of the wavefront such as that which occurs through ischemic and infarcted areas. Bretylium causes an initial transient release of catecholamines which may improve the phase 0 characteristics of the depressed Purkinje fibers of infarcted areas, reducing the difference in conduction times between normal and infarcted tissue.

2.28 *Temporarily withhold CPR:* CPR should be temporarily stopped to defibrillate the patient. This should only be a short delay as the patient will be without circulation and breathing during this time period. If unnecessary delays are encountered in preparing for defibrillation, CPR should be reinitiated until defibrillation can be readily performed.

2.29 *Defibrillate using 360 joules:* Defibrillation is the only definitive therapy for ventricular fibrillation. It should be performed as soon as possible because successful resuscitation is more likely the sooner defibrillation is performed following the onset of ventricular fibrillation. A higher dosage is indicated here to improve chances for successful defibrillation. When a lower dosage is successful in converting ventricular fibrillation, but the patient reverts into this dysrhythmia, the lower dosage may be employed. When lower dosages have not been successful, a higher dosage may be applied.

2.30 *Sinus tachycardia:* This dysrhythmia has all the characteristics of (normal) sinus rhythm, but the rate is over 100 per minute.

2.31 *Check for a pulse:* Each time definitive therapy is instituted, the pulse should be checked. This should be done regardless of the ECG rhythm because many factors such as loose ECG electrodes influence the rhythm seen. The pulse is a true evaluation of circulation, whereas the ECG shows only the electrical activity of the heart.

2.32 *Discontinue CPR:* Because the patient now has a palpable pulse and satisfactory blood pressure, it can be assumed that vital organs are being perfused adequately. Chest compressions may, therefore, be discontinued. If the victim is still apneic or has an insufficient ventilatory rate, however, continue assisted ventilations (rescue breathing).

2.33 *Lidocaine, 1-mg/kg bolus IV push:* This patient would need a dose of 55 mg. Since the patient was in ventricular fibrillation, the fibrillation threshold of the myocardium is probably lower. Additionally, many medications administered during resuscitation stimulate cardiac electrical activity and may lower the fibrillation threshold. Lidocaine raises the fibrillation threshold and discourages reentry; its use may prevent the patient from slipping back into ventricular tachycardia or fibrillation. Lidocaine should be administered routinely following successful termination of ventricular fibrillation. Do not wait for ventricular ectopic activity such as PVCs to develop before giving lidocaine.

An important note is that lidocaine bolus administration may not be indicated if the conversion occurs shortly following previous lidocaine bolus administration. In those cases, a lidocaine infusion may be all that is needed to sustain therapeutic levels.

2.34 *Lidocaine infusion at 2 to 4 mg/minute:* Since the half-life of lidocaine in the central compartment is less than 10 minutes, a single bolus of lidocaine will maintain therapeutic levels for only a short time. To sustain adequate levels of lidocaine in the central compartment, a continuous IV infusion must be administered after the bolus dose(s).

SCENARIO 3

3.01 *Begin CPR:* Because the patient has been in cardiac arrest for several minutes, it is important to reestablish breathing and circulation to maintain patient viability. CPR will provide oxygen-enriched blood to maintain function of the vital organs.

3.02 *Identify the ECG rhythm:* Treatment protocols vary depending on the condition. Dysrhythmias such as ventricular tachycardia or ventricular fibrillation can be treated at once with defibrillation, whereas other conditions such as asystole or electromechanical dissociation (EMD) require pharmacological intervention. Obtain an ECG reading as soon as possible. It can be determined by either the "quick-look" paddles of the defibrillator or by attaching the patient to the ECG monitor leads. Some prefer the expediency of the paddles; others prefer to monitor the patient continuously using the monitor leads.

3.03 *Asystole:* Asystole is the total absence of cardiac electrical activity. Since there is no depolarization of the myocardial cells, the heart does not contract and there is no cardiac output. Asystole may occur in cardiac arrest as a primary event or it may follow ventricular fibrillation; in the latter instance, it is usually due to a hypoxic and acidotic myocardium. Asystole may also be seen with complete AV block when there is no escape pacemaker. Treatment of asystole is directed at stimulating electrical and mechanical activity of the heart as well as eliminating hypoxia and acidosis. Asystole should be confirmed in at least two ECG leads.

3.04 *Continue CPR:* Since there is no cardiac output, CPR should be performed. This will provide oxygenated blood to the cells and circulate medications which are administered. The effectiveness of CPR should be checked periodically by determining if a pulse is generated with cardiac compressions. If no pulse is generated, the depth of compression should be increased and the hand position of the rescuer doing compressions should be checked.

3.05 *Establish an IV lifeline:* In general, an IV lifeline provides the most effective route for medication administration in cardiac arrest. Lidocaine, epinephrine, and atropine can, however, be effectively administered via an endotracheal tube.

3.06 *Administer epinephrine, 0.5 to 1.0 mg:* Epinephrine is used to elevate perfusion pressures generated during chest compression, to improve myocardial contractility, stimulate spontaneous contractions, and to make ventricular fibrillation more susceptible to cardioversion.

Because sodium bicarbonate is of questionable value in cardiac arrest, it is no longer recommended in the early cardiac arrest sequence. More recent data suggest that bicarbonate does not enhance the outcomes of defibrillation and may produce undesirable shifts in acid–base balance and in the oxyhemoglobin dissociation curve. If used at all, bicarbonate should only be used after more proven interventions have been employed. Remember that acidosis in cardiac arrest is often at least partly due to hypoxia. As long as the patient is hypoxic, she will continue to have anaerobic metabolism and acidosis. This further emphasizes the need to deliver the highest possible concentrations of oxygen to patients in cardiac arrest.

3.07 *Intubate the trachea:* An endotracheal tube should be placed for optimal patient ventilation and oxygenation. This allows direct access to the trachea for medication administration and suctioning and seals the airway to prevent aspiration. It is also the easiest device to maintain once it is in place.

3.08 *Administer atropine, 1.0 mg IV push:* Since asystole may be caused by high levels of parasympathetic tone, atropine may be an effective treatment. Its vagolytic action blocks the effects of acetylcholine and may allow the heart to return to its intrinsic rate or allow the sympathetic nervous system to accelerate heart rate. Higher dosages (1 mg) are used to treat asystole because it shortens the time required for achieving a therapeutic response. Atropine can also be administered via endotracheal route. Atropine administration (1.0 mg) can be repeated in 5 minutes.

3.09 *Administer epinephrine, 0.5 to 1.0 mg IV push:* Epinephrine is used to elevate perfusion pressures generated during chest compression, to improve myocardial contractility, stimulate spontaneous contractions, and to make ventricular fibrillation more susceptible to cardioversion. Epinephrine administration may be repeated once every 5 minutes. Epinephrine can also be administered via endotracheal route.

3.10 *Increase the rate of ventilations and attach an oxygen supply line and reservoir device to the bag-valve-mask device:* When using a ventilatory adjunct during resuscitation, the ventilation rate can be safely increased to at least one ventilation every 3 seconds (20 per minute). This rate may need to be increased depending upon the patient's PaCO$_2$.

The highest possible concentration of oxygen should be used during resuscitation. To deliver 100% oxygen, the bag-valve-mask device must receive 100% oxygen via the supply line and there must be a reservoir which accumulates adequate volumes of oxygen between ventilations. Subsequently, each time the bag is emptied and refilled, it draws from that 100% oxygen in the reservoir rather than drawing from ambient (room) air that contains only 21% oxygen.

3.11 *Sodium bicarbonate (1 mEq/kg):* Sodium bicarbonate is used to treat metabolic acidosis. This patient would require a dose of 45 mEq. Many medications do not work in an acidotic medium. Remember that acidosis in cardiac arrest is often at least partly due to hypoxia. As long as the patient is hypoxic, she will continue to have anaerobic metabolism and acidosis. This further emphasizes the need to deliver the highest concentration of oxygen to patients in cardiac arrest.

3.12 *Ventricular fibrillation:* This chaotic ventricular rhythm occurs when multiple areas of the ventricles depolarize and repolarize in a totally uncoordinated fashion. Since there is no organized depolarization of the ventricles as a chamber, the ventricles do not contract in a uniform fashion. There is no cardiac output with this dysrhythmia because the ventricles are quivering rather than contracting. Ventricular fibrillation is the most common mechanism of cardiac arrest that results from myocardial ischemia or infarction.

3.13 *Temporarily withhold CPR:* CPR should be temporarily stopped to defibrillate the patient. This should only be a short delay as the patient will be without circulation and breathing during this time period. If unnecessary delays are encountered in preparing for defibrillation, CPR should be reinitiated until defibrillation can be readily performed.

3.14 *Defibrillate using 200 joules:* Since the only definitive treatment for ventricular fibrillation is defibrillation, the patient should be defibrillated as soon as possible. Previously it was taught that CPR should be performed for at least 2 minutes before defibrillation, while medications such as epinephrine and bicarbonate were given and circulated. It is now thought that defibrillation is more likely to be successful the sooner it is provided following the onset of ventricular fibrillation.

3.15 *(Normal) sinus rhythm:* This rhythm has P waves of normal configuration and contour preceding each QRS complex and the rate is between 60 and 100 per minute. QRS complexes have a normal duration and configuration. This rhythm is generally associated with a palpable pulse and usually provides adequate cardiac output.

3.16 *Check for a pulse:* Each time definitive therapy is instituted, the pulse should be checked. This should be done regardless of the ECG rhythm because many factors such as loose ECG electrodes influence the rhythm seen. The pulse is a true evaluation of circulation, whereas the ECG shows only the electrical activity of the heart.

3.17 *Discontinue CPR:* Because the patient now has a palpable pulse and satisfactory blood pressure, it can be assumed that vital organs are being perfused adequately. Chest compressions may, therefore, be discontinued. If the victim is still apneic or has an insufficient ventilatory rate, however, continue assisted ventilations (rescue breathing).

3.18 *Lidocaine, 1-mg/kg bolus IV push:* This patient would need a dose of 45 mg. Since the patient was in ventricular fibrillation, the fibrillation threshold of the myocardium is probably lower. Additionally, many medications administered during resuscitation stimulate cardiac electrical activity and may lower the fibrillation threshold. Lidocaine raises the fibrillation threshold and discourages reentry; its use may prevent the patient from slipping back into ventricular tachycardia or fibrillation. Lidocaine should be administered routinely following successful termination of ventricular fibrillation. Do not wait for ventricular ectopic activity such as PVCs to develop before giving lidocaine.

3.19 *Lidocaine infusion at 2 to 4 mg/minute:* Since the half-life of lidocaine in the central compartment is less than 10 minutes, a single bolus of lidocaine will maintain therapeutic levels for only a short time. To sustain adequate levels of lidocaine in the central compartment, a continuous IV infusion must be administered after the bolus dose(s).

SCENARIO 4

4.01 *Begin CPR:* Because the patient has been in cardiac arrest for several minutes, it is important to reestablish breathing and circulation to maintain patient viability. CPR will provide oxygen enriched blood to maintain function of the vital organs.

4.02 *Ventricular fibrillation:* This chaotic ventricular rhythm occurs when multiple areas of the ventricles depolarize and repolarize in a totally uncoordinated fashion. Since there is no organized depolarization of the ventricles as a chamber, the ventricles do not contract in a uniform fashion. There is no cardiac output with this dysrhythmia because the ventricles are quivering rather than contracting. Ventricular fibrillation is the most common mechanism of cardiac arrest that results from myocardial ischemia or infarction.

4.03 *Defibrillate using 200 joules:* Since the only definitive treatment for ventricular fibrillation is defibrillation, the patient should be defibrillated as soon as possible. Previously it was taught that CPR should be performed for at least 2 minutes before defibrillation, while medications such as epinephrine and bicarbonate were given and circulated. It is now thought that defibrillation is more likely to be successful the sooner it is provided following the onset of ventricular fibrillation.

4.04 *Establish an IV lifeline:* In general, an IV lifeline provides the most effective route for medication administration in cardiac arrest. Lidocaine, epinephrine, and atropine can, however, be effectively administered via an endotracheal tube.

4.05 *Administer epinephrine 0.5 to 1.0 mg:* Epinephrine is used to elevate perfusion pressures generated during chest compression, to improve myocardial contractility, stimulate spontaneous contractions, and to make ventricular fibrillation more susceptible to cardioversion.

Because sodium bicarbonate is of questionable value in cardiac arrest, it is no longer recommended in the early cardiac arrest sequence. More recent data suggest that bicarbonate does not enhance the outcomes of defibrillation and may produce undesirable shifts in acid–base balance and in the oxyhemoglobin dissociation curve. If used at all, bicarbonate should only be used after more proven interventions have been employed. Remember that acidosis in cardiac arrest is often at least partly due to hypoxia. As long as the patient is hypoxic, she will continue to have anaerobic metabolism and acidosis. This further emphasizes the need to deliver the highest possible concentrations of oxygen to patients in cardiac arrest.

4.06 *Administer atropine, 1.0 mg IV push:* Since asystole may be caused by high levels of parasympathetic tone, atropine may be an effective treatment. Its vagolytic action blocks the effects of acetylcholine and may allow the heart to return to its intrinsic rate or allow the sympathetic nervous system to accelerate heart rate. Higher dosages (1 mg) are used to treat asystole because it shortens the time required for achieving a therapeutic response. Atropine can also be administered via endotracheal route. Atropine administration (1.0 mg) can be repeated in five minutes.

4.07 *Check for a pulse:* Each time definitive therapy is instituted, the pulse should be checked. This should be done regardless of the ECG rhythm because many factors such as loose ECG electrodes influence the rhythm seen. The pulse is a true evaluation of circulation, whereas the ECG shows only the electrical activity of the heart.

4.08 *Defibrillate using 200 to 300 joules:* Since the only definitive treatment for ventricular fibrillation is defibrillation, the patient should be defibrillated as soon as possible. Previously it was taught that CPR should be performed for at least 2 minutes before defibrillation, while medications such as epinephrine and bicarbonate were given and circulated. It is now thought that defibrillation is more likely to be successful the sooner it is provided following the onset of ventricular fibrillation.

4.09 *Check for a pulse:* Each time definitive therapy is instituted, the pulse should be checked. This should be done regardless of the ECG rhythm because many factors such as loose ECG electrodes influence the rhythm seen. The pulse is a true evaluation of circulation, whereas the ECG shows only the electrical activity of the heart.

4.10 *Electromechanical dissociation (EMD):* EMD is a condition characterized by organized electrical activity on the ECG without effective myocardial contraction (no palpable pulse). EMD may result from failure of the calcium transport system, which is essential for coupling of the electrical event of depolarization with the mechanical event of contraction. Treatment is directed at effecting contraction of the ventricles. Medications such as epinephrine are used because of their ability to increase myocardial contractility.

It is important to rule out other conditions that may mimic EMD because the therapy for each of these is different. These conditions include hypovolemia, myocardial rupture, and cardiac tamponade. Fluid challenges with IV fluids or antishock trousers may indicate the correct etiology.

4.11 *Continue CPR:* Since there is no cardiac output, CPR should be performed. This will provide oxygenated blood to the cells and circulate medications that are administered. The effectiveness of CPR should be checked periodically by determining if a pulse is generated with cardiac compressions. If no pulse is generated, the depth of compression should be increased and the hand position of the rescuer doing compressions should be checked.

4.12 *Administer epinephrine, 0.5 to 1.0 mg IV push:* Epinephrine is used to elevate perfusion pressures generated during chest compression, to improve myocardial contractility, stimulate spontaneous contractions, and to make ventricular fibrillation more susceptible to cardioversion. Epinephrine administration may be repeated once every 5 minutes. Epinephrine can also be administered via endotracheal route.

4.13 *Check for a pulse:* Each time definitive therapy is instituted, the pulse should be checked. This should be done regardless of the ECG rhythm because many factors such as loose ECG electrodes influence the rhythm seen. The pulse is a true evaluation of circulation, whereas the ECG shows only the electrical activity of the heart.

4.14 *Sodium bicarbonate, 1 mEq/kg, IV push:* This patient would require a dose of 68 mEq. Because sodium bicarbonate is of questionable value in cardiac arrest, it is no longer recommended in the early cardiac arrest sequence. More recent data suggest that bicarbonate does not enhance the outcomes of defibrillation and may produce undesirable shifts in acid–base balance and in the oxyhemoglobin dissociation curve. If used at all, bicarbonate should only be used after more proven interventions have been employed. Remember that acidosis in cardiac arrest is often at least partly

due to hypoxia. As long as the patient is hypoxic, she will continue to have anaerobic metabolism and acidosis. This further emphasizes the need to deliver the highest possible concentrations of oxygen to patients in cardiac arrest.

Bicarbonate would be considered at this point, however, since more proven measures have already been taken and were unsuccessful. A dose of 1 mEq/kg is indicated. One-half of the original dose may be given every 10 minutes as indicated.

4.15 *Ventricular fibrillation:* This chaotic ventricular rhythm occurs when multiple areas of the ventricles depolarize and repolarize in a totally uncoordinated fashion. Since there is no organized depolarization of the ventricles as a chamber, the ventricles do not contract in a uniform fashion. There is no cardiac output with this dysrhythmia because the ventricles are quivering rather than contracting. Ventricular fibrillation is the most common mechanism of cardiac arrest that results from myocardial ischemia or infarction.

4.16 *Defibrillate using 360 joules:* Defibrillation is the only definitive therapy for ventricular fibrillation. It should be performed as soon as possible because successful resuscitation is more likely the sooner defibrillation is performed following the onset of ventricular fibrillation. A higher dosage is indicated here to improve chances for successful defibrillation. When a lower dosage is successful in converting ventricular fibrillation, but the patient reverts into this dysrhythmia, the lower dosage may be employed. When lower dosages have not been successful, a higher dosage may be applied.

4.17 *Idioventricular rhythm:* This dysrhythmia is characterized by beats of ventricular origin. QRS complexes are wide (over 0.12 second), bizarre in configuration, not preceded by P waves, and are associated with T waves oriented opposite to the QRS direction. The rhythm is usually regular and the rate is typically between 20 and 40 per minute.

4.18 *Administer epinephrine, 0.5 to 1.0 mg IV push, or atropine, 0.5 to 1.0 mg:* Epinephrine may be effective in restoring adequate cardiac output in idioventricular rhythm by increasing cardiac rate and contractility. Since an idioventricular rhythm may result from complete AV block, atropine can also be used to increase heart rate. The effectiveness of atropine is based on its ability to relieve sinoatrial block, thus restoring sinus rhythm. Atropine is more likely to be effective when P waves are present.

4.19 *Ventricular fibrillation:* This chaotic ventricular rhythm occurs when multiple areas of the ventricles depolarize and repolarize in a totally uncoordinated fashion. Since there is no organized depolarization of the ventricles as a chamber, the ventricles do not contract in a uniform fashion. There is no cardiac output with this dysrhythmia because the ventricles are quivering rather than contracting. Ventricular fibrillation is the most common mechanism of cardiac arrest that results from myocardial ischemia or infarction.

4.20 *Defibrillation using 360 joules:* Defibrillation is the only definitive therapy for ventricular fibrillation. It should be performed as soon as possible because successful resuscitation is more likely the sooner defibrillation is performed following the onset of ventricular fibrillation. A higher dosage is indicated here to improve chances for successful defibrillation. When a lower dosage is successful in converting ventricular fibrillation, but the patient reverts into this dysrhythmia, the lower dosage may be employed. When lower dosages have not been successful, a higher dosage may be applied.

4.21 *Sinus rhythm with run(s) of ventricular tachycardia:* The underlying rhythm has a P wave of normal contour preceding each QRS complex with a rate between 60 and 100 per minute. The ectopic beats appear to be of ventricular origin; the QRS complex is wide (over 0.12 second), bizarre, without preceding P waves, and associated with T waves of opposite orientation. Because the ectopic beats appear as consecutive beats of three or more PVCs, they qualify as a run of ventricular tachycardia.

4.22 *Discontinue CPR:* Because the patient now has a palpable pulse and satisfactory blood pressure, it can be assumed that vital organs are being perfused adequately. Chest compressions may, therefore, be discontinued. If the victim is still apneic or has an insufficient ventilatory rate, however, continue assisted ventilations (rescue breathing).

4.23 *Sinus rhythm progressing to ventricular tachycardia:* The underlying rhythm has a P wave of normal contour preceding each QRS complex with a rate between 60 and 100 per minute. The ectopic beats appear to be of ventricular origin; the QRS complex is wide (over 0.12 second), bizarre, without preceding P waves, and associated with T waves of opposite orientation. The second premature beat falls on the ''vulnerable period'' of the preceding cycle T wave, precipitating a continuous run of premature ventricular contractions (PVCs); this is referred to as R-on-T-phenomenon.

4.24 *Deliver a precordial thump:* Precordial thumps have been shown to be effective in evoking ventricular depolarization and resumption of synchronous myocardial contraction. The technique is most commonly used to restore sinus rhythm in the setting of monitored (recent onset) ventricular fibrillation or tachycardia.

4.25 *Ventricular tachycardia:* This dysrhythmia is characterized by beats of ventricular origin; the QRS complex is wide (over 0.12 second), bizarre, without preceding P waves, and associated with T waves of opposite orientation. The rhythm is usually regular and the rate is generally between 100 and 250 per minute.

4.26 *Defibrillate using up to 360 joules:* Patients who are pulseless and in ventricular tachycardia should be managed the same as if they were in ventricular fibrillation in order to simplify treatment protocols, facilitate use of external defibrillators, and avoid delays involved with synchronization.

4.27 *Sinus rhythm with a PVC:* The underlying rhythm has a P wave of normal contour preceding each QRS complex and the rate is between 60 and 100 per minute. The ectopic beat appears to be of ventricular origin; the QRS complex is wide (over 0.12 second), bizarre,

without preceding P waves, and is associated with T waves of opposite orientation. A (full) compensatory pause follows the early beat.

4.28 *Check for a pulse:* Each time definitive therapy is instituted, the pulse should be checked. This should be done regardless of the ECG rhythm because many factors such as loose ECG electrodes influence the rhythm seen. The pulse is a true evaluation of circulation, whereas the ECG shows only the electrical activity of the heart.

4.29 *Lidocaine, 1-mg/kg bolus IV push:* This patient would need a dose of 68 mg. Since the patient was in ventricular fibrillation, the fibrillation threshold of the myocardium is probably lower. Additionally, many medications administered during resuscitation stimulate cardiac electrical activity and may lower the fibrillation threshold. Lidocaine raises the fibrillation threshold and discourages reentry; its use may prevent the patient from slipping back into ventricular tachycardia or fibrillation. Lidocaine should be administered routinely following successful termination of ventricular fibrillation. Do not wait for ventricular ectopic activity such as PVCs to develop before giving lidocaine.

4.30 *Lidocaine infusion at 2 to 4 mg/minute:* Since the half-life of lidocaine in the central compartment is less than 10 minutes, a single bolus of lidocaine will maintain therapeutic levels for only a short time. To sustain adequate levels of lidocaine in the central compartment, a continuous IV infusion must be administered after the bolus dose(s).

4.31 *(Normal) sinus rhythm:* This rhythm has P waves of normal configuration and contour preceding each QRS complex and the rate is between 60 and 100 per minute. QRS complexes have a normal duration and configuration. This rhythm is generally associated with a palpable pulse and usually provides adequate cardiac output.

SCENARIO 5

5.01 *Monitored witnessed ventricular fibrillation:* This chaotic ventricular rhythm occurs when multiple areas of the ventricles depolarize and repolarize in a totally uncoordinated fashion. Since there is no organized depolarization of the ventricles as a chamber, the ventricles do not contract in a uniform fashion. There is no cardiac output with this dysrhythmia because the ventricles are quivering rather than contracting. Ventricular fibrillation is the most common mechanism of cardiac arrest that results from myocardial ischemia or infarction.

Ventricular fibrillation is considered ''monitored'' when the rescuer witnesses the onset of fibrillation and is able to intervene immediately. Immediate treatment consists of a precordial thump and defibrillation. These treatments precede CPR in monitored ventricular fibrillation because the patient should not yet be so acidotic that other measures are needed before these can terminate the fibrillation.

5.02 *Deliver a precordial thump:* Precordial thumps have been shown to be effective in evoking ventricular depolarization and resumption of synchronous myocardial contraction. The technique is most commonly used to restore sinus rhythm in the setting of monitored (recent onset) ventricular fibrillation or tachycardia.

5.03 *Defibrillate using 200 joules:* Since the only definitive treatment for ventricular fibrillation is defibrillation, the patient should be defibrillated as soon as possible. Previously it was taught that CPR should be performed for at least 2 minutes before defibrillation, while medications such as epinephrine and bicarbonate were given and circulated. It is now thought that defibrillation is more likely to be successful the sooner it is provided following the onset of ventricular fibrillation.

5.04 *Electromechanical dissociation (EMD):* EMD is a condition characterized by organized electrical activity on the ECG without effective myocardial contraction (no palpable pulse). EMD may result from failure of the calcium transport system, which is essential for coupling of the electrical event of depolarization with the mechanical event of contraction. Treatment is directed at effecting contraction of the ventricles. Medications such as epinephrine are used because of their ability to increase myocardial contractility.

It is important to rule out other conditions that may mimic EMD because the therapy for each of these is different. These conditions include hypovolemia, myocardial rupture, and cardiac tamponade. Fluid challenges with IV fluids or antishock trousers may indicate the correct etiology.

5.05 *Begin CPR:* Because the patient is in cardiac arrest, it is important to reestablish breathing and circulation to maintain patient viability. CPR will provide oxygen enriched blood to maintain function of the vital organs.

5.06 *Epinephrine, 0.5 to 1.0 mg IV push:* Epinephrine is used to elevate perfusion pressures generated during chest compression, to improve myocardial contractility, stimulate spontaneous contractions, and to make ventricular fibrillation more susceptible to cardioversion. Epinephrine administration may be repeated once every 5 minutes.

5.07 *Intubate the trachea:* An endotracheal tube should be placed for optimal patient ventilation and oxygenation. This allows direct access to the trachea for medication administration and suctioning, and seals the airway to prevent aspiration. It is also the easiest device to maintain once it is in place.

5.08 *Sodium bicarbonate, 1 mEq/kg, IV push:* This patient would require a dose of 73 mEq. Because sodium bicarbonate is of questionable value in cardiac arrest, it is no longer recommended in the early cardiac arrest sequence. More recent data suggest that bicarbonate does not enhance the outcomes of defibrillation and may produce undesirable shifts in acid–base balance and in the oxyhemoglobin dissociation curve. If used at all, bicarbonate should only be used after more proven interventions have been employed. Remember that acidosis in cardiac arrest is often at least partly due to hypoxia. As long as the patient is hypoxic, he will continue to have anaerobic metabolism and acidosis. This further emphasizes the need to deliver the highest possible concentrations of oxygen to patients in cardiac arrest.

Bicarbonate would be considered at this point, however, since more proven measures have already been taken and were unsuccessful. A dose of 1 mEq/kg is indicated. One-half of the original dose may be given every 10 minutes as indicated.

5.09 *Epinephrine, 0.5 to 1.0 mg IV push:* Epinephrine is used to elevate perfusion pressures generated during chest compression, to improve myocardial contractility, stimulate spontaneous contractions, and to make ventricular fibrillation more susceptible to cardioversion. Epinephrine administration may be repeated once every 5 minutes. Epinephrine can also be administered via endotracheal route.

5.10 *Ventricular fibrillation:* This chaotic ventricular rhythm occurs when multiple areas of the ventricles depolarize and repolarize in a totally uncoordinated fashion. Since there is no organized depolarization of the ventricles as a chamber, the ventricles do not contract in a uniform fashion. There is no cardiac output with this dysrhythmia because the ventricles are quivering rather than contracting. Ventricular fibrillation is the most common mechanism of cardiac arrest that results from myocardial ischemia or infarction.

5.11 *Defibrillation using 200 to 300 joules:* Since the only definitive treatment for ventricular fibrillation is defibrillation, the patient should be defibrillated as soon as possible. Previously it was taught that CPR should be performed for at least 2 minutes before defibrillation, while medications such as epinephrine and bicarbonate were given and circulated. It is now thought that defibrillation is more likely to be successful the sooner it is provided following the onset of ventricular fibrillation.

5.12 *Sinus tachycardia with frequent PVCs:* The underlying rhythm has a P wave of normal contour preceding each QRS and the rate is over 100 per minute. The ectopic beats appear to be ventricular in origin; the QRS complexes are wide (over 0.12 second), bizarre, not preceded by a P wave, and associated with an S-T segment and T-wave oriented opposite to the QRS. Since the ectopic beats occur more often than six per minute, they are referred to as "frequent" PVCs.

5.13 *Administer lidocaine, 1-mg/kg bolus IV push:* This patient would need a dose of 72 mg. Since the patient was in ventricular fibrillation, the fibrillation threshold of the myocardium is probably lower. Additionally, many medications administered during resuscitation stimulate cardiac electrical activity and may lower the fibrillation threshold. Lidocaine raises the fibrillation threshold and discourages reentry; its use may prevent the patient from slipping back into ventricular tachycardia or fibrillation. Lidocaine should be administered routinely following successful termination of ventricular fibrillation. Do not wait for ventricular ectopic activity such as PVCs to develop before giving lidocaine.

5.14 *Lidocaine infusion at 2 to 4 mg/minute:* Since the half-life of lidocaine in the central compartment is less than 10 minutes, a single bolus of lidocaine will maintain therapeutic levels for only a short time. To sustain adequate levels of lidocaine in the central compartment, a continuous IV infusion must be administered after the bolus dose(s).

5.15 *Lidocaine, 0.5 mg/kg or a 50 to 100 mg IV bolus:* With breakthrough ventricular ectopy, an additional lidocaine bolus is administered. The rate of lidocaine infusion may also be increased. If the ventricular ectopy persists after the above therapy, additional boluses of lidocaine can be administered up to a total dose of 225 mg.

5.16 *(Normal) sinus rhythm:* This rhythm has P waves of normal configuration and contour preceding each QRS complex and the rate is between 60 and 100 per minute. QRS complexes have a normal duration and configuration. This rhythm is generally associated with a palpable pulse and usually provides adequate cardiac output.

SCENARIO 6

6.01 *Ventricular fibrillation:* This chaotic ventricular rhythm occurs when multiple areas of the ventricles depolarize and repolarize in a totally uncoordinated fashion. Since there is no organized depolarization of the ventricles as a chamber, the ventricles do not contract in a uniform fashion. There is no cardiac output with this dysrhythmia because the ventricles are quivering rather than contracting. Ventricular fibrillation is the most common mechanism of cardiac arrest that results from myocardial ischemia or infarction.

6.02 *Temporarily withhold CPR:* CPR should be temporarily stopped to defibrillate the patient. This should only be a short delay as the patient will be without circulation and breathing during this time period. If unnecessary delays are encountered in preparing for defibrillation, CPR should be reinitiated until defibrillation can be readily performed.

6.03 *Defibrillate using 200 joules:* Since the only definitive treatment for ventricular fibrillation is defibrillation, the patient should be defibrillated as soon as possible. Previously it was taught that CPR should be performed for at least 2 minutes before defibrillation, while medications such as epinephrine and bicarbonate were given and circulated. It is now thought that defibrillation is more likely to be successful the sooner it is provided following the onset of ventricular fibrillation.

6.04 *Defibrillate using 200 to 300 joules:* Since the only definitive treatment for ventricular fibrillation is defibrillation, the patient should be defibrillated as soon as possible.

6.05 *Defibrillate with up to 360 joules:* When treating ventricular fibrillation (or ventricular tachycardia without a pulse), a third shock should be immediately administered if the first two shocks fail to defibrillate successfully. The third defibrillation should be delivered with up to 360 joules.

6.06 *Asystole:* Asystole is the total absence of cardiac electrical activity. Since there is no depolarization of the myocardial cells, the heart does not contract and there is no cardiac output. Asystole may occur in cardiac arrest as a primary event or it may follow ventricular fibrillation; in the latter instance, it is usually due to a hypoxic and acidotic myocardium. Asystole may also be seen with complete AV block when there is no es-

cape pacemaker. Treatment for asystole is directed at stimulating electrical and mechanical activity of the heart as well as eliminating hypoxia and acidosis.

Because this patient has evidenced ventricular fibrillation within the past few minutes, it may be reasonable to suspect that he is still having this dysrhythmia. Since fine ventricular fibrillation can masquerade as asystole, it is necessary to confirm that this is asystole rather than fibrillation by checking the rhythm in at least two different ECG leads. Additionally, this rhythm is not very distinct, it may or may not be asystole. However, *at this point* in the scenario it does not really matter whether it is ventricular fibrillation or asystole, as the treatment is the same.

6.07 *Establish an IV lifeline:* In general, an IV lifeline provides the most effective route for medication administration in cardiac arrest. Lidocaine, epinephrine, and atropine can, however, be effectively administered via an endotracheal tube.

6.08 *Epinephrine 0.5 to 1.0 mg:* Epinephrine is used to elevate perfusion pressures generated during chest compression, to improve myocardial contractility, stimulate spontaneous contractions, and to make ventricular fibrillation more susceptible to cardioversion.

Because sodium bicarbonate is of questionable value in cardiac arrest, it is no longer recommended in the early cardiac arrest sequence. More recent data suggest that bicarbonate does not enhance the outcomes of defibrillation and may produce undesirable shifts in acid–base balance and in the oxyhemoglobin dissociation curve. If used at all, bicarbonate should only be used after more proven interventions have been employed. Remember that acidosis in cardiac arrest is often at least partly due to hypoxia. As long as the patient is hypoxic, he will continue to have anaerobic metabolism and acidosis. This further emphasizes the need to deliver the highest possible concentrations of oxygen to patients in cardiac arrest.

6.09 *Atropine, 1.0 mg IV push:* Since asystole may be caused by high levels of parasympathetic tone, atropine may be an effective treatment. Its vagolytic action blocks the effects of acetylcholine and may allow the heart to return to its intrinsic rate or allow the sympathetic nervous system to accelerate heart rate. Higher dosages (1 mg) are used to treat asystole because it shortens the time required for achieving a therapeutic response. Atropine can also be administered via endotracheal route. Atropine administration (1.0 mg) may be repeated in five minutes.

6.10 *Sodium bicarbonate, 1 mEq/kg, IV push:* This patient would require a dose of 86 mEq. Because sodium bicarbonate is of questionable value in cardiac arrest, it is no longer recommended in the early cardiac arrest sequence. More recent data suggest that bicarbonate does not enhance the outcomes of defibrillation and may produce undesirable shifts in acid–base balance and in the oxyhemoglobin dissociation curve. If used at all, bicarbonate should only be used after more proven interventions have been employed. Remember that acidosis in cardiac arrest is often at least partly due to hypoxia. As long as the patient is hypoxic, he will continue to have anaerobic metabolism and acidosis. This further emphasizes the need to deliver the highest possible concentrations of oxygen to patients in cardiac arrest.

Bicarbonate would be considered at this point, however, since more proven measures have already been taken and were unsuccessful. A dose of 1 mEq/kg is indicated. One-half of the original dose may be given every 10 minutes as indicated.

6.11 *Idioventricular rhythm:* This dysrhythmia is characterized by beats of ventricular origin. QRS complexes are wide (over 0.12 second), bizarre in configuration, not preceded by P waves, and are associated with T waves oriented opposite to the QRS direction. The rhythm is usually regular and the rate is typically between 20 and 40 per minute.

6.12 *Epinephrine, 0.5 to 1.0 mg, or atropine, 0.5 to 1.0 mg IV push:* Epinephrine may be effective in restoring adequate cardiac output in idioventricular rhythm by increasing cardiac rate and contractility. Since an idioventricular rhythm may result from complete AV block, atropine can also be used to increase heart rate. The effectiveness of atropine is based on its ability to relieve sinoatrial block, thus restoring sinus rhythm. Atropine is more likely to be effective when P waves are present.

6.13 *Defibrillation using 360 joules:* Defibrillation is the only definitive therapy for ventricular fibrillation. It should be performed as soon as possible because successful resuscitation is more likely the sooner defibrillation is performed following the onset of ventricular fibrillation. A higher dosage is indicated here to improve chances for successful defibrillation. When a lower dosage is successful in converting ventricular fibrillation, but the patient reverts into this dysrhythmia, the lower dosage may be employed. When lower dosages have not been successful, a higher dosage may be applied.

6.14 *Fine ventricular fibrillation:* This chaotic ventricular rhythm occurs when multiple areas of the ventricles depolarize and repolarize in a totally uncoordinated fashion. Since there is no organized depolarization of the ventricles as a chamber, the ventricles do not contract in a uniform fashion. There is no cardiac output with this dysrhythmia because the ventricles are quivering rather than contracting. Ventricular fibrillation is the most common mechanism of cardiac arrest that results from myocardial ischemia or infarction.

Fine ventricular fibrillation exists when the waves have low amplitude; a more coarse form, with waveforms of greater amplitude, often precedes it when fibrillation is of recent onset. Fine fibrillation will often need treatment with epinephrine, oxygen, and bicarbonate to correct anoxia and acidosis before it can be successfully defibrillated.

6.15 *Lidocaine, 1-mg/kg:* This patient would need 86 mg. Lidocaine is now recommended for ventricular fibrillation that is resistant to defibrillation, since it may improve the response to electrical therapy. Among the positive effects of lidocaine in ventricular fibrillation is that it raises the fibrillation threshold and blocks reentry. Lidocaine can be administered by both endotracheal and intravenous routes.

6.16 *Defibrillation using 360 joules:* Defibrillation is the only definitive therapy for ventricular fibrillation. It should

be performed as soon as possible because successful resuscitation is more likely the sooner defibrillation is performed following the onset of ventricular fibrillation. A higher dosage is indicated here to improve chances for successful defibrillation. When a lower dosage is successful in converting ventricular fibrillation, but the patient reverts into this dysrhythmia, the lower dosage may be employed. When lower dosages have not been successful, a higher dosage may be applied.

6.17 *Administer bretylium, 5-mg/kg IV bolus:* This patient would require a dose of about 430 mg. Bretylium and lidocaine are used for refractory ventricular fibrillation. These medications may be effective in raising the fibrillation threshold and preventing reentry. Epicardial mapping studies indicate that ventricular fibrillation may result from the presence of more than one activation line passing across the myocardium at the same time. This event may result from a conduction delay of the normal wavefront such as that which occurs through ischemic and infarcted areas. Bretylium causes an initial transient release of catecholamines, which may improve the phase 0 characteristics of the depressed Purkinje fibers of infarcted tissues, reducing the difference in conduction times between normal and infarcted tissues. If 5 mg/kg is not effective, the dose may be increased to 10 mg/kg. Some may prefer to use repeated doses of lidocaine, which may be given in 0.5-mg/kg boluses every 8 minutes to a total dose of 3 mg/kg.

6.18 *Defibrillation using 360 joules:* Defibrillation is the only definitive therapy for ventricular fibrillation. It should be performed as soon as possible because successful resuscitation is more likely the sooner defibrillation is performed following the onset of ventricular fibrillation. A higher dosage is indicated here to improve chances for successful defibrillation. When a lower dosage is successful in converting ventricular fibrillation, but the patient reverts into this dysrhythmia, the lower dosage may be employed. When lower dosages have not been successful, a higher dosage may be applied.

6.19 *Second degree AV block, Mobitz II:* This AV conduction defect is characterized by the presence of normal P waves which are not each followed by a QRS complex. The ratio of P waves to QRS complexes may remain constant (2:1, 3:1, 4:1, etc.) or vary. The P-P interval is regular and the P-R interval is constant for all conducted beats. The atrial rate is usually normal, but the ventricular rate depends on the number of impulses conducted to the ventricles. Mobitz II is indicative or more serious cardiac conduction problems and is more likely to progress to complete AV block than Mobitz I. Treatment is directed at increasing heart rate to maintain adequate cardiac output. Atropine and isoproeterenol are the initial treatments, followed by a permanent pacemaker.

6.20 *Atropine, 0.5 to 1.0 mg IV push:* A slow heart rate may be the result of vagal stimulation. Atropine's vagolytic action is likely to be effective in relieving the slow heart rate in these cases.*

---

*If you elected to administer atropine in question 6.22, disregard these answers as you have already given the total (2.0 mg) dosage of atropine.

6.21 *Atropine, 0.5 to 1.0 mg IV push:* A slow heart may be the result of vagal stimulation. Atropine's vagolytic action is likely to be effective in relieving the slow heart rate in these cases.*

6.22 *Isoproterenol 2 to 10 µg/minute IV infusion:* Because of its beta stimulating properties, isoproterenol may be a useful treatment for bradycardia or AV block. Isoproterenol increases heart rate and increases myocardial contractility. The cost of these benefits is increased myocardial oxygen consumption.

6.23 *(Normal) sinus rhythm:* This rhythm has P waves of normal configuration and contour preceding each QRS complex and the rate is between 60 and 100 per minute. QRS complexes have a normal duration and configuration. This rhythm is generally associated with a palpable pulse and usually provides adequate cardiac output.

6.24 *Ventricular bigeminy:* Sinus beats alternate with premature ventricular contractions (PVCs). The ectopic beats have QRS complexes which are wide (over 0.12 seconds), bizarre, not preceded by P waves, and associated with T waves oriented in an opposite direction; these are followed by a (full) compensatory pause. When ectopic beats alternate with normal beats, the rhythm is referred to as a bigeminy; this is ventricular bigeminy because the premature beats are of ventricular origin.

6.25 *Lidocaine, 1-mg/kg bolus IV push:* This patient would need a dose of 85 mg. Since the patient was in ventricular fibrillation, the fibrillation threshold of the myocardium is probably lower. Additionally, many medications administered during resuscitation stimulate cardiac electrical activity and may lower the fibrillation threshold. Lidocaine raises the fibrillation threshold and discourages reentry; its use may prevent the patient from slipping back into ventricular tachycardia or fibrillation.

   Discontinue the isoproterenol infusion: The isoproterenol infusion should be discontinued because there is no longer any indication for its use and it may be precipitating the PVCs now observed.

6.26 *Lidocaine infusion at 2 to 4 mg/minute:* Since the half-life of lidocaine in the central compartment is less than 10 minutes, a single bolus of lidocaine will maintain therapeutic levels for only a short time. To sustain adequate levels of lidocaine in the central compartment, a continuous IV infusion must be administered after the bolus dose(s).

6.27 *(Normal) sinus rhythm:* This rhythm has P waves of normal configuration and contour preceding each QRS complex and the rate is between 60 and 100 per minute. QRS complexes have a normal duration and configuration. This rhythm is generally associated with a palpable pulse and usually provides adequate cardiac output.

SCENARIO 7

7.01 *Ventricular bigeminy progressing to ventricular tachycardia:* Sinus beats alternate with premature ventricular contractions (PVCs) initially. The ectopic beats have QRS complexes which are wide (over 0.12 second), bizarre, not preceded by P waves, and associated with T waves oriented in an opposite direction; these are followed by a (full) compensatory pause. When ectopic beats alternate with normal beats, the rhythm is referred to as a bigeminy; this is ventricular bigeminy because the premature beats are of ventricular origin. The PVCs occur during the T wave of the preceding cycle, finally precipitating a continuous run of ventricular beats (ventricular tachycardia).

7.02 *Check for a pulse:* This should be done regardless of the ECG rhythm because many factors such as loose ECG electrodes influence the rhythm seen. The pulse is a true evaluation of circulation, whereas the ECG shows only the electrical activity of the heart.

7.03 *Deliver unsynchronized countershock using 50 joules:* When hypotension, pulmonary edema, or unconsciousness is present, an unsynchronized countershock should be administered to avoid the delay associated with synchronization. Although this patient has a pulse, he is "unstable" because he has hypotension, shortness of breath, and chest pain and is unconscious. Had the patient been stable, a precordial thump could have been employed prior to cardioversion. The initial recommended level of countershock is 50 joules.

7.04 *Ventricular tachycardia:* This dysrhythmia is characterized by beats of ventricular origin; the QRS complex is wide (over 0.12 second), bizarre, without preceding P waves, and associated with T waves of opposite orientation. The rhythm is usually regular and the rate is generally between 100 and 250 per minute.

7.05 *Deliver unsynchronized countershock using 100 joules:* When hypotension, pulmonary edema, or unconsciousness is present, an unsynchronized countershock should be administered to avoid the delay associated with synchronization. This patient is classified as "unstable" because he has hypotension, shortness of breath, and chest pain and is unconscious. If the initial countershock is unsuccessful, a second countershock using 100 joules should be used.

7.06 *Deliver unsynchronized countershock using 200 joules:* When hypotension, pulmonary edema, or unconsciousness is present, an unsynchronized countershock should be administered to avoid the delay associated with synchronization. This patient is classified as "unstable" because he has hypotension, shortness of breath, and chest pain and is unconscious. If the second countershock is unsuccessful, a third countershock using 200 joules is indicated.

7.07 *Deliver unsynchronized countershock using up to 360 joules:* When hypotension, pulmonary edema, or unconsciousness is present, an unsynchronized countershock should be administered to avoid the delay associated with synchronization. This patient is classified as "unstable" because he has hypotension, shortness of breath, and chest pain and is unconscious. When three previous attempts at countershock have been unsuccessful, the next attempt may use up to 360 joules.

7.08 *Lidocaine 1 mg/kg IV push and lidocaine infusion at 2 to 4 mg/minute:* Since the half-life of lidocaine in the central compartment is less than 10 minutes, a single bolus of lidocaine will maintain therapeutic levels for only a short time. To sustain adequate levels of lidocaine in the central compartment, a continuous IV infusion must be administered after the bolus dose(s).

SCENARIO 8

8.01 *(Normal) sinus rhythm with multiform (multifocal) PVCs:* The underlying rhythm has a P wave of normal configuration preceding each QRS complex; the rate is between 60 and 100 per minute. The ectopic beats have QRS complexes which are wide (over 0.12 second), bizarre, not preceded by P waves, and associated with T waves oriented in an opposite direction; these are followed by a (full) compensatory pause. Since the ectopic beats have different configurations, they are referred to as "multiform" PVCs.

8.02 *Acute myocardial infarction (MI):* The suspicion of acute myocardial infarction is based primarily on the patient's history. If the history is consistent with acute MI, the patient should be treated accordingly. Signs and symptoms of acute MI include chest pain, dyspnea, weakness, pallor, diaphoresis, anxiety, nausea, and vomiting.

8.03 *Eliminating the ventricular ectopy:* PVCs are a signal of enhanced ventricular automaticity. Especially in the presence of myocardial ischemia, ectopy may lead to ventricular tachycardia or fibrillation. Lidocaine is the treatment of choice for this problem, though bretylium and procainamide may also be useful.
  Relieving hypoxia: Cellular hypoxia will occur any time circulation to the tissues is impaired. Treatment is directed toward raising oxygen delivery to the tissues via high inspired concentrations (100%) of supplemental oxygen.

8.04 *Ventricular tachycardia or fibrillation:* PVCs are a signal of enhanced ventricular automaticity. Especially in the presence of myocardial ischemia, ectopy may lead to ventricular tachycardia or fibrillation.

8.05 *5% Dextrose in water:* The preferred IV solution for use in acute MI is generally 5% dextrose in water. This solution is the preferred medium for diluting medications given by IV infusion and avoids the sodium, which may be harmful to patients in heart failure.

8.06 *Morphine sulfate, 2 to 5 mg slow IV push:* Morphine is used to relieve the chest pain and anxiety associated with MI; it also limits catecholamine activity by these actions. Morphine sulfate increases venous capacitance and reduces systemic vascular resistance, thereby reducing myocardial workload and oxygen consumption.
  Lidocaine, 1 mg/kg: Lidocaine is used to raise the fibrillation threshold and prevent reentry and ventricular ectopy. Lidocaine may be administered prophylactically in acute myocardial ischemia or infarction to prevent life-threatening ventricular dysrhythmias, which may or may not be preceded by so-called "warning dysrhythmias."

8.07 *Lidocaine:* Whenever bolus lidocaine is administered, it should be followed by a continuous IV infusion of at least 2 to 4 mg of lidocaine per minute.

8.08 *Sinus bradycardia:* This rhythm has all the characteristics of (normal) sinus rhythm, but the rate is less than 60 per minute (albeit, so slightly).

SCENARIO 9

9.01 *Complete (3rd degree) AV block:* Complete AV block is characterized by normal P waves which are not related to QRS complexes; P waves appear to "march through" the QRS complexes as P-R intervals are totally inconsistent from one cycle to the next. The atrial rhythm (P-P interval) and ventricular rhythm (R-R intervals) are each regular but unrelated to (independent of) each other. The atrial rate exceeds the ventricular rate. QRS complexes may appear as junctional or ventricular in origin, depending on the escape mechanism driving the ventricles. When a junctional escape rhythm exists, the ventricular rate is usually 40 to 60 per minute; ventricular escape rhythms effect a ventricular rate of 20 to 40 per minute usually, precipitating potentially lethal reductions in cardiac output. Treatment is directed at increasing the heart rate to maintain adequate cardiac output. Atropine and isoproterenol are the immediate therapies; permanent pacemaker insertion is required for long-term treatment.

9.02 *Increasing the heart rate:* Complete AV block often results in an insufficient heart rate to afford adequate tissue perfusion. Treatment is directed at increasing the heart rate to maintain adequate cardiac output. Atropine and isoproterenol are the immediate therapies; permanent pacemaker insertion is required for long-term treatment.
  Eliminating the hypoxia: Cellular hypoxia occurs any time circulation to the tissues is reduced. Treatment is directed at increasing tissue oxygenation via high inspired concentrations (100%) of supplemental oxygen.

9.03 *Asystole:* Asystole is the total absence of cardiac electrical activity. Since there is no depolarization of the myocardial cells, the heart does not contract and there is no cardiac output. Asystole may also be seen with complete AV block when there is no escape pacemaker. Treatment for asystole is directed at stimulating electrical and mechanical activity of the heart as well as eliminating hypoxia and acidosis.

9.04 *Atropine, 0.5 to 1.0 mg IV push:* A slow heart rate may be the result of vagal stimulation. Atropine's vagolytic action is likely to be effective in relieving the slow heart rate in these cases.

9.05 *Atropine, 0.5 to 1.0 mg IV push:* A slow heart rate may be the result of vagal stimulation. Atropine's vagolytic action is likely to be effective in relieving the slow heart rate in these cases.

9.06 *Isoproterenol 2 to 10 μg/minute IV infusion:* Because of its beta stimulating properties, isoproterenol may be a useful treatment for bradycardia and AV block. Isoproterenol increases heart rate, and increases myocardial contractility. The cost of these benefits is increased myocardial oxygen consumption.

9.07 *(Normal) sinus rhythm:* This rhythm has P waves of normal configuration and contour preceding each QRS complex and the rate is between 60 and 100 per minute. QRS complexes have a normal duration and configuration. This rhythm is generally associated with a palpable pulse and usually provides adequate cardiac output.

9.08 *Morphine sulfate, 2 to 5 mg slow IV push:* Morphine has several favorable effects for the treatment of acute MI. It is used to relieve the chest pain and anxiety associated with MI; it also limits catecholamine activity by these actions. Morphine sulfate increases venous capacitance and reduces systemic vascular resistance, thereby reducing myocardial workload and oxygen consumption.

9.09 *A permanent pacemaker:* Complete AV block may be associated with block above or below the bundle of His bifurcation. In the setting of acute MI, block below the AV junction suggests extensive myocardial damage which often produces life-threatening reductions in heart rate; this necessitates insertion of a permanent pacemaker for definitive therapy.

SCENARIO 10

10.01 *Ventricular tachycardia:* This dysrhythmia is characterized by beats of ventricular origin; the QRS complex is wide (over 0.12 second), bizarre, without preceding P waves, and associated with T waves of opposite orientation. The rhythm is usually regular and the rate is generally between 100 and 250 per minute.

10.02 *Establish an IV access:* In general, an IV lifeline provides the most effective route for medication administration.

10.03 *Lidocaine, 1-mg/kg IV push:* This patient would need a dose of 80 mg. Lidocaine raises the fibrillation threshold and discourages ventricular ectopic activity and re-entry; its use may prevent the patient from slipping into ventricular fibrillation. As the patient is conscious with ventricular tachycardia, the treatment is less aggressive.

10.04 *Lidocaine, 0.5 mg/kg IV push:* This patient would need a dose of 40 mg. In a patient with ventricular tachycardia who has a pulse and is stable, the revised standards suggest that, if the initial dose of lidocaine is not successful in terminating this dysrhythmia, lidocaine at 0.5 mg/kg be given every 8 minutes until the ventricular tachycardia resolves or the dose reaches 3 mg/kg.

10.05 *Procainamide, 20 mg/minute, slow IV push:* Procainamide is an effective agent for suppressing ventricular ectopy. It is recommended when lidocaine is contraindicated or when lidocaine fails to suppress recurrent ventricular tachycardia (as well as PVCs). In urgent situations, up to 20 mg/minute may be administered to a total dose of 1 gm. It also would be acceptable to administer repeat doses of lidocaine at 0.5 mg/kg every 8 minutes.

10.06 *Check for a pulse:* Each time definitive therapy is instituted, the pulse should be checked. This should be done regardless of the ECG rhythm because many factors such as loose ECG electrodes influence the rhythm seen. The pulse is a true evaluation of circulation, whereas the ECG shows only the electrical activity of the heart.

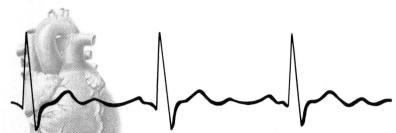

Appendix

Additional Changes in the Advanced Cardiac Life Support Standards

The following are among the additional changes in the ACLS guidelines.

1. Medication administration via peripheral veins during resuscitation is considered less effective

Growing evidence suggests that during resuscitation (even when CPR is being performed effectively) peripheral IV sites are less effective for delivering medications to the heart. The following are the reasons:

(1) There is a significant delay in the arrival time of medications to the heart when peripheral sites are used.

(2) Peak drug levels are less when medications are administered via peripheral veins than when administered via central veins.

To overcome this problem, it is now recommended that during cardiac arrest the antecubital fossa is the peripheral vein of choice. Additionally, when medications are administered via this IV site, the health care professional should either elevate the arm or administer an IV solution bolus chaser to assist the medication in reaching the heart.

2. During resuscitation efforts, arterial blood gases are no longer used to determine dosage for sodium bicarbonate administration

It appears that there will be greater emphasis on interpreting arterial blood gases during the course of resuscitation. However, the focus will be on PaO_2 and $PaCO_2$ levels. In the past, when arterial blood gases were avail-able, sodium bicarbonate replacement was determined by using the arterial blood gases and GOLDEN RULES I, II, and III. The new standards no longer recommend the use of arterial blood gases to determine the amount of sodium bicarbonate replacement during the course of resuscitation. The only recommendation that currently exists is that bicarbonate should be administered when "first-line treatments" have been unsuccessful; at which point, bicarbonate may be administered initially at a dosage of 1 mEq/kg and may be repeated at ten minute intervals at a dosage of 0.5 mEq/kg (half the initial dose).

3. Torsades de Points, a unique ventricular dysrhythmia

Ventricular tachycardia, which is characterized by a "successive growth then recession of QRS amplitude in reference to the baseline," is referred to as Torsades de Points. It is important to recognize this condition as it requires different treatments than more typical forms of ventricular tachycardia. While a number of electrophysiologic mechanisms have been suggested as the cause of Torsades de Points, re-entry is widely believed to be the most likely culprit. Special attention should be paid to the length of the QT interval of complexes preceding the tachycardia. Long QT intervals are suggestive of this condition. They represent delayed ventricular repolarization. Possible causes of Torsades de Points include congenital disorders; antiarrhythmics such as: Group 1A: Quinidine, disopyramide, procainamide, aprindine; Group 1B: Lidocaine, mexiletine, tocainide; antianginals: Prenylamine; Psychotropics: Tricyclic antidepres-

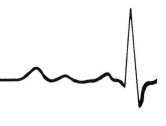

sants, phenothiazines, tetracyclics; Cerebrovascular disease: Strokes, carotid endarterectomies, neck surgery, intracranial lesions; Organophosphates; Liquid protein diets; Electrolyte disorders: Hypokalemia, hypomagnesemia, hypocalcemia; Cardiac disease; Bradycardia, mitral valve prolapse, coronary heart disease.

Conventional treatment used for ventricular dysrhythmias is largely ineffective and may be deleterious in Torsades de Points. Initial therapy consists of identifying and removing (or correcting) underlying causes such as offending drugs or electrolyte imbalances. Direct therapy is aimed at reducing the QT interval by accelerating the heart rate with either electrical pacing, atropine, or a catecholamine infusion such as isoproterenol.

Catecholamines have been found to increase the heart rate and shorten repolarization, thus eliminating the conditions necessary for re-entry. If overdrive pacing is used, it should be initiated at a rate of 130 to 150 and then decreased to a rate which can prevent the recurrence of Torsades de Points. Other suggested therapies include IV magnesium sulfate and lidocaine. Immediate cardioversion may be necessary when the patient is hemodynamically unstable. Quinidine-like drugs are contraindicated.

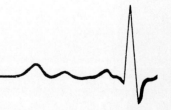